Handbook of
African American Health

Anthony J. Lemelle • Wornie Reed • Sandra Taylor
Editors

Handbook of African American Health

Social and Behavioral Interventions

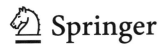 Springer

Editors
Anthony J. Lemelle
Department of Sociology
John Jay College
CUNY, NY, USA
alemelle@jjay.cuny.edu

Wornie Reed
Department of Sociology
Virginia Tech
Blacksburg, VA, USA
wornie@vt.edu

Sandra Taylor
Department of Sociology and Criminal
Justice, Clark Atlanta University
Atlanta, GA, USA
staylor@cau.edu

ISBN 978-1-4419-9615-2 (hardcover)   ISBN 978-1-4419-9616-9 (eBook)
ISBN 978-1-4614-8571-1 (softcover)
DOI 10.1007/978-1-4419-9616-9
Springer New York Heidelberg Dordrecht London

Library of Congress Control Number: 2011933567

Preface

In 2010, the USA made a major stride in the history of its public health services. Under the leadership of President Barak Obama, a compressive reform of health care moved through Congress passing its legislative hurdles. This legislative accomplishment occurred as the authors of this handbook completed their manuscripts. Senior Editor Teresa Krauss and Editorial Director Bill Tucker at Springer Science + Business Media approached the editors of the *Handbook of African American Health* several months before and asked that we specifically focus manuscripts on evidence-based outcomes. We all knew about the growth of literature addressing health disparities. In 2008, the National Institutes of Health had called for a conference to share leading knowledge about the status and prevention intervention work to assist in the reduction of health disparities (National Institutes of Health, 2008). Health disparity has been a considerable problem that was obstinate, particularly among African Americans. The editors have included 18 chapters that we believe offer innovative knowledge that relates to social and behavioral interventions. In this preface, we explain the political context for sharing some leading perspectives on health interventions for African Americans. We then provide an overview of the chapters in the handbook.

The passage of Obama's healthcare proposal in 2010 clearly demonstrates US political exceptionalism. Technically speaking, Congress passed bill H.R. 3590, the Patient Protection & Affordable Care Act (PPAC) and Obama signed the legislation into law on March 23. On March 30, Obama signed a separate bill, H.R. 4872, The Health Care & Education Reconciliation Act. There were differences in the House and Senate versions of H.R. 3590 and H.R. 4872 resolved those differences (Ardito, 2010). The exceptionalism is getting the healthcare reform through a contentious Congress, before Obama's signature was dry, oppositional leadership began repeating the mantra, we cannot afford it. We can see this exceptionalism by first going back to Obama's campaign proposal for healthcare reform. Next, we would need to see how the congressional leadership brought the reform through Congress. Finally, we need to know what came out of the process and its significance for the African American population.

Healthcare Reform Proposal

During the Obama presidential campaign, he and his running mate, Joe Biden, issued a report that gave details of the healthcare crisis (Obama & Biden, 2008). The problem was that healthcare costs increased at alarming rates (Himmelstein & Woolhandler, 2008); millions of US citizens had no healthcare coverage (The Henry J. Kaiser Family Foundation, 2009); and there was significant underinvestment in prevention and public health (Lambrew, 2008, April). Obama and Biden reported an increase in the cost of health insurance premiums – over the previous 8 years, they doubled. Moreover, co-pays increased and deductibles thwarted access to care. Increasingly, insurance companies limited physician visits and allowable hospital days. Medical errors and iatrogenic infections were rising. In an age of digital communication, many healthcare providers continued to rely on costly paper-based recordkeeping and information services (Obama & Biden, 2008). Rising healthcare costs increased the number of adults and children without healthcare coverage or the ability to pay healthcare costs. Obama and Biden detailed it, "Eighty percent of the uninsured are in working families" (Obama & Biden, 2008). However, even when employers provided healthcare for employees, the increasing cost that had become a burden for many firms – particularly small businesses. Many poor health conditions are preventable through diet, exercise, immunizations, and screenings. Nonetheless, Obama and Biden observed, "… less than 4 cents of every healthcare dollar is spent on prevention and public health" (Lambrew, 2008, April; Obama & Biden, 2008).

For African Americans healthcare social forces increased their vulnerability to disparate health outcomes. In fact, many social scientists remarked about unique mobility experience among African Americans (Steinberg, 2007). Clearly, there is a relationship between socioeconomic status – that is, social integration – and health (Williams & Collins, 1995). There is little doubt that greater African American integration into society would decrease health disparities (Ruffin, 2008). Distinguished sociologist Richard Alba describes the likelihood of greater social integration for minorities in the future (Alba, 2010). With healthcare reform, increased minority integration that Alba observes would support reductions in African American health disparities. This would be exceptional. Alba stresses demographic shifts in the labor market that would transform neighborhoods into more integrated ones. Moreover, the demographic shifts would also change the way labor markets are populations in terms of racial and ethnic organization. Given this, according to Alba, we should expect greater contact among populations – we would likely to see increases in intermarriage, mixed-race populations, and greater cultural sentiment reflecting greater social integration (Alba, 2010). There is little doubt that Alba's projections, which he bases on historical demographic trends, are forthcoming. Even less doubt that such developments would reduce health disparities. Nevertheless, these developments are not without risks. Therefore, Alba cautions:

> Only enlightened public policy can address the large educational gaps that will leave larger and larger proportions of young people behind. Only with affirmative action in some form can we hope to keep African Americans from slipping – yet again – behind the children of more recent immigrants… Eradicating racial inequalities is more utopian hope than practical goal. The vague anticipation that a future majority made up of minorities will, in a democratic society, find a way to overturn the existing racial order doesn't take into account the ongoing process of assimilation. This will produce a multiracial mainstream majority, including at a minimum many Asians and light-skinned Latinos, who along with whites will resist radical change. (Alba, 2010, p. 60)

Healthcare reform would likely need additional modifications in the near future. The social forces that Alba describes will help to ameliorate health disparities. As it stands, in the near future, we could expect improved efficiency in the healthcare system that will lower costs, improvement in delivery of care that increases prevention and better manages chronic conditions, and a reorganization of the market structure that would help manage and regulate payment, catastrophic illness outcomes, and health insurance accessibility and affordability. Nonetheless, African Americans social statuses will challenge competition for healthcare equality. Most significant is the relationship between African American residential locations, poverty, and the distribution of healthcare resources. We would likely need to think about some affirmative action in these matters.

Recently, economic sociologist William Julius Wilson reminded us that concentrated poverty among African Americans is a major impediment to the overall health of this social aggregate (Wilson, 2008, 2009). Even if we were to reach public health goals including comprehensive benefits, affordable premiums, co-pays and deductibles, simplified paperwork, easy enrollment, portability and choice, and quality and efficiency, we would still need additional assistance among the poor. Wilson aptly states our challenge:

> The economic situation for many African Americans has now been further weakened because not only do they tend to reside in communities that have higher jobless rates and lower employment growth – for example, places like Detroit or Philadelphia – but also they lack access to areas of higher employment growth. As the world of corporate employment has relocated to America's suburban communities, over two-thirds of employment growth in metropolitan areas has occurred in the suburbs, many of the residents of our inner-city ghettos have become physically isolated from places of employment and socially isolated from the informal job networks that are often essential for job placement. (Wilson, 2009, p. 10)

In the details of Wilson's studies, he elaborates covariates between cultural and structural social forces in the production of concentrated poverty. These social forces are the salient ones explaining health disparities that African Americans experience. In the terms of public health, Wilson shows the fragmentation of family life, out of wedlock births, and negative health outcomes are particularly a production of concentrated poverty (Wilson, 2009). Moreover, Wilson shows that policy decisions also have a disparate affect on health outcomes when it comes to African Americans, particularly poor African Americans (Wilson, 2008). Therefore, Alba and Wilson are both correct; we must affirmatively keep these social forces in mind as we experience exceptional demographic and social transformations.

Lessons Learned from Healthcare Reform's Political Exceptionalism

Massachusetts's Governor Deval Patrick supported the presidential campaign of Obama as Senator Obama had supported the gubernatorial campaign of Patrick. Obama might not have made the most convincing presentations for healthcare reform during his presidential campaign – for example; he had to debate Senator Hilary Clinton, a dean of healthcare policy, where the presentation was less than stellar. Nonetheless, Obama became a leading healthcare policy wonk (Cohn, 2010). Massachusetts implemented the plan in 2006. The central feature of Massachusetts health reform was a promise to reduce bureaucratic costs. The way to accomplish this was the single-payer option in the policy. Single-payer means government-run healthcare (Cohn, 2010, p. 16). Most, even the political right, recognized the cost of care was uncontrollable by the 1970s; nonetheless, the right sought a market-based solution (Cohn, 2010). The left preferred government intervention. The left compromised over the years. Eventually, healthcare conversations resulted in the Clinton proposal. Clintoncare promoted the idea "to give everybody insurance but to make it private insurance, with consumers shopping around for the best plans" (Cohn, 2010, p. 16). The nation did not take well to Clintoncare because many would have to shift their existing coverage to regulated health plans. Clintoncare met its defeat in 1994. It took 10 years for the conversation to change, the new idea suggested that individuals with good healthcare coverage – the kind that good jobs provide – would keep that coverage while others would buy their own, some using subsidies. In short, healthcare coverage would become "a regulated marketplace where everybody could buy affordable coverage regardless of preexisting conditions" (Cohn, 2010, p. 16). It is not completely clear, but some in Massachusetts claimed that 97% of the state had healthcare coverage by 2009 (Gruber, 2008).

A regulated marketplace would have been exceptional – in the sense that it retains market force as the underlying engine of the proposed system (Himmelstein & Woolhandler, 2009). Harvard Medical School health-policy researchers and physicians, David Himmelstein and Steffie Woolhandler, reveal how the reform gave "tax-funded windfalls that brought private insurers and hospitals on board" and it, "proved far more expensive than politicians forecast – costing the state $1.3 billion this fiscal year [2009], according to the state's report to its bondholders" (Himmelstein & Woolhandler, 2009, p. 14). Moreover, there were other problems with the Massachusetts reform.

To some extent, Obamacare includes some of these deficiencies. This is the case since Obamacare was unable to convince Congress or the US citizenry about the importance for having a public option. Many among the US left expected nothing less than for Obama fully to support a single-payer structure. This position might have been ambitious – the administration likely early on recognized this credulity. Nonetheless, Himmelstein and Woolhandler correctly observe the importance of a single-payer system that is necessary to reduce bureaucratic costs. However, there are other, perhaps even more pernicious effects. Himmelstein and Woolhandler detect canceling-out outcomes when they write:

> Indeed, Massachusetts's reform has actually increased bureaucratic costs; the new insurance exchange (similar to that touted by President Obama and Senate Finance Committee chair Max Baucus) has added 4% to insurers' already high overhead… Facing yawning budget deficit and desperate to stay the course on the 2006 reform plan, Patrick has slashed funding to safety-net providers such as Cambridge Health Alliance (CHA) and Boston Medical Center (BMC) (né Cambridge City and Boston City Hospitals)… At CHA – a Harvard affiliate that operates three hospitals, 21 community clinics and more psychiatric beds than all of Boston's big teaching hospitals combined – the cuts will shutter one hospital, six clinics, the area's only inpatient detox unit and nearly half of the psychiatric wards. (Himmelstein & Woolhandler, 2009, p. 15)

Massachusetts's healthcare-problems stand for less care availability for the poor, when African Americans – including Latin(a)o African Americans – exist in greater concentrated poverty. Moreover, the larger fiscal crisis results in diminished funds for clinics and hospitals in areas of concentrated poverty around the country. For example, Himmelstein and Woolhandler remark on Chicago cuts resulting in loss of half the outpatient clinics, where the only central city hospital closed – other public hospitals there face major shortfalls; they find similar conditions in Detroit, Philadelphia, New Orleans, and New York (Himmelstein & Woolhandler, 2009). Insofar as African Americans are concerned, if we consider health disparities as pernicious, then the words of Himmelstein and Woolhandler are profound, "The pernicious market signals in medical care don't reflect consumer preferences or invisible hands; they arise largely from government policy" (Himmelstein & Woolhandler, 2009, p. 16).

Obama's comprehensive healthcare reform required partnership from various stakeholders. The Executive Branch had its players, including chief of staff Rahm Emanuel, and Vice President Biden. The Senate Finance Committee was a major stakeholder. A few of the other stakeholders included major unions, particularly the Service Employees International Union (SEIU), Department of Health and Human Services, White House Office of Health Reform, Pharmaceutical Research and Manufacturers of America, American Hospital Association, House Energy and Commerce Committee, and the House Ways and Means Committee. There was a need to exercise premier diplomatic skills on the part of all the stakeholders to accomplish their goals. It is entirely amazing that the nation accomplished its initial goal despite modifications resulting from bureaucratic and political processes. However, as some in the healthcare reform field remarked along the way, spot on universal healthcare reform would remain an incremental exercise.

Speaker of the House, Nancy Pelosi, demonstrated brilliant political skill as she worked with the so-called Tri-Com to get the legislation passed. The Tri-Com was composed of three powerful congressional committees: George Miller's Education and Labor Committee, Charles Rangel's Ways and Means Committee, and Henry Waxman's House Energy and Commerce Committee (Cohn, 2010). However, in addition to the management of her Tri-Com allies, Pelosi had to convince Maine Republican Olympia Snowe and others among the moderate-right – she found some successes, in other cases, she was not as successful. However, she achieved more than the 218 votes needed – she got 220. Nonetheless, the public option did not survive the process. Both Obama and Pelosi favored it. The Tri-Com leadership also favored it. The right would not hear of it. They produced a powerful brand to resist what they viewed as government takeover of healthcare. They created brands that they could stamp on moments in the discourse: erroneous claims about jail-time penalties for those without insurance, death panels for euthanizing the frail elderly, government sponsored abortions, and socialism. Senator Joe Lieberman's leadership eventually dashed any hopes for accomplishment of a public option. In the Senate, Majority Leader Harry Reid also faced major challenges. In some instances, he felt betrayal. Nevertheless, Pelosi's brilliance was particularly associated with her timing. Had she not forced the votes, the outcome would have been less propitious.

The incremental nature of the reform is disappointing for many on the left. Nevertheless, as leading healthcare commentator Jonathan Cohn concluded:

> They inherited a crusade that liberals launched in the early twentieth century and carried to completion – transforming life for tens of millions of Americans, reorganizing the most dysfunctional part of the US economy, and proving that the United States can at least make a serious effort to solve its biggest problems. They were lucky, yes. They were also good. (Cohn, 2010, p. 25)

Healthcare reform provides enduring hope for the possibility of overcoming health disparities. As Himmelstein and Woolhandler recognized, it will require political will that will likely consist of incremental successes. This is the lesson we learned from healthcare reform. Therefore, this handbook is an effort to meet the urgency that Wilson warns us about in his studies of concentrated poverty. There too, we noticed the importance of political action to impact structural and cultural forces leading to health disparities. These conditions are ones that establish the environment of our collective work to extend human success over eventual morbidity and mortality.

The *Handbook* includes eight sections. Section 1 presents two chapters. Anthony J. Lemelle, Jr. discusses selected concepts, operations, and theories that are important for social and behavioral interventions among African Americans. He proposes more systematic approaches to intervention work that use marketing knowledge in network social work. In Chap. 2, Cynthia Hudley argues the failure of just focusing on individual decisions when studying health disparities; she stresses the importance of environmental and structural predictors of health disparities. For Hudley, there are ethical reasons for doing the latter in context of limited resources and the need for resource mobilization. Hudley gives an evidence-based multidimensional model of cultural competence to use in health interventions.

Section 2 considers fundamental intervention needs. Angela J. Hattery and Earl Smith wrote Chap. 3. They demonstrate the political economy of an intersectional condition of inequality. Under such conditions, class, gender, and race stratification affect nutrition. They discuss "food deserts" under conditions of class, gender, and race strain. They recommend evidence-based policy interventions on the political economy. Raegan A. Tuff and Billy Hawkins note the importance of physical activity at an early age to promote life-course health in Chap. 4. They provide a template for multi-component physical activity approaches that enhance family participation and take place in schools and after-school programs that are likely to become successful among Black youth.

Section 3 raises major lifestyle considerations. Jane A. Allen, Donna M. Vallone, and Amanda K. Richardson tackle mass media campaigns. Their work here specifically addresses smoking prevention and cessation. However, we can quickly see how media campaigns are useful for other health-disparity effects among the underserved. They present model campaigns that are applicable for health promotion. These campaigns successfully diffused innovation.

Section 4 contains important interventions for children. Co-editor Wornie Reed discusses the pernicious condition of lead poisoning on African American children in Chap. 6. He reports where the lead-poison contaminants reside in environments often inhabited by African Americans. He explains pathological correlates of lead-poison contaminants. Finally, he discusses treatment and prevention evidence. Reed stresses that lead poisoning is completely preventable. Duane E. Thomas, Elizabeth M. Woodburn, Celine I. Thompson, and Stephen S. Leff wrote Chap. 7. They point to high rates of violence among African American youth. They recommend Phenomenological Variant of Ecological Systems Theory (PVEST) as a guide for intervention strategies. They then present a variety of interventions that diffuse different competencies for the reduction of violence. For example, they present an intervention to reduce bullying among youth. Moreover, they present an intervention for strengthening family ties.

Chapter 8, written by Von E. Nebbitt, Andridia Mapson, and Ajita Robinson, is an impressive and important contribution to understanding adolescents living under distressful housing conditions of concentrated poverty – that is, those residing in public housing. They empirically identify structural effects from public housing environments that associate with depression in minority youth. Their social and behavioral work is from a multisite study in major US cities. One of their major findings is, "African American males in urban public housing experience heightened depressive symptoms relative to their female counterpart." Donna Shambley-Ebron wrote Chap. 9. She studied rites of passage interventions for the prevention of HIV/AIDS incidence and prevalence among African American girls. Her concept of cultural guidance through African American churches is promising, not just in terms of the HIV/AIDS pandemic but for other sexually transmitted infections, including emergent infectious agents.

Section 5 discusses urgent interventions for African American women. Paula Braveman wrote Chap. 10 about Black and White disparities in birth outcomes. The chapter is among the most important in the *Handbook*. She shows, "These patterns suggest an 'environmental' cause, in the broadest sense of environment – some factor(s) in the social or physical environment to which black women are exposed when they are born and raised in the USA – rather than a genetic cause." Braveman stresses the importance of social solutions for social causes. In addition, she promotes the importance of paying more attention to neighborhoods – much like in the works of Richard Alba and William Julius Wilson that this preface mentioned earlier. Sarah Gehlert, Eusebius Small, and Sarah Bollinger contributed Chap. 11 where they argue the significance of multiple-level interventions for breast cancer prevention and treatment. This chapter is a major contribution. The authors show the importance of thinking about various dimensions of individual existence. Important dimensions for disease acquisition include psychological, social, biological, and access to care. They show experiences with these dimensions might change across the life course. To assist with breast cancer intervention strategies they present the Center for Interdisciplinary Health Disparities Research at the University of Chicago. The intervention includes psychosocial, psychotherapeutic, social support, and patient advocacy techniques.

Section 6 concerns critical interventions for African American men. Benjamin P. Bowser contributes Chap. 12. He is concerned with risky sexual behaviors among African American men. In a meticulous and lucid chapter, Bowser shows the importance of theory for developing prevention interventions that reduce African American male sexual risks. He shows African American males represent a unique and underserved aggregate. In addition, lack of theory produces the impossibility of empirically testing outcomes for their prevention effectiveness. Bowser shocks us with one of his findings, "In this 60 article review of the literature since 2000, 12 new theory-based studies of HIV prevention intervention efforts among African Americans were found. Only two focused specifically on HIV prevention among black men; seven focused on men and women and three were specifically on women."

Armon R. Perry, Michael A. Robinson, Rudolph Alexander, Jr., and Sharon E. Moore wrote Chap. 13. They discuss the significance of incarceration and reentry of African American males. The chapter represents the importance of multicultural consciousness in social work training. Social workers are key stakeholders in prevention interventions, different class, gender, and racial backgrounds would likely impact clinical approaches. In this study, for example, we sense the Afrocentric threads of social work practice. The authors show Afrocentricity is an effective producer of family cohesion; family cohesion – broadly speaking to include "fictive" families – reduces some effects of reentry trauma. Michael A. Robinson, Armon R. Perry, Sharon E. Moore, and Rudolph Alexander, Jr. wrote Chap. 14, which addresses suicide among African American males. The authors demonstrate the importance of community building as an intervention strategy. They introduce the elements of effective community building, including mentorship, support groups, and familial supports. They effectively distinguish forms of suicide showing subtle differences comparing African American males to other males from different racial and ethnic aggregates. One contribution of this chapter is its articulation of racialized social stressors that presumably predicts increased suicidal ideation.

Section 7 presents chapters on clinical interventions for healthy communities. Wornie Reed, Ronnie Dunn, and Kay Colby present an intervention for increasing cultural competency among medical care providers. They present results from the Urban Cancer Project that used a video-based approach for assisting in culturally competent prevention intervention work with health providers. The African American cultural themes include mistrust of the medical system, ethno-medical beliefs and fears, daily living issues, and spirituality. They demonstrate effectiveness of the intervention using a repeated measure. Marlyn Allicock, Marci Campbell, and Joan Walsh present a comprehensive overview of cancer reduction interventions working with African American churches in Chap. 16. The chapter is exceptional for introducing readers to solid empirical and theoretical work in the subfield of cancer prevention intervention. The authors describe many of the effective interventions including Body & Soul, Eat for Life, and The Witness Project. They connect communication theory to mind–body–spirit connection in intervention work. The chapter also describes the Wellness for African Americans Through Churches (WATCH) intervention. In addition, the authors provide information on modes of health communication that includes tailoring and targeting print and video materials.

Margaret Shandor Miles, Suzanne Thoyre, Linda Beeber, Stephen Engelke, Mark A. Weaver, and Diane Holditch-Davis wrote Chap. 17. It discusses nursing support interventions for African American preterm mothers living in rural communities. The authors show the possibility of subtle distress from preterm deliveries. For example, preterm mothers might experience post-trauma stress from memories of their infants' illness and hospitalization. These feelings and their consequences might continue long after discharge. They present the Preterm Maternal Support Intervention. The purpose of the intervention is to improve psychological well-being, support mothers in developing relationships with their babies, guiding them in reducing daily stress, and strengthening their ability to identify and use family support and community health resources. The authors describe the Guided Discovery pedagogy that eschews pedantic communication.

Marcia J. Wilson, Bruce Siegel, Vickie Sears, Jennifer Bretsch, and Holly Mead wrote Chap. 18. It represents a beautiful and comprehensive closing chapter for the *Handbook*. The authors explain steps and activities required for the development of interventions that address healthcare disparities. They are particularly concerned about formal healthcare institutions such as hospitals. They explain a collaborative intervention for quality of life improvements among cardiac care minorities – Expecting Success: Excellence in Cardiac Care project. The project's purpose was to reduce disparities in cardiac care through quality improvement techniques. They conclude by sharing lessons learned from Expecting Success. The chapter provides hopeful visions for health disparity amelioration conditioned by US exceptionalism.

Anthony J. Lemelle
New York, NY

References

Alba, R. (2010). Achieving a more integrated America. *Dissent, 57*(3), 57–60.

Ardito, S. C. (2010). U.S. healthcare reform: A follow-up. *Searcher, 18*(8). Retrieved from http://www.infotoday.com/searcher/oct10/Ardito.shtml

Cohn, J. (2010). How they did it: The inside account of health care reform's triumph. *New Republic, 241*(9), 14–25.

Gruber, J. (2008). Symposium: Health care: Incremental universalism for the United States: The states move first? *Journal of Economic Perspectives, 22*(4), 51–68.

Himmelstein, D. U., & Woolhandler, S. (2008). Health policy placebos. *Nation, 286,* 6–8.

Himmelstein, D. U., & Woolhandler, S. (2009). Healthcare lifeboats: Washington should reconsider launching a national plan based on the Massachusetts model. *Nation, 288*(16), 14–16.

Lambrew, J. M. (2008, April). A wellness trust to prioritize disease prevention, Brookings Institution: The Hamilton Project Discussion Paper Available from http://www.brookings.edu/papers/2007/04useconomics_lambrew.aspx

National Institutes of Health. (2008). *The science of eliminating health disparities.* Paper presented at the National Institutes of Health Summit, Washington, D.C.

Obama, B., & Biden, J. (2008). Barack Obama and Joe Biden's plan to lower health care costs and ensure affordable, accessible health coverage for all. Retrieved from www.barackobama.com/pdf/issues/HealthCareFullPlan.pdf

Ruffin, J. (2008). *Opening ceremony plenary session.* Paper presented at the National Institutes of Health Summit: The science of eliminating health disparities, National Center on Minority Health and Health Disparities.

Steinberg, S. (2007). *Race relations: a critique.* Stanford, CA: Stanford.

The Henry J. Kaiser Family Foundation. (2009). The uninsured: A primer, Supplemental data tables Available from http://www.kff.org/uninsured/7451.cfm

Williams, D. R., & Collins, C. (1995). U.S. socioeconomic and racial differences in health: Patterns and explanations. *Annual Review of Sociology, 21*, 349–386.

Wilson, W. J. (2008). The political and economic forces shaping concentrated poverty. *Political Science Quarterly, 123*(4), 555–571.

Wilson, W. J. (2009). *More than just race: being black and poor in the inner city* (1st ed.). New York: Norton & Company.

Contents

Contributors

Rudolph Alexander, Jr. Department of Social Work,
Ohio State University, Columbus, OH, USA
alexander.2@osu.edu

Jane A. Allen American Legacy Foundation, Washington, DC, USA
jallen@legacyforhealth.org

Marlyn Allicock Department of Nutrition, Gillings School of Global Public Health,
University of North Carolina at Chapel Hill, Chapel Hill, NC, USA
allicock@email.unc.edu

Linda Beeber School of Nursing, University of North Carolina
at Chapel Hill, Chapel Hill, NC, USA
beeber@email.unc.edu

Sarah Bollinger George Warren Brown School of Social Work,
Washington University in St. Louis, St. Louis, MO, USA
sbolling@dom.wustl.edu

Benjamin P. Bowser Department of Sociology and Social Services,
California State University, East Bay, San Francisco, CA, USA
benjamin.bowser@csueastbay.edu

Paula Braveman Department of Family and Community Medicine,
Center on Social Disparities in Health, San Francisco, CA, USA
braveman@fcm.ucsf.edu

Jennifer Bretsch School of Public Health and Health Services,
George Washington University, Washington, DC, USA
canjxb@gwumc.edu

Marci Kramish Campbell Department of Nutrition, Gillings School of Global
Public Health, University of North Carolina, Chapel Hill, NC, USA
campbel7@email.unc.edu

Kay Colby Public Health Television, Inc., Cleveland OH, USA
kaycolby@publichealthtv.com

Ronnie Dunn Department of Urban Studies, Cleveland State University,
Cleveland, OH, USA
r.dunn@csuohio.edu

Stephen Engelke Division of Neonatology, Department of Pediatrics, School of Medicine, East Carolina University, Greenville, NC, USA engelkes@ecu.edu

Sarah Gehlert GeorgeWarren Brown School of Social Work, Washington University, St. Louis, MO, USA sgehlert@wustl.edu

Angela J. Hattery Women and Gender Studies, George Mason University, Fairfax, VA, USA ahattery@gmu.edu

Billy Hawkins Department of Kinesiology, University of Georgia, Athens, GA, USA bhawk@uga.edu

Diane Holditch-Davis School of Nursing, Duke University, Durham, NC, USA diane.hd@duke.edu

Cynthia Hudley Department of Education, Gervirtz School, University of California, Santa Barbara, CA, USA hudley@education.ucsb.edu

Stephen S. Leff The Children's Hospital of Philadelphia and The Philadelphia Collaborative Violence Prevention Center, Philadelphia, PA, USA leff@email.chop.edu

Anthony J. Lemelle Department of Sociology, John Jay College, City University of New York, NY, USA alemelle@jjay.cuny.edu

Andridia Mapson School of Social Work, Howard University, Washington, DC, USA amapson@howard.edu

Holly Mead School of Public Health and Health Services, George Washington University, Washington, DC, USA holly.mead@gwumc.edu

Margaret Shandor Miles School of Nursing, University of North Carolina at Chapel Hill, Chapel Hill, NC, USA mmiles@email.unc.edu

Sharon E. Moore Raymond A. Kent School of Social Work, University of Louisville, Louisville, KY, USA semoor02@louisville.edu

Von E. Nebbitt School of Social Work, Howard University, Washington, DC, USA vnebbitt_@howard.edu

Armon R. Perry Kent School of Social Work, University of Louisville, Louisville, KY, USA arperr01@louisville.edu

Wornie Reed Department of Sociology, Virginia Tech, Blacksburg, VA, USA wornie@vt.edu

Amanda K. Richardson American Legacy Foundation, Washington, DC, USA
arichardson@legacyforhealth.org

Michael A. Robinson School of Social Work, The University of Alabama,
Tuscaloosa, Alabama
mrobinson4@sw.ua.edu

Ajita Robinson Graduate School of Education and Human Development,
George Washington University, Washington, DC, USA
ajita@gwmail.gwu.edu

Vickie Sears School of Public Health and Health Services,
George Washington University, Washington, DC, USA
blocked email

Donna Shambley-Ebron College of Nursing, University of Cincinnati,
Cincinnati, OH, USA
donna.shambley-ebron@uc.edu

Bruce Siegel School of Public Health and Health Services,
George Washington University, Washington, DC, USA
siegelmd@gwu.edu

Eusebius Small George Warren Brown School of Social Work,
Washington University in St. Louis, St. Louis, MO, USA
esmall@mail.uh.edu

Earl Smith Department of Sociology, Wake Forest University
smithea@wfu.edu

Duane E. Thomas Graduate School of Education,
University of Pennsylvania, Philadelphia, PA, USA
duanet@gse.upenn.edu

Celine I. Thompson Graduate School of Education,
University of Pennsylvania, Philadelphia, PA, USA
celinet@design.upenn.edu

Suzanne Thoyre School of Nursing, University of North Carolina
at Chapel Hill, Chapel Hill, NC, USA
thoyre@email.unc.edu

Raegan A. Tuff Public Health, Department of Health Promotion and Behavior,
University of Georgia, Athens, GA, USA
rtuff@uga.edu

Donna M. Vallone American Legacy Foundation, Washington, DC, USA
dvallone@americanlegacy.org

Joan Walsh Department of Nutrition, Gillings School of Global Public Health,
University of North Carolina at Chapel Hill, Chapel Hill, NC, USA
walshj@email.unc.edu

Mark A. Weaver Family Health International, Durham, NC, USA
mweaver@fhi.org

Marcia J. Wilson Center for Health Care Quality, The George Washington University, Washington, DC, USA
marcia.wilson@gwumc.edu

Elizabeth M. Woodburn University of Delaware and The Philadelphia Collaborative Violence Prevention Center, Philadelphia, PA, USA

Part I
Background of Social and Behavioral Health Disparities Interventions Among African Americans

Chapter 1
Conceptual, Operational, and Theoretical Overview of African American Health Related Disparities for Social and Behavioral Interventions

Anthony J. Lemelle

Introduction

The purpose of this handbook is to share information about evidence-based approaches for the reduction of health disparities in the USA. It brings information about intervention research that affects African Americans. For this project, there are three initial concepts: African Americans, health disparities, and intervention. This chapter reviews selected literature to provide definitions and framing. In this process, the chapter offers conceptual, operational, and theoretical reconsiderations.

African Americans and Health Disparities

There are at least three conceptual, empirical, historical problems associated with the concept African American. The literature on African Americans (1) generally divides the concept of African American as an externally imposed identity, internally developed identity, or as an identity that comes from processes of social reaction, internalization, and identification (Cross, 1991; Hacker, 1992). Moreover, (2) the concept has different meanings across time (Yancey, 2003). For example, colored, Negro, black, and African American are terms that recent history used to identify African Americans. Social scientists usually distinguish between ethnicity and race; nonetheless, throughout US history, colloquially US Americans have understood the notion of US Americans from Africa as referring to a racial group. In fact, some scholars make it clear that black and white distinctions represent *the* racial classes in the USA (Marx, 1998; Steinberg, 2007). Moreover, (3) we can quickly discern the nomenclature equivocation within the term African American; immigrants from Botswana living in the USA and having US citizenship would become confused with descendants of slaves whose cultural characteristics marginally survived experiences with the transatlantic slave trade and US organized slavery (Fullilove, 1998). From a scientific standpoint, the concept becomes virtually meaningless. Imagine that we conceptualized the term to mean anyone with at least one-drop of African blood (Lemelle, 2007); the confusion would escalate since we know that "biracial" experience is different in some ways from uniracial experience.

A.J. Lemelle (✉)
Department of Sociology, John Jay College,
City University of New York, NY, USA
e-mail: alemelle@jjay.cuny.edu

A.J. Lemelle et al. (eds.), *Handbook of African American Health: Social and Behavioral Interventions*, DOI 10.1007/978-1-4419-9616-9_1, © Springer Science+Business Media, LLC 2011

One way around some of the confusion is to recognize racial/ethnic classification as pragmatic political constructs. For example, the U.S. Census Bureau provides the following definition:

> The concept of race as used by the Census Bureau reflects self-identification by people according to the race or races with which they most closely identify. These categories are sociopolitical constructs and should not be interpreted as being scientific or anthropological in nature. Furthermore, the race categories include both racial and national-origin groups. The racial classifications used by the Census Bureau adhere to the October 30, 1997, Federal Register Notice entitled, "Revisions to the Standards for the Classification of Federal Data on Race and Ethnicity" issued by the Office of Management and Budget (OMB) (U.S. Census Bureau, 2000).

Moreover, when the Census Bureau refers to African Americans, agents also use the term black. The official definition is, *"Black or African American.* A person having origins in any of the Black racial groups of Africa. It includes people who indicate their race as "Black, African Am., or Negro," or provide written entries such as African American, Afro American, Kenyan, Nigerian, or Haitian" (U.S. Census Bureau, 2000). Speaking generally, given the scientific imprecision of the Census Bureau's definition, this handbook adheres to its definition. The most salient aspect of the definition is its reliance on self-identification. In addition to categorical problems with the concept, some of which were worth mentioning above; there are problems with self-identification. For one thing, there is within-group variation among individuals that self-indentify. Moreover, there is likely variation in social reaction associated with other social inequalities, particularly in terms of racial/ethnic group self-identification. For example, subcategories of assets, education, gender, income, and wealth might affect health outcomes triggered by cognition and/or institutional organization and practice (Braveman, 2005, 2006; Braveman, Cubbin, Egerter, & Marchi, 2006; Pollack et al., 2007). One consequence of African American social status has been attempts of conflate it with other status categories. For example, some scholars might understand African American inequality as having more to do with class and not race. Such propositions have found much debate in public health and the social sciences (Ochs, 2006). It is likely that the African American concept includes dimensions of race, class, gender, sexual orientation, and political ideology – i.e., various health policy perspectives. In addition, there are possibly other dimensions of the concept that public health would have a need to address.

However, this essay highlights selected important features of African American healthcare experiences that researchers often associate with health disparities. It discusses an ecological perspective where social strain is highly connected to health disparities. Therefore, it introduces the overall need for the diffusion of evidence-based interventions to ameliorate strain.

What Are Health Disparities?

There are many definitions of health disparities. Paula Braveman listed "six selected definitions of health disparities, inequalities, or equity in previous literature, in chronologic order of publication" (Braveman, 2006, pp. 173–175). One of the strongest definitions in her list reads:

> Equity means that people's needs, rather than their social privileges, guide the distribution of opportunities for well-being. In virtually every society in the world, social privilege is reflected by differences in socioeconomic status, gender, geographical location, racial/ethnic/religious differences and age. Pursuing equity in health means trying to reduce avoidable gaps in health status and health services between groups with different levels of social privilege. (Braveman, 2006, p. 173; World Health Organization et al., 1996, p. 1)

The advantage of that definition is that it "explicitly refers to comparisons among more and less socially advantaged groups; [w]ide range of social groups (e.g., by race/ethnicity/religion, gender, disability, sexual orientation) are included, not only socioeconomically disadvantaged, [and the] [m]easurement implications are more clear" (Braveman, 2006, p. 173).

Braveman also lists three "examples of definitions of health disparities currently used by U.S. agencies" (Braveman, 2006). Those examples are broad definitions. One of the most attractive among the three is the Centers for Disease Control and Prevention's definition from *Healthy People 2010*:

> Health disparities include "differences … by gender, race or ethnicity, education or income, disability, geographic location, or sexual orientation." "Compelling evidence of large and often increasing racial/ethnic disparities demand national attention." "Racial and ethnic minority populations" [the racial/ethnic groups of concern] are: American Indian & Alaska Native, Asian American, black or African American, Hispanic or Latino, and Native Hawaiian and Other Pacific Islander. (Braveman, 2006, p. 176)

Research to eliminate health disparities is essentially social engineering science related to health inequality. In this way, it is important to realize that the work is not merely interdisciplinary but requires trans-disciplinary approaches. From this section, we can understand health inequality contain the elemental propositions below.

Elemental Definition for Confronting Health Inequality

1. A particular kind of difference in health outcome

   (a) Difference where specific social aggregates historically experienced *persistent* social disadvantage or discrimination

   - Disadvantage refers to an aggregate's relative position in a social hierarchy determined by lack of wealth, power, and/or prestige
   - Historical aggregation of persistent social disadvantage refers to aggregates like those in poverty, those receiving less income for similar occupational roles, some racial and/or ethnic minorities, certain aggregates of sexual minorities, and others classifiable under the rule
   - Social disadvantage typically, however, not necessarily, is shaped by administrative, educational, governmental, institutional, political, public, public health, social, and other forms of policies

2. Health disparities include differences between aggregates with the most advantage in a specified category and the others in that specified category
3. Eliminating health disparities refers to pursuing equity; that is, the elimination of health inequalities

The elemental definition for confronting health inequality recognizes that health inequality is a social product. Health disparities are not necessary. It is possible to avoid them. Moreover, they are unfair. Equality would mean equal availability, equal utilization, and equal quality of care; these equalities are fractions where the denominator is need.

African American Identity and Self-theory

Below this chapter would link health disparity to learning interventions. Specifically, the elimination of health disparities is a global literacy campaign. However, thinking about and doing such campaigns need more conversation. There is a need to discuss effective communication and the diffusion of communications when thinking about health promotion campaigns. For the moment, therefore, this section links identity (that is, the self) to performance (that is, the role) so we can consider the importance of becoming an African American as one role that requires a minimum range of scripts; it is one subunit of a global self. In the definition of African American, this manuscript adopted self-identification of race and ethnicity as the rule for African American identification. This section provides more detail about the theory of identity and social learning. It first explains analytical dimensions of identity that would help in understanding rational choice of healthy behaviors. In this sense, it begins with a definition of a social self.

Social self. Social psychologists have come to understand early conceptions of the self by James ([1892] 1968) and Mead and Morris (1934) as more complicated than they elaborated. Nonetheless, they understood the self as an organized structure. Self means that an individual has the capacity to make itself an object while engaging in social relationships. Therefore, humans come to know themselves, that is, the self, through patterned interaction with others. According to this theory, social interaction forms identity; social interaction influences the behavior of a social player since the player would strive to perform roles given the expectations of their interaction network. The complication is that an individual potentially plays many roles. Some of the roles might overlap or conflict with other roles. Therefore, social psychology began to conceptualize theories of multiple selves. For example, Burke stressed the importance of understanding multiple selves (Burke, 1980). Following this line of theory development, social psychologists tied subunits of the self to positions in the social structure (for an excellent example, see, Stryker, 1968). This theory helps us to understand African American identity and our tasks for eliminating health disparities among them. Ultimately, we must understand identities as motives to accomplish a goal. However, first, it is important to understand how individuals rank identities in their interactions, since individuals must put unique parts of multiple identities in operation during social situations. Moreover, after invoking an identity, others must agree with the attribution and must grant acceptance. Even more, a player must make a commitment to the identity to accomplish social expectation. African American status is an identity, a social self, with social role expectations.

Consequential Rankings of Identity: African Americans and the Salience Hierarchy

When African Americans interact in society, their interactions are largely relationships with other identities in the social organization. Some of the relationships are between African Americans and other racial and ethnic groups. For example, interactions are relationships between African Americans and European Americans. Even more, some interactions are within African American groups. For example, some relationships are between black females and males. Moreover, the relationships could become increasingly complex. For example, relationships between African Americans and institutions where there is racialization. Imagine, in the latter example that some African Americans use a community where all the physicians are European American. We could not think of the many relational ways human beings name difference. A relational analysis would require that we systematically think about these relationships because these relationships are the main ingredient of identification. An individual African American could equally have a relationship with the self where the individual entertains a self-debate about its view of African American, and puts into operation another set of behaviors associated with the modified conception. Those relationships potentially produce distinct identities that would require putting into operation other lines of action; and, as we shall see below, other motivations for action. Individuals must make a decision about which identities to deploy in their arsenal of possible identities. Usually this decision is an invocation. In this case, the individual gives out an identity. Identity theorists have written a great deal about this process. However, we might consider modifying the theory and consider that a powerful group could draw out a quasi-symbolic identity. The latter case implies different physiological processes. For example, under conditioning situations, a person might hear a bell and begin to salivate – primarily an autonomic nervous system function, or, a person might become hungry, push a button, and expect a waiter to bring his meal – primarily a somatic nervous system function. This distinction is likely important when we think about prevention intervention strategies for the elimination of health disparities since such interventions are set in competitive situations.

Given the variations mentioned in the paragraph above, identity theorists remarked that we should think about the hierarchy of salience and commitment to identity. Hierarchy of salience has to do with the chance for a behavioral outcome that a player associates with an identity in terms of the many likely identities that an individual could call upon. One way to guess an identity an individual is likely to put into operation is to rank the identities. In scientific terms, a researcher could express the identities' probabilities. Nonetheless, some researchers could qualitatively express the rank order. A striking example of calling on identity might be to imagine an African American substance-injecting male. Imagine this male is attending a drug use rehabilitation services center. Which identity would the typical drug user call to mind? What mind-frame would that individual most likely put into operation? Alternatively, imagine if the drug user has gone to church on Sunday and imagine the church is largely African American and practices Pentecostalism. This would likely change the hierarchy of salience. In the former case, the individual would likely assume the identity of drug addict. The important identity for social exchange in the rehabilitation services venue is drug addiction. In the latter situation, the top of the ranking would likely become African American status since Pentecostalism heavily serves African Americans and it rewards shunning devilment – drug addiction is a major satanic spirit in the view of many practicing Pentecostalism.

African American Identity and Group Relations

There are many definitions of African American identity. Earlier the chapter accounted for a small fraction of this variation. Below the chapter considers selected important African American group experiences. Conceptually, we could treat the African American identity category as an aggregate or we could treat the identity category as a group. It might be best to treat the African American category as a group. For instance, Kurt Lewin's concept of life-space is helpful in understanding the importance of group membership. Lewin argued that individuals' psychological activities occur within the psychological field that he called the life-space. The life-space consists of all past, present, and future events that assists in influencing and shaping individuals. Each of the events contributes to behavioral responses in particular situations. In addition, the life-space also contains an individual's needs in social interaction with the psychological environment (Lewin, Gentile, & Miller, 2009). Health behaviors intimately connect to life space. Moreover, performing health behaviors are group situations. Lewin defined the group in the following way:

> It is today widely recognized that a group is more than, or, more exactly, different from, the sum of its members. It has its own structure, its own goals, and its own relations to other groups. The essence of a group is not the similarity or dissimilarity of its members, but their interdependence. A group can be characterized as a "dynamical whole"; this means that a change in the state of any subpart changes the state of any other subpart. The degree of interdependence of the subparts of members of the group varies all the way from a loose "mass" to a compact unit. It depends, among other factors, upon the size, organization, and intimacy of the group. (Lewin, 1997, p. 68)

Social psychologists recognize that individuals are typically members of many groups. In fact, more often than not, the groups overlap. For example, church, family, leisure, school, and work groups might be typical organizations that individuals have regular associations with in the USA. The potency of a group depends on how much a particular group influences an individual's behavior. Social situations determine the measure of group potency. For example, when an individual is at home, the family likely is the most potent group when compared to when the individual is at the office. At the office, perhaps, like-minded colleagues are the most potent group. If an individual is an African American construction worker, perhaps the group of African American construction workers on a particular construction site is the most potent group. In addition, Lewin recognized that groups have meaning for individuals. "If a person is not clear about his belongingness or if he is not well established within his group, his life-space will show the characteristics of an unstable ground" (Lewin, 1997, p. 69).

Groups are instrumental in the sense that individuals use groups to gain some need. Individual needs could be emotional, mental, physical, or spiritual ones. However, to gain a need, the individual would establish a goal and then use affiliate groups to accomplish the goal. Therefore, to attack a group is to attack the individual members' goals; it is similar to attacking an individual. Therefore, group members would likely resist such attacks against the group. This is simply because attacks that decrease the status of a group reflect on the statuses of individuals that belong to the group. Lewin demonstrated that the more status an individual has in a group the more freedom the individual has to move within the group. This would influence the life-space of the individual. Therefore, Lewin shows how much health means to the life-space of individuals (Lewin, 1997; Lewin et al., 2009; Lewin & Gold, 1999).

When it comes to group life, the preferential outcome for an individual is to gain as much freedom as possible without losing group affiliation. This means that an individual would have to balance individual needs with group needs. African American cultural practices, therefore, are integral to its health practices.

The African American Self and Motive

Individuals apparently choose subunits of the global-self based on situational conditions for social advantage. Identity theorist Peter Burke, for example, argued that "identities are meanings a person attributes to the self as an object in a social situation or social role" (Burke, 1980, p. 18). Others in a social organization also have the power to attribute identities to a person. An individual can only come to understand self-meanings through interaction with others in situations. That is, the individual must learn the meaning through conversations with others. In this game, the player must accomplish the unification between an identity and the role performance. The player must meet the expectations of the group confirming the adequacy of the performance. Given this, the performance becomes a significant communication when an individual properly performs it. The identity is a name and a performance that implies alternative names and performances in a social group. For example, for an individual to self-attribute the identity mother, implies that the identity is not father, brother, or sister. What is a good mother? Let us presume that the identity includes a role of nursing her infants. We do not expect the other identities to do so. When the infant becomes hungry, we would expect the mother to nurse the infant. Therefore, mothers give the gift of feeding the young; the motivation of the mother is to feed the infant. The motivation of society is to provide for the survival of the young. In this sense, a mother identity has a goal, narrowly defined here, as providing nurturance for children for the larger goal of social survival.

The paragraph above means that "identities provide motivation by acting as agents for the 'meaningful' classification and naming of social objects" (Burke, 1980, p. 22). However, Burke offers the following caveats:

> [T]he classification system that is used operates to classify identities relative to other identities in some sort of semantic space. The meaning (and therefore action implications) of an identity is given by its particular location in the semantic space, and that location is fixed relative to other identities. Identities located close together would have very similar action implications, while identities located more distantly from each other would have very different action implications. In this sense, as Stryker (1968) pointed out, the action implications are the meanings of an identity. But, just as identities have action implications, acts and performances have identity implications (Hull & Levy, 1979; Burke, 1980, p. 22)

How is an identity associated with lines of action? Typically, in the view of many identity theorists, the lines of action are associated with an image. For one problem, individuals are always in a process of becoming. Therefore, there are past and present images of the self. An individual that was alive in 1968, that dramatic year, would certainly not have the same self-image in 2011.

This gloss of identity theory is a brief one. It provides some ideas about how we might think about African American identities in our struggle against health disparities. However, recall that an important element of this perspective is the saying that humans possess the unique ability to make objects of the self. This means that identities are reflexive – "[I]dentities influence performances and these performances are assessed by the self for the kind of identity they imply" (Burke, 1980, p. 20). Therefore, the physician, researcher, and social worker also possess an ability to make an object of their identity and this objectification affects their behavior. Seldom in health disparity studies is self-objectification of researchers' identities examined. Typically, studies treat the relational aspects of health disparities as separate studies where the researcher conceives the mind of the researcher as objective, the researcher considers the mind of the physician as expert and professional, and the researcher considers the mind of the subject as deficient. Such downward comparison is measurable. This is likely an important emergent goal for identity theorists to demonstrate empirically ranking that occurs when we deploy identity names, that is, labels, in public health occupations. We should develop measures of the potential such labeling has to contribute to the creation of stress in consumers of public health.

Bridging and Framing

We are now in the position to "bridge" African American identity to other theories that would provide a frame in our work for the elimination of health disparities. The previous sentence introduces two new concepts in this chapter: bridge and frame. I am using these concepts in the sense that identity theorist Stryker has defined them (Stryker, 2008). Stryker explains that in social and behavioral studies, "A frame specifies a manageable set of general assumptions and concepts assumed important in investigating particular social behaviors… but it does not specify the connections between and among the concepts/variables" (Stryker, p. 17). A theory helps us more in terms of predictive power. Stryker continues, "[A] theory provides a testable explanation of empirical observations, making use of relationships among the concepts provided by the frame" (Stryker, p. 17). A frame is a step that would help us in the production of researchable theory. Stryker then explains building bridges and the importance of them when he writes:

> If single frames and theories cannot provide full explanations of any social behavior, capacity to bridge to other frames and theories becomes an important criterion in evaluating them. Relating ideas across theoretical and research traditions helps avoid intellectual chaos in a field in which specialized theories dealing with specialized topics seem unrelated to one another. Building bridges requires knowledge of ideas with implications beyond particular segments, implying a need for communication across segments. Communication across segments increases the probability of encountering ideas that can generate novel insights unavailable if communication is limited to persons sharing the same ideas. (Stryker, 2008, p. 21)

Stryker has an initial interest in building bridges between identity theory and other microtheories explaining identity commitment, competing identification, and identity management. However, this chapter wants to bridge identity theory to ecological structures where African American identities are likely highly salient in health-related situations. To do so, the chapter briefly glosses the ecological perspective. The idea is to tie ecologies to social and human capital models that help us to understand network structures that potentially communicate diffusion of health promotion.

The Ecological Frame

Influences of the environment on self-perception are important ways for thinking about the elimination of health disparities. The ecological perspective concerns studying human populations in the framework of their cultural characteristics, physical setting, and the organization of its space (that is, its capacity and scope). Ecological frames are thick and complex because ecology is difficult. There are so many layers to human organization. Nonetheless, an advantage to thinking about ecology in pursuit of the elimination of health disparities is that it does justice to reciprocal causation; thereby, it presents greater accuracy corresponding to reality. For example, if health researchers are thinking about eliminating behaviors that promote sexually transmitted infection as one element of a health promotion campaign, they might need to think about the social control of sex in a community as well as individual characteristics of barrier use and promiscuity. The way we think about these research strategies is important enough to think about them in some general detail.

Urie Bronfenbrenner and his colleagues contribute a life of research in this area (Bronfenbrenner, 1986, 2000, 2005a, 2005b; Bronfenbrenner, Friedman, & Wachs, 1999; Bronfenbrenner, Morris, Lerner, & Damon, 2006). Ecological health researchers typically focus on five dimensions of organization: (1) intrapersonal qualities, (2) interpersonal relations, (3) organizational characteristics, (4) community organization, and (5) public policy.

Intrapersonal issues associates with the observation that individuals can change their attitudes, beliefs, information base, and skill sets. Such change could contribute to behavioral change. Individuals can also change their identities; or at least, the meanings and requirements of their identities. There are behavioral models that might apply to health intervention work. For example, health belief, social learning, stages of change, and theory of reasoned action are a few. These models each contain a function for human choice and determination.

Interpersonal relations are typically relationships with coworkers, family, friends, and neighbors; that is more intimate relationships, or relationships with significant others. Bronfenbrenner's work is heavily concerned with such relationships. He calls them proximal ones and has a concern about proximal processes. This section will describe proximal processes in detail below. However, proximal relations are ones that are part of the daily routine, where the relationships with the environment are immediate and happen over an extended period. There are a number of health intervention models for working on interpersonal behaviors. For example, network, social support, and aspects of marketing approaches would function in interpersonal situations.

Participation, Relevance, and Selection in Daily Health Routines

Organizations can influence health outcomes and health outcomes can influence them. Typically, health researchers think about organizational change for the maintenance of organizational capacity and scope. Below is a general framework for thinking about the organization of structures that might promote efficient change to impact the health outcomes of large populations. Perhaps it is prudent to introduce a new idea about combining principle of participation, principle of relevance, and issue selection into our thinking about organizational structures. We typically find these three concepts in community organizing literature. Dorothy Nyswander has contributed to this conceptual framework (2006; 1942). The principle of participation refers to learning by doing. The principle of relevance refers to meeting the population where it is. Issue selection cautions health researchers to select projects that communities find important. In one sense, it has to do with ranking the identification of a problem based on its salience for group identities. Problems that appear potent for the community are preferred above problems that the health researcher finds vital. We could quickly discern that in the context of historical US racialization, African Americans would likely find "racism" a major problem. This is not to say that African Americans would not find improvement in race relations over time; that is, they would likely report decreasing "racism" in society.

If racialization is a major problem among African Americans, it becomes a candidate for intervention. Typically, we would think the most appropriate place for a racialization intervention would occur in the organizational process. Since racialization is a process of ranking and sorting to engineer inequality of treatment and outcome, we recognize its effectiveness embedded in social organization.

This hunch needs additional conceptual consideration and empirical verification. However, we should first explore the idea before we attempt to validate it. In the process of exploring this idea, we might design studies that introduce counter-racialization strategies. For example, we might think of the counter-racialization phenomena in the terms of dosing. Therefore, we might imagine what dosage of which instruction decreases racialized outcomes. The viewpoint that major structures like class, gender, and race are untreatable by public health workers requires interrogation. These structures of inequality are likely social disease and, ecologically speaking, they spread greater disease.

Community and Proximal Relations

Another dimension of these proximal relations happens in community. In the community, there is face-to-face interaction with primary groups. These interactions are where identity takes place. This chapter discussed the identity theory aspect of identification above. In that description, identity occurs in a competitive situation where identity salience emerges from a rational choice process. Community provides mediating structures contributing to identity choice and commitment, while also contributing to other resources, not the least of which is social support. Resource management can assist in community health development through coalition building and coordination. Moreover, community health organizers can initiate educational campaigns through community organization. For example, health workers could establish and measure empowerment campaigns that stress learning by doing through community organization. Such campaigns are literacy ones, however, the function is not to lecture a community about proper health practices. Rather, the purpose is to present the competitive outcomes of health choices available in the environment and facilitate resources for students to teach themselves about health promotion (Freire, 1983).

Social policy refers to governance policies that promote the US creed of social justice for its citizenry. Such policies have typically targeted the reduction of some diseases and infectious agents. From a modern ecological perspective, powerful individuals and groups made and enforced choices resulting in the unequal distribution of outcomes. This means that social organization preceded ecological outcomes. There has been considerable advancement of ecological theories. In fact, ecological models are ones that we should likely consider as emergent ones. Those models tackle conditions and processes of human development. That is, many of the early studies addressed childhood development. Earlier, the chapter mentioned that Bronfenbrenner's work is important to the field. In fact, Bronfenbrenner now refers to the model as the bioecological model. The chapter next explains this formulation.

Bioecological Model

Earlier the chapter mentioned proximal processes. They conceptually and operationally refer to the devices that result in biopsychological development. In this frame, biopsychological development is never ending in the individual; therefore, stages of development are observable throughout the life course (Bronfenbrenner & Morris, 1998). The bioecological model has two major propositions. Bronfenbrenner and Pamela Morris reported them first in 1998 as follows:

> *Proposition I.* Human development takes place throughout life through processes of progressively more complex reciprocal interaction between an active, evolving biopsychological human organism and the persons, objects, and symbols in its immediate external environment. To be effective, the interaction must occur on a fairly regular basis over extended periods of *time*. Such enduring forms of interaction in the immediate environment are referred to as *proximal processes* (Bronfenbrenner & Morris, 1998, p. 996). (Quoted in Bronfenbrenner, 2000, p. 130).

Intensity of interaction and repetition, that is, potency and consistent dosing, are essential to ecological outcomes. Inconsistent and occasional strain likely would contribute much less ecological influence when compared to structural strain.[1] Bronfenbrenner reported the second proposition:

> *Proposition II.* The form, power, content, and direction of the proximal processes effecting development vary systematically as a joint function of the characteristics of the developing *person*: the *environment* – both immediate and more remote – in which the processes are taking place; the nature and the *developmental outcomes* under consideration; and the social continuities and changes occurring over *time* through the life course and the historical period during which the person has lived. (Bronfenbrenner, 2000, p. 130)

Underdevelopment of health is interdependent on both propositions. Taken together, the model contains consideration of the process, person, context, and time; therefore, Bronfenbrenner refers to it as the *Process–Person–Context–Time* model (PPCT). To Proposition I he adds a corollary, accounting for affective attachment, "The developmental power of proximal processes is substantially enhanced when they occur within the context of a relationship between persons who have developed a strong emotional attachment to each other" (Bronfenbrenner, 2000, p. 130). For example, strong emotional ties between parent and child reduce strain, thereby increasing healthy development. Strain is normal physiological response to situations or stimuli that individuals perceive as dangerous. In the parent–child relationship, strong emotional ties reduce negative health effects in parents as well as in children. For example, children require unusual attention, which is a stressor. Greater emotional ties increase capacity to pay attention. Therefore, according to empirical findings in Bronfenbrenner and his colleagues' work, strong emotional ties between parent and child are mutually rewarding for development. Moreover, they produce self-control in the child. Locus of control becomes more internal (Rotter offers important details related to this sentence, 1975). The child then learns to "defer immediate gratification in the interest of pursuing and achieving longer-range goals. The process through which this transition is achieved is called internalization" (Bronfenbrenner, 2000, p. 130).

General Hypotheses

We have bridged several frames and theories in this section. It covers a great deal of empirical work. Nonetheless, we are at a point where it is possible to see the kinds of hypotheses with higher explanatory power that we might suggest from the ecological frame, particularly, the bioecological model. For one, we expect the environmental context produces variation in the Process. For example, we expect covariance between individual characteristics and socioeconomic status to produce variation in health development. Specifically, African American identity and low socioeconomic status have the greatest impact on health disadvantage. Moreover, we expect that health-development produces variation in African American identity and low socioeconomic status. That is, the more health development, the more social development among those with African American identity and those that identify as African American from lower socioeconomic statuses.

Bronfenbrenner introduces the terms dysfunction and competence. These terms assist in designing studies that measure health disparities. According to the bioecological model, the central hypothesis is:

> The greater developmental impact of proximal processes … in disadvantaged or disorganized environments is expected mainly for outcomes reflecting developmental *dysfunction*. By contrast, for outcomes reflecting developmental *competence*, proximal processes are posited as likely to have greater impact in more advantaged and stable environments. … The term "dysfunction" refers to the recurrent manifestation of difficulties on the

---

[1] Strain refers to stress from actions or force that deforms a social organization. In short, strain produces unexpected public health outcomes. Strain implies capricious application of policies. Major structural strains are class, gender, and race. They imply capricious treatment in social organization. Disorganization and disadvantage imply strain.

part of the developing person in maintaining control and integration of behavior across a variety of situations, whereas "competence" is defined as the further development of abilities – whether intellectual, physical, socioemotional, or combinations of them.

Proximal processes provide for choice, whether the choice comes from health care providers or consumers. Naturally, our social and behavioral interventions would require that health promoters enter corrections where choice is doable. In addition, we would need to use the cheapest cost for the most interventional potency – given that we are working with large populations. Moreover, we would need to have precise strategies for interventional diffusion at the cheapest cost. Ideas for change are competitive, competition is not perfect, and therefore we need to think about marketing strategies given civilized competition. We would also need innovative ways to think about measuring comparisons between health dysfunction and competence in context of ecological strains. The chapter now turns to this latter problem and discusses it in the context of African American identity. It will suggest a relational approach to some variable constructions and this relational approach would allow for a discussion of entering at interventional openings, and specific strategies for the diffusion of innovation.

Background of the African American Experience: Identity and Strain

This section glosses the social experience of African Americans with widespread diffusion of marginalization and discrimination against African Americans. The section raises a concern that African American identity is a major stressor requiring tackling in order to reduce and eliminate African American health disparities. To aid in the elucidation, the section discusses William Cross's identity conflict theory of Nigrescence. Nigrescence is a theory of black identity formation in the context of US racialization. This strategy helps us to see unique intervention needs for African Americans. It assists us in understanding the possibility that generic models of health promotion might fail stigmatized identities; it would also help seeing how stigmatize populations might internalize stigma and how that internalization might strain health promoting locus of control. Moreover, interrogating strain in this way, sensitize us to the ways racialization as a sorting mechanism constitutes an association between social statuses and identity, and ultimately mental health (Schwartz & Meyer, 2010). While these effects might be additive, as Schwartz and Meyer suggest in their empirical tests of between- and within-group variation associated with social stress theory, we might also think that racialized sorting is constitutive of strain.

Brief History of African American Social Status as an Identity Strain

African American experience in the USA is replete with experiences of inequality. After 1776, there were likely free people of African descent. Nonetheless, most African Americans were slaves. Even free people of color suffered differential social status. The USA did not allow for the political representation of African Americans. Moreover, early US society excluded African Americans from many other rights, for examples, the society did not allow them to read, write, or enter into contract. In fact, there were separate laws for African Americans and these discriminations affected the organization of family and the inheritance of property. Since marriage is contractual, it precluded African American participation. Following the Civil War, presidential proclamation and constitutional amendments outlawed organized plantation slavery – the USA outlawed the importation of slaves in 1808. Nonetheless, sections of the nation reconstituted black servitude through a number of discriminatory practices, notwithstanding resistance by blacks that they learned during slavery (Bauer & Bauer, 1942). In addition, the federal government compromised African American civil rights by yielding to campaigns of states' rights. By 1896, "separate but equal" laws prevailed. Despite the fact that the Supreme Court repealed these laws in the 1950s, the society continued to marginalize African Americans in virtually every aspect of human existence. For example, the society would regularly riot against African Americans. To control them, miniature race riots in the form of lynching became widespread throughout the nation (Ginzburg, 1988). It was not until the 1960s that blacks retaliated through riot. However, blacks mobilized during the 1950s to eliminate social disparities.

US society continued its harassment of African Americans. For example, in the labor market, employers routinely paid lower wages to African Americans for the same or similar work than they paid most European Americans (Bonacich, 1975). In health, also, US society traditionally marginalized African Americans resulting from racialization. An example of the inequality was the life and death of Dr. Charles Richard Drew. In the 1940s, Drew developed a technique to separate blood plasma from whole blood. The technique extended the shelf life of blood ready for transfusions. In addition, that technique made it possible for his discovery that blood transfusions did not require blood typing since plasma contains no red blood cells. Therefore, physicians could use plasma alone in transfusion procedures. The international community quickly recognized Drew and applied his work to national war efforts. For example, he was involved in Great Britain's first blood bank. Nonetheless, he was destitute since the medical profession paid black researchers considerably lower wages than white researchers and the profession paid black physicians considerably less than they paid white physicians. Drew died from injuries incurred in 1950 from an automobile accident while traveling related to his professional responsibility. The African American folklore is that Drew required a transfusion but the hospital denied him stemming from social racialization.

One consequence of the history glossed in this section is that African American experience with discrimination, marginalization, and racialization contributes to the overall degradation of their social category. The degradation of the social category strains the identity. Therefore, researchers concerned about interventions to reduce health disparities might have a need to acknowledge African American identity as an ecological stressor.

Nigrescence

William Cross's theory of Nigrescence is about individuals developing black identity that represents a "sense of people hood" (Bridges, 2010), that is, social capital embedded in social networks (Cross, 1991). The reason for discussing Nigrescence in this section is to draw a connection between African American identities as one social stressor where we find within-group variation. Group social agency changes within-group variation overtime. Cross's theory of Nigrescence also helps us to see this agency effect – that is, intervention effect – because Nigrescence theory revisions have been necessary overtime. Furthermore, Nigrescence theory is an example of "structural group disadvantage" (Schwartz & Meyer, 2010) that influences conceptual models of independent, mediator, and outcome variations operating ecologically.[2] Given Cross's theory, we are able to

---

[2] There are two technical background details related to this discussion. One has to do with early work on ecological fallacies. This would become clearer below since a great deal of research has rehabilitated ecological approaches. Nonetheless, the work of W.S. Robinson might interest some health disparity intervention researchers (Robinson, 1950). Herbert Blalock responded by suggesting the necessity of including aggregate, ecological, data in social research studies while cautioning such designs must be conceptually sound (Blalock, 1979). Moreover, Davis and his colleagues suggested the importance of including both individual and aggregate level data in research designs (Davis, Spaeth, & Huson, 1961). A second technicality has been with the validity and reliability of outcome measures of disparities. For example, a mental health outcome that compares groups with advantages to groups with disadvantages, that is, between group differences. Brown and his colleagues present a lucid discussion of this problem (Brown et al., 1999).

conceptualize the importance of identification and how identity contains variations in stress. This is considerably different from "structural disadvantage" that many researchers working on health disparities study. The difference is the opportunity to think about variation in identification produces variation in stress levels. This latter proposition is more sensitive to variation vis-à-vis coping among the structurally disadvantaged, given equality of resources or the relative lack of resources.

There are five stages for African American development contextualized as adaptive development after experience with racialized conquer and historical debasement. The stages are pre-encounter, encounter, immersion–emersion, internalization, and internalization-commitment. Pre-encounter refers to individual rejection of black culture and virtually full acceptance of a racialization culture that includes its social norms and roles. Encounter refers to eye-opening experiences with social inconsistency between civil rights and the social structure of racialization; in short, the individual becomes aware of the oppression of black culture. Immersion–emersion refers to individual saturation of African American culture while simultaneously rejecting the culture of racialization. Internalization alludes to individual acceptance of African legacy that includes acknowledging attitudes, beliefs, traditions, and values of other cultures. Internalization-commitment observes self-esteem, tolerance of social and cultural difference, while continuing internalization of black identity (Cross, 1991; Cross et al., 2001; Vandiver, Cross, Worrell, & Fhagen-Smith, 2002; Vandiver, Fhagen-smith, Cokley, Cross, & Worrell, 2001; Worrall & Pratt, 2004; Worrell, Cross, & Vandiver, 2001; Worrell, Schaefer, Cross, & Fhagen-Smith, 2006; Worrell, Vandiver, Cross, & Fhagen-Smith, 2004).

Cross and his colleagues revised Nigrescence theory. The revisions maintain the important point for our work here. Most notably, structural group disadvantage is fundamentally identification. Moreover, within the organization of hierarchical identification, there is simultaneously learning, that is, development, and human agency. Therefore, at the social psychological level of analysis, when it comes to health disparities, we can expect individual and social change initiated through learning by individuals. If this were not the case, the symbolic interaction perspective in social psychology is bogus. Below this would become clearer. For the moment, it should be clear that even if we read Cross as moralistic rather than scientific, it has little consequence on the conceptual framework. Therefore, Nigrescence theory's change is because of observations that are more appropriate in the pre-encounter, immersion-emersion, and internalization stages of identity. In the pre-encounter stage, race has insignificant strength and nationalism has significant strength. Cross and his colleagues conceptualized a pre-encounter mis-education identity where the individual internalizes negative stereotypes about black Americans; notably, they are criminal, lazy, promiscuous, and violent. Furthermore, the pre-encounter self-hatred identity holds more intense negative views about African Americans when compared to merely internalizing negative stereotypes. The individual presents anti-black self-hatred attitudes and beliefs (Worrell et al., 2001).

The revision includes two identities forming a Manichean belief system for the immersion-emersion stage of identity. Intense black involvement identity is where everything black is good. Anti-white identity views everything white as bad. This revision is largely categorical and not substantive. The revision of internalization consists of two dimensions. Black Nationalism is an African-centered identity that eschews degrading other identities. Multicultural inclusive identity acknowledges cultures of non-black groups while simultaneously believing in the importance of black identity.

These identities are all constitutive of social strain. Perspectives concerning them might rank their categorical intensities differently. For example, if a researcher conceptualizes the USA as a heavily racialized society where continuing racialization is prevalent, as perhaps sociologist Joe Feagin, political scientist Andrew Hacker, or historian and political scientist Manning Marable and his colleagues might (Feagin, 2004; Hacker, 1992; Marable, Steinberg, & Middlemass, 2007), then the most intense identity stressor would become those in Cross's internalization-commitment category. On the other hand, researchers with colorblind perspectives, like linguist John McWhorter or economist Thomas Sowell (McWhorter, 2000; Sowell, 1981), might consider a solution to an identity stressor problem to be assimilation, where the closer an African American identifies with Cross's pre-encounter orientation, there we would find diminishing identity strain. In this view, one that we might call a relational view since it conceptualizes identities as structures in relationship to other structures, that is, as symbolic interaction. Thinking in this way eliminates the possibility of conceptualizing stress as a variable outside of identity structure. Instead, social and behavioral researchers might consider stress as inextricable from the identity category, which is another part of structure, as are the gender, geographic location, economic, and sexual orientation stressors. Given this, we might ask who is an African American. Part of that answer here is that an African American identity in the USA is a social stressor. Who is an African American? The answer is, a person living under conditions of irregular strain. This does not elide between groups or within group variation. The next section discusses how conceiving of the possibility that identities are social stressors assist us in thinking of the possibility that virtually all health disparity finds its origin in socio-ecological stress.

Who Is African American?

One way to think about racial and ethnic categorizations is to think of them as language to serve some social function. In the preceding, this chapter glossed the impression of the scientific category, African American. One solution that the manuscript takes is to adopt the U.S. Census Bureau's definition, which is self-identification. We saw this identification is complex through Cross's theory of Nigrescence. In this section, the manuscript suggests that the African American identity is a structural disadvantage based on its stressor content. If this view is correct, then not only is the social stressor a mediating variable, the person that internalizes the African American identity embodies the social stressor associated with it. That is, the identity is not merely a variable; rather, its content contains strain. This section first glosses stressor theory. Next, it considers how social and behavioral health disparity research might model health disparity in the context of various structural stressors. The latter will reveal the complexity of stressors; however, the section would highlight identity and social capital stressors.

Stressor Theory

In an analysis of mental health disparities research, Sharon Schwartz and Ilan H. Meyer wrote:

> There are many pathways through which social disadvantage can translate into health disparities, including exposure to deleterious physical and social environments and limited access to adequate health care. Recently, the social stress model has gained predominance as an explanatory frame… Social stressors, particularly those related to prejudice and discrimination, have been invoked to explain disparities in diverse mental and physical health outcomes… (Schwartz & Meyer, 2010, p. 1111)

Schwartz and Meyer go on to show that social stress theory implies a meditational model. The main effect in the model is that persons with lower social standing, that is, disadvantaged social status, results in greater health disparities. In that model, there are three variables: the independent variable is disadvantaged social status, the mediating variable is stress, and the outcome variable is health disparity. Nonetheless, there are three ways that health disparity researchers working with social stress theory conceptualize the relationship. The first is within group analyses. In it, structural group disadvantage is independent but likely subsidiary and leads to stressors that are determinative of the health disparity criterion. The second model is between group analyses. In such models, the researcher recognizes health disparity if the association between structural group disadvantage and stress is substantial and the mediating stress substantially reduces the main effect between structural group disadvantage and health disparity (Schwartz & Meyer, 2010, p. 1112). Below, this section proposes an African American identity stressor model that departs from typical patterns of analyses.

However, before leaving Schwartz and Meyer, the section glosses important grounds of social stress theory that they highlight.

Schwartz and Meyer add some cautionary notes that health-disparity intervention researchers should note. When researchers observe a difference between populations, it is not necessarily a health disparity. For example, finding higher rates of venereal infection in promiscuous individuals is a difference. However, finding higher rates of venereal infection in monogamous African Americans than in monogamous European Americans is a disparity. Therefore, Schwartz and Meyer point out that, health disparity refers to an "inequality in health due to social factors or allocation of resources."

When studying stressors associated with social disadvantage, the concern is for the social group; therefore, typically analyses are concerned with "average effects." These average effects betray individual differences. For example, among African Americans a segment of the population might not have experienced any disease conditions that disproportionately affect them. However, structural group disadvantage researchers have assumptions about the spread of disease that the model implies. For one thing, contagion is communicative and occurs in networks. In addition, that communication operates among healthy subpopulations of African Americans. Therefore, health disparities are ecological where one major aspect of it has to do with social capital. Moreover, there are dimensions of health disparities that deal with other forms of capital, including cultural, financial, and human. For this reason, we can map our interventions in productive ways using empirical and theoretical knowledge based on experience with competitive markets, networks, social support, systems of communication, and diffusion of innovative practices. In this way, intervention researchers become culture-makers that can make new ways of health promotion. It does little good for researchers endlessly to recite health disparities from scientific studies without pragmatism. Pragmatic orientations insist that social and behavioral science can improve health outcomes in ways that are economically, politically, and socially possible. Parsimony requires work at the aggregate level. However, this is not the only reason for adopting an aggregate level approach to the elimination of health disparities. More importantly, healthy societies require a group approach. Social groups generate knowledge about healthy living and they disseminate the knowledge as groups to educate other groups. It is impractical to think that individuals do this work. Health interventions are groups, that is, clusters, of individuals working together to accomplish healthy living goals.

Schwartz and Meyer also caution that structural group disadvantage researchers interested in social stressors are not primarily concerned about specific disorders. They typically are concerned about omnibus health outcomes. For example, researchers would focus on venereal infection rather than a specific and relatively rare strain of syphilis, for instance, *Treponema pallidum*, in the USA (Mitchell et al., 2006). This does not preclude observations of specific variations of disease. Insofar as this is concerned, such focusing issues are problematic for social and behavioral interventions. This is particularly relevant when health educators and researchers must form collaborative alliances with community collaborators. The definition of disease affects the rates of disease; that is, structural disorder. The more distant a social aggregate is from influencing a social problem's nomenclature, the higher is that aggregate's likely association in presenting the pathological condition. One outcome of this is that educators and researchers often play the roles of lecturing communities with structural group disadvantages. One deleterious effect of such relationships is their risk of diminishing trust between the players in the health promotion competition.

African American Identity Stressor Model

Pragmatic complications that are implications from the discussion above suggest that researchers might modify approaching some health disparities, particularly when studying African Americans. For example, there might be a need to increase conversations concerning the conceptualization of stressors. We have enough evidence to know that major inequalities associate with major categories of structural group disadvantages. We also know of a possibility that some racial/ethnic categories, like African American, are codes for racialization. Therefore, Fig. 1.1 presents an alternative conceptualization of stressors that assumes it flows from social factors and allocation of resources.

The main effect for the African American identity stressor model is the composite African American identity disadvantage stressors. Here, we would consider that identification with the group is a major social stressor given the context of US discrimination, racialization, and unequal health outcomes. There is within-group variation among African Americans. For example, we would suspect sexual orientation variation. There is within-group variation among alternative sexual orientation of African Americans. For example, we would suspect differences among young African American lesbians and elderly African American lesbians. Researchers could treat each of these subgroup variations in the same manner they treat the major category, African American. That is, a researcher could recode those demographic characteristics as dummy variables in their analyses. Likewise, such recodes allow for comparison (control) groups. For example, if collaboration would like to compare black and white aggregates, it is possible to create dummy variables for each of the two characteristics. This would create identity variables as metaphors representing average characteristics of the structure of racialization in the population. Path a in Fig. 1.1 is a representation of the main effect. If there is no difference between the structurally disadvantaged African Americans compared to other aggregates or selected privileged aggregates in the population, then we must stop the analysis since there would be no disparity.

A relatively great deal of literature has developed on socioeconomic characteristics as predictors of health disparities (Braveman, 2005; Braveman et al., 2006; Braveman, Cubbin, Marchi, Egerter, & Chavez, 2001; LaVeist, 2005; Williams, Adler, Marmot, McEwen, & Stewart, 1999; Williams, Mohammed, Leavell, & Collins, 2010). For example, Duncan et al. reported wealth and recent family income association was strongest in association study with mortality (Duncan, Daly, McDonough, & Williams, 2002). Williams et al. reported socioeconomic status associates with health disparities across racial groupings. They found that race is associated with multiple dimensions of social inequality (Williams et al.). Williams et al. described higher disease rates for blacks compared to whites that are pervasive and persistent over time (Williams et al.). In addition, researchers found such persistent conditions associated with generic conditions. For example, Verna Keith et al. reported that race, socioeconomic status, and gender influence mental health among black women (Keith, Brown, Scheid, & Brown, 2010). Relin Yang et al. found African American patients were less likely to undergo operations for invasive ductal and lobular breast carcinoma. In addition, low socioeconomic status predicted less likelihood to have operations and patients presenting with larger tumors. Some studies contradict the race and socioeconomic association with certain disease conditions. For example, Lisa Signorello et al. found difference in diabetes prevalence rates among African Americans compared to whites likely reflects differences in risk factors such as socioeconomic status (Signorello et al., 2007).

Given the above, researchers might conclude the importance of including a measure of socioeconomic status disadvantage. Issues of multicollinearity might require caution. Nonetheless, a standard measure of socioeconomic status or some combined measures, for example, level of schooling, father's income when a respondent was 16, or researchers might use some other relevant variables to measure socioeconomic status. These decisions would necessarily depend on the research question, past research practices, and trial and error while working with the data. For illustrative purposes, Fig. 1.1 includes socioeconomic status disadvantage and geographic location stressors (Jung Hoon, Sunderland, Kendall, Gudes, & Henniker, 2010). Other variables could be included in the model, for example, gender. Unidentified vertical solid lines in the figure connect these variables; the important statistical fact about them is that they co-vary with each other. Links d, e, and f represent those covariates.

African American identity stressor model

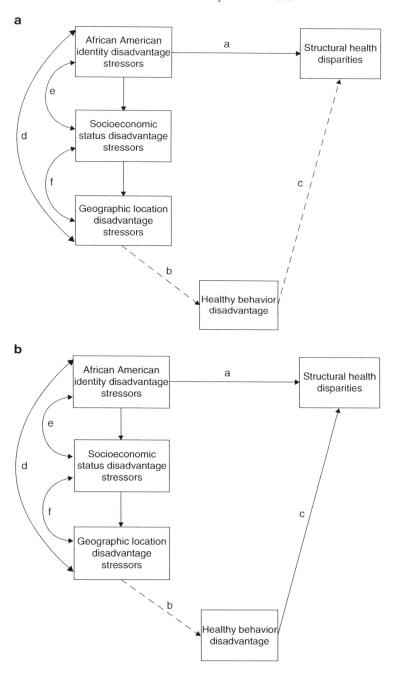

Fig. 1.1 African American identity stressor model. Note: The *single-arrow solid line* is a main effect. *Vertical solid lines* between exogenous predictors are logical paths where the order is inconsequential. *Broken lines* are mediating effects. *Double arrows* indicate covariance

The model includes a mediator, namely behavioral disadvantage. The literature indicates different kinds of behavioral disadvantages. One disadvantage is a lack of trust of the public health system. Therefore, conditions of trust might need interventions. One quick response to lack of trust is to ridicule the distrustful until some sign of change in attitude becomes apparent. Another response is to lecture the distrustful hoping to transform them with reason. These ways of transforming trust might not change attitudes, behaviors, and beliefs as effectively as other ways of communicating with distrustful populations. Below, for example, the chapter reviews some selected aspects of diffusion theory. We learn there that spreading new attitudes, beliefs, and behaviors, that is, contagion, is more effective when target individuals has close ties with adopters of the new attitudes, beliefs, and behaviors. Reciting that African Americans do not trust public health agents does little to advance transformation. Many factors could account for lack of trust, for example, experiences over the life course would affect behavior. Before describing Fig. 1.1 panels in additional detail, this section briefly glosses some ways ecology could affect attitudes, beliefs, and behaviors. For example, ecological insults could affect activities of daily living and these might affect health outcomes. There is no requirement that the insult effect is immediate. It might influence behavior over time. On the other hand, the effect could have immediate consequences.

James S. Jackson and his colleagues studied race and unhealthy behaviors where they used longitudinal data from the Americans' Changing Lives study that the Survey Research Center, Institute for Social Research, University of Michigan collected (2010). The authors report the following:

> Compared with Americans of European descent, Black Americans have greater physical health morbidity and mortality at every age. For example, Black women are twice as likely as White women to die of hypertensive cardiovascular disease. In addition, Blacks have a lower average life expectancy (70 years) than Whites do (77 years), with Black men having a life expectancy of only 66 years. Although the causes of these differences are debated, what is notable is how consistently these physical health disparities favor non-Hispanic Whites over Blacks. … We theorize that, over the life course, coping strategies that are effective in "preserving" the mental health of Blacks may work in concert with social, economic, and environmental inequalities to produce physical health disparities in middle age and late life. (Jackson, Knight, & Rafferty, 2010, p. 933)

Jackson et al. show how different bioecological experiences might change behaviors of individuals. For one thing, the behavioral change could follow shortly after an experience. On the other hand, the behavioral change could occur after so many dosages of an experience, that is, after intense reinforcement. Even more, the behavior change could uniquely relate to an experience with well-being effects but with life course detrimental effects. Jackson et al. demonstrate that particular ecological stresses result in behavioral changes among African Americans. They refer to these as "stress response." For example, negative life events produce more consumption of "comfort food" among many African Americans, particularly among African American women. Comfort foods are high in fats and carbohydrates, bio-psycho-physiological research shows they reduce feelings of anxiety (cited by Jackson et al., 2010; Dallman, Akana et al., 2003; Dallman, Pecoraro et al., 2003). Use of such foods or other unhealthy behavior, like smoking cigarettes or using illicit drugs, might hide depression. For example, if we were to compare self-reported depression among blacks and whites, whites in less stressful ecologies might report more depression. However, this might find explanation in self-medication that abates depression while contributing to long-term unhealthy effects.

When researchers move from the conceptual definition to the operational definition of a variable in a study, often the concept and the indicator are incompatible. For example, in thinking about ecological stressors among African Americans, it is possible to think of at least three ways to make them operational. The researcher could have an objective indicator, for example, the researcher could reason that an experience with unemployment is a stressor. The researcher might reason that if they ask the people they are studying what stresses them, rank order those responses, and then sum them, they could report those experiences as an indicator of life stressors. Finally, a researcher could ask others, including those not being studied what is a life stressor and sum those responses from individuals included in a study to estimate life stressors. Researchers might think about this carefully. For example, in some health disparity research among low female and black socioeconomic groups, they reported seeing someone beaten on the streets or in their homes as major stressors (Fullilove & Fullilove, 1994). Among incarcerated men and women, witnessing a prison rape might represent the most salient stressor (Mariner & Human Rights Watch, 2001). When we use middle-class measures of social stressors, we run the risk of bias and might miss the opportunity to identity conditions that would likely mediate behavior.

The fact that life course experience might greatly affect health outcomes is important. In fact, we would not necessarily know where in the life course an influence triggers behavioral change. Nonetheless, we know that bioecological insults might lie dormant for many years and their consequences might erupt at another stage of the life course. For example, Steven Haas and Leah Rohlfsen (2010) report a number of "life course influences on racial/ethnic disparities in health." Here is a selected list of some they considered "*critical* or *sensitive*" that they report:

- Barker (1998) hypothesizes that poor maternal nutrition during gestation results in fetal growth retardation, which alters the structure and function of tissues associated with insulin, blood pressure, and lipid regulation, increasing the risk of adult cardiovascular disease and diabetes.
- Empirically, those experiencing socioeconomic disadvantage in childhood have worse adult health outcomes including increased risk of various disabling chronic diseases (Wannamethee & Whincup, 1996) and higher mortality rates (Smith & Hart, 1997).
- Childhood SES is also associated with low physical functioning at midlife (Guralnik, Butterworth, Wadsworth, & Kuh, 2006) as well as functional health trajectories (Haas, 2008).
- There is debate as to the relative influence of early life and adult SES. Some researchers suggest that the impact of childhood SES is limited to that of a determinant of more proximal adult SES (Marmot, Shipley, Brunner, & Hemingway, 2001).
- Others suggest that the impact of childhood and adult SES varies by underlying disease process (Lawlor, Ebrahim, & Smith, 2005).
- Those who experience poor childhood health have increased risk of chronic disease and work-limiting disability (Blackwell, Hayward, & Crimmins, 2001; Colley, Douglas, & Reid, 1973; Haas, 2008; Kuh & Wadsworth, 1993; Ye & Waite, 2005).
- Evidence from the 1946 British cohort study links birth weight, physical growth, and cognitive development to physical performance in midlife (Kuh et al., 2002, 2006).
- Childhood health has been shown to have significant impacts on trajectories of functional limitation in the USA (Haas, 2008; Haas & Rohlfsen, 2010, p. 241).

Haas and Rohlfsen remark, "the *cumulative insults* approach thus posits that there are social, environmental, and behavioral exposures over the life course which alters an individual's risk of disease in addition to any critical/sensitive period effects" (Haas & Rohlfsen, 2010, p. 241). There is evidence of life course determinants of racial/ethnic disparities in functional health disparities. These disparities likely influence behaviors at moments in the life course. Some of them would come from feelings of hopelessness among some African Americans. Others might come from feelings of distrust. Yet, others might come from feelings that others do not care. Therefore, health behavior disadvantage is a complicated mediator that affects disparate outcomes.

The two panels A and B represent different ways researchers might think about a stressor model. These are merely examples and there are other ways to think about modeling variation. The main effect is the same in both panels. That is, both show that African American status is a social stressor that correlates with other social stressors. Structural health disparities are associated with these stressors.

In Panel A, health behavior disadvantage is a mediator of the three groups of stressors. Path A*b* represents this and these relationships and path A*c* represents measure changes of structural health disparities. A number of studies that generally conform to its pattern influence this thinking. For examples, the following studies might fit this paradigm. Albert et al. examined illness beliefs about heart failure among black and white cohorts. Health failure beliefs were less accurate among African Americans. They cautioned health care providers to consider the causes of the differences particularly in terms of the ways they teach about, use pedagogy materials, and engage patients' family members in educating about heart failure (Albert, Trochelman, Meyer, & Nutter, 2010). Fuller-Thompson et al. studied how education and income affects activities of daily living among elderly black and white in the U.S. Education and income explains disability by socioeconomic status. Reductions in racialized health disparities require more understanding of the mechanisms where lower income and education are associated with functional outcomes in older persons (Fuller-Thomson, Nuru-Jeter, Minkler, & Guralnik, 2009). Hajat et al. found that stress – measured by cortisol models – mediates the relationship between socioeconomic status and race and cardiovascular disease (Hajat et al., 2010). Jung Hoon et al. studied the distribution through e-health of chronic disease by geographic location and socioeconomic status. The authors associate geographical variation with Internet accessibility, Internet status, and chronic diseases. They found significant disparities in access to health information among socioeconomically disadvantaged areas (Jung Hoon et al., 2010). Karlamangla et al. found an association between coronary heart disease and socioeconomic slopes. Disparities in cardiovascular risk in the USA are primarily associated with socioeconomic status; however, race and ethnicity affects some disparate outcomes (Karlamangla, Merkin, Crimmins, & Seeman, 2010). Pan et al. studied the relationship between poverty and childhood cancer. They found that medium and high poverty counties had lower age-adjusted incidence of childhood cancer rates when compared to low poverty counties. However, they found a race effect when they stratified the sample. The researchers found associations among whites but not among blacks (Pan, Daniels, & Zhu, 2010). Quinn et al. reported that housing stressors and socioeconomic status affect respiratory outcomes for children and behavioral and biological characteristics mediate the respiratory outcomes (Quinn, Kaufman, Siddiqi, & Yeatts, 2010).

In panel B, the three groups of stressors mediate health behavior disadvantage; path B*b*. represents that relationship. Health behavior disadvantage, path B*c*, has a direct effect on structural health disparities. A number of studies might fit this model. The following, for examples, are candidates. Denney et al. examined smoking levels by socioeconomic status. The smoking behavior is an important mediator for education-mortality (Denney, Rogers, Hummer, & Pampel, 2010). Fry-Johnson et al. examined black infant mortality disparities among blacks and whites. They defined resilient counties as those with low black infant mortality scores. They found a stratum that was unusually resilient. They reported uneven outcomes. Black infant mortality in the resilient stratum exceeded US black infant mortality and black infant mortality in the resilient stratum was less than the matching white infant mortality (Fry-Johnson, Levine, Rowley, Agboto, & Rust, 2010). Grana et al. examined the association between the physical environment and personal health behavior among high school children – specifically drug use. They compared students attending alternative high school to students attending regular high school. They reported alternative high school students from schools with high disrepair were more likely to use illicit controlled substances. Regular high school students from schools with high disrepair were more likely to smoke cigarettes (Grana et al., 2010). Hertweck et al. compared two groups of students from different socioeconomic conditions; one group of college students and youth from a teen clinic to investigate the relationship between exposure to community violence and depressive symptoms. They found exposure to community violence contributed to depression in both groups (Hertweck, Ziegler, & Logsdon, 2010). Kamphuis et al. studied how neighborhood perceptions and objective neighborhood features affects behavior – notably, amount of physical exercise. They reported comparisons between higher and lower socioeconomic statuses. Lower statuses are more likely to see their neighborhoods as unattractive and unsafe. Their perception is associated with lower levels of physical activity (Kamphuis et al., 2010). Kim et al. studied association between race, socioeconomic status, and health outcomes through access to resources. They observe that benefiting from early detection leads to better survival. Typically, health providers diagnose ovarian cancer at advanced stages. The researchers found no racial difference in stage of diagnosis. However, they found racialization in mortality and survival outcomes. They observed socioeconomic differences between black and white women. "[B]lack women were less likely to be married, less educated, more frequently used genital powder, had tubal ligation, and resided in higher poverty census tracts" (Kim, Dolecek, & Davis, 2010).

Thinking Intervention

The ecology of health is complex and in market-driven societies, like the USA, it might be prudent to start with the obvious. Throughout this chapter, it promoted the idea that behavioral, policy, and social choices are set in competitive situations. Competitive situations imply some stress; this is not what the chapter means by use of the terms stressor and strain. These latter terms mean disadvantage and inequity in the game of life. They mean that something unfair is systematic in the game. In other words, competition is imperfect. If competition was nearly perfect, individuals and groups would follow the rules inherent in the US Creed, it would reflect the systematic organization of life where the distribution of freedom and justice maximally serves the population despite differences in group affiliation, identity, or personality. In market economies, players come to the market as a competitive player. They bring assets and invest those to earn a profit beyond their initial investment. When Bronfenbrenner conceptualizes competence, he implies competitive imaging that guides behavior, which then contributes to development. Similarly, when economic sociologists and network analysts tell, "[t]he market production equation predicts profit" (Burt, 1992, p. 57), we realize these ideas of human exchange are premiere for the consciousness of democracy. The gloss below addresses social science knowledge about social capital and innovative diffusion.

Development is the production of competence. Once we find increasingly competent ways of doing things, we must share the innovations with others for them to become effective. For example, if we discover a treatment for the management of breast cancer, one requiring taking two pills each day, our innovation requires informing the population about it, getting them to accept that cancer is treatable, adopting the procedure, and taking the medicine. Therefore, "[d]iffusion is the process through which an *innovation*, defined as an idea perceived as new, spreads via certain communication channels over time among the members of a social system" (Rogers, 2004, p. 13). Typically, we understand diffusion as a process that we can observe and track. However, the way we observe and how we track it might yield variant competence. Many health professionals rely on the Rogers's diffusion model. Therefore, the next section briefly glosses it and then the chapter turns to a discussion of some findings from network research that might help our diffusion efforts.

Rogers's diffusion model. Social life means living within a social system. Social capital means, "that the people who do better are better connected" in a social system (Burt, 1999, p. 48). We should distinguish between social and human capital, too. Human capital means that people that do better in a social system enjoy higher income, get to the top faster, and are typically leaders in their fields. This advancement presumably happens through competition where people who are more attractive for roles, have greater skills, and employers consider more smart have greater competence. Of course, competition is not perfect, imperfect competition is unhealthy; that is, it is incompetent for the system. All incompetence would require study and treatment. Once an effective treatment is discoverable, we must diffuse the innovation. Innovations experience different rates of adoption, therefore, we must keep an accounting of the rate of adoption. Rogers points out five characteristics that determine an innovations rate of adoption: relative advantage, compatibility, complexity, trialability, and observability. He defines these in the following way:

> Relative advantage is the degree to which an innovation is perceived as better than the idea it supersedes. It does not matter so much if an innovation has a great deal of objective advantage. What does matter is whether an individual perceives the innovation as advantageous. Compatibility is the degree to which an innovation is perceived as being consistent with the existing values, past experiences, and needs of potential adopters. Complexity is the degree to which an innovation is perceived as difficult to understand and use. Trialability is the degree to which an innovation may be experimented with on a limited basis. Observability is the degree to which the results of an innovation are visible to others. (Rogers, 2002, p. 990)

Rogers adds that most individuals buy innovations based on their perception of their associates with equal social standing; that is, their peers, or those associates sharing social equivalence. Diffusion is a social process in which individuals spread, through talking to one another, acceptance and belief in innovation. The process has five mental stages and five adoption categories. The mental stages begin with knowledge of an innovation, then the individual must form an attitude about the innovation, next the individual must make a decision to accept or reject the innovation. If the individual accepts the innovation, they must implement it, and the final stage in the mental process is to confirm that decision (Rogers, 2002). The five-adopter categories have to do with accepting an innovation. Once individuals experience exposure to innovations, they become one of the following: innovators, early adopters, early majority, late majority, and laggards (Rogers, 2003). Some might view several of these labels as less than efficient, perhaps pejorative. Nonetheless, there is empirical work showing that the categorical memberships could not happen by chance. Rogers presents us with strategies for diffusing preventive innovations:

1. Change the perceived attributes of preventive innovations. As mentioned previously, the relative advantage of a preventive innovation needs to be stressed (Lock & Kaner, 2000).
2. Utilize champions to promote preventive innovations. A champion is an individual who devotes his/her personal influence to encourage adoption of an innovation. Goodman and Steckler (1989) found that champions for health ideas were often middle-level officials in an organization.
3. Change the norms of the system regarding preventive innovations through peer support. Changing norms on prevention is a gradual process over time, but can be accomplished (Kaner, Lock, McAvoy, Heather, & Gilvarry, 1999; Keller & Galanter, 1999).
4. Use entertainment–education to promote preventive innovations. Entertainment–education is the process of placing educational ideas (such as on prevention) in entertainment messages (Singhal & Rogers, 1999).
5. Activate peer networks to diffuse preventive innovations. Previously, we mentioned that diffusion is a social process of people talking about the new idea, giving it meaning for themselves, and then adopting. Anything that can be done to encourage peer communication about a preventive idea, such as training addiction counselors in new addiction treatment techniques, thus encourages adoption (Martin, Herie, Turner, & Cunningham, 1998).

One effective method for the diffusion of innovation has been to identify popular opinion leaders, train them in preventive health interventions, and deploy them in communities where disease incidence and prevalence is high. Imagine if there is a high rate of an infectious disease in selected neighborhoods in any given metropolitan area. Also, imagine hand washing with a sanitizing agent reduces its incidence. Finally, for this hypothetical, imagine that residents typically eat out at local restaurants five times weekly. A prevention intervention player might decide using an innovative diffusion by targeting restaurants to educate residents about sanitizing hands. The social worker might ask those that frequent certain restaurants to name people that they hold in high esteem, that is, who are community leaders whose opinion they respect. From this list, the researcher might rank those the community agreed were important opinion leaders, contact, hire, and train them in an intervention process. Finally, the social worker might deploy them. The intervening would want to maintain an accounting of change in the community. If over time, the infectious disease rate decreases, it is safe to imagine that the intervention was one factor in the decrease of infections (Singhal & Rogers, 1999; Wohlfeiler, 1998). Such interventions might improve with considerable detail.

For example, imagine if there had been a bridge to other communities at the time of the intervention. Therefore, the community where the intervention applied would find a decrease in the infectious agent. The destination of the bridge would experience increasing incidence. Moreover, imagine the intervention agency computed incidence at the metropolitan level, where those without the disease in a given amount of time was the denominator reflecting the metropolitan disease-free population. At the same time, imagine a highly and racially stratified metropolitan area where African Americans resided in a particular and different county in the same metropolitan area where there total population was 6% of the total metropolitan population. Next, imagine their county incidence rate over a 2-year period was an astounding 3,800 per 100,000 – that is, 3.8% incidence rate. To complicate our hypothetical, imagine the African Americans resided in relatively lower socioeconomic conditions than one could expect by chance. Therefore, it might result in less health coverage, fewer visits to health providers, less health-related social support, and other effects of lower socioeconomic status (Williams et al., 2010; Williams & Collins, 1995, 2004). Moreover, it would result in fewer in the population eating out each week. What does this mean for diffusion of innovation?

One answer to this question is we would need new thinking about how to approach the elimination of health disparities for African Americans. We could use similar technologies to accomplish it. However, we would need to increase our ecological innovative diffusions. In the latter hypothetical, for example, we would need intense intervention for researchers computing incidence and prevalence statistics. There is also intervention need for social work agencies executing the intervention. For example, imagine the intervention agency hired popular opinion intervention staff from the metropolitan area the staff was 93% European American. That organization would need to provide leadership for targeting the county with the 3.8% incidence rate. What dysfunction is causing the agency's oversight? Is it racialization, sexual orientation stratification, or some other feature of the regimentation of humans? Is it intellectual incompetence? Is it a sense of cultural superiority? Is it a combination of these factors along with other factors? Therefore, the prevention intervention would need a simultaneous intervention. All of the interventions would likely need heavy dosing. For example, just pulling a research team together and doing an intervention on diversity would likely produce incompetent results. On the other hand, an intervention that weekly asks agencies to account for their hiring selection practices after an initial intervention would likely produce increased development. The message in this paragraph is that eliminating health disparities require simultaneous multiple innovative diffusions. As we can imagine, startup funds are expensive. Nonetheless, we are thinking about the flow of communication to social groups. Work done in that field can reduce our overall costs. Below are some more efficient ways that we might consider doing this kind of work.

Diffusion and Network Models

Ronald Burt has done considerable work refining diffusion in his studies of contagion (Burt, 1990, 1992, 1999, 2000, 2007, 2010; Burt, Jannotta, & Mahoney, 1998; Burt & Ronchi, 1994). In this section, the chapter presents commentary on network structure and contagion, equivalence, cohesion, parsimonious selection of opinion leaders, – or rather, broker-leaders, structural holes, and the strength of weak ties. The purpose of this section is to add additional ways to think about organizing innovative diffusion. The section primarily reports research findings from Burt and his colleagues.

In public health work, belief and behavior are important because good health depends on competent development. Competent development is the term Bronfenbrenner defined earlier in the chapter.

In the bioecology, at the person interaction level, Burt has called the person ego. The person with whom the ego interacts, Burt has called alter. We will use these names to talk about network relations. Ego likely base interactions on three conditions: cohesion, structural equivalence, and contagion. Contagion refers to the spread of innovative diffusion. Cohesion and structural equivalence are the network conditions that predict contagion. The strength of relationship between ego and alter is cohesion. The greater the interaction between ego and alter, the greater the sentiment. Greater sentiment and frequent interaction increases cohesion. The more cohesion the more likely alter's adoption of an innovation will influence ego's adoption. In addition to talking to alter, ego makes an assessment of the cost and benefits of adoption. Recall from above, Rogers observed that adoption is social, largely based on intensity of relationships rather than being based on scientific knowledge (Burt, 1999, p. 39).

Equivalence applies to ego and alter sharing similar relationships with other people. Contagion by equivalence happens because of competition. The social crux of the relationship is, according to Burt, "The more similar ego's and alter's relations with other persons, the more likely that ego will quickly adopt any innovation perceived to make alter more attractive as the object or source of relations" (1999, p. 39). This revises Rogers's conceptualization of contagion of intervention by adding more specificity to our understanding of recruiting and deploying popular opinion leaders. To explain its contribution requires a great deal of detail. Therefore, the next pages will follow Burt's leadership and draw a modified network sociogram to help visualize how opinion leaders might affect ego's adoption. For Burt, "Opinion leaders defined by function (people whose conversations make innovations contagious)" is important. Therefore, that instrumental category of opinion leader is important for health promotion among African Americans (Burt, 1999, p. 47). Moreover, the section will ultimately discuss weakly equivalent alters as important for eliminating communicative redundancy in diffusion projects. "These opinion leaders are not leaders with superior authority or leaders with the sense of being more attractive such that they are individuals that others want to imitate" (Burt, p. 47). Instead, Burt quotes King and Summers (1970, p. 44), "In most contexts, the notion of an opinion leader dominating attitudes or behavior in his social network overstates the power of interpersonal communication" (Burt, p. 47).

Figure 1.2 is a hypothetical network sociogram. The dots refer to individuals, more specifically those requiring some form of public health intervention. They might be individuals that work at a community health agency, clinic, or hospital; on the other hand, they might represent healthcare consumers, or preventive healthcare clients. The solid lines connect pairs of individuals that have strong relationships. Dashed lines connect individuals with weak relationships. Strong relationships contain three elements: strong affection between the individuals, they see one another often, and they have known one another for many years. Weak relationships lack one of these elements, either completely or substantially (Burt, 1992, 1999; Burt, Bartkus, & Davis, 2009). The figure shows three groups, A, B, and C. Group A contains five members. The relationships are all strong. Moreover, there is cohesion and equivalence among the individuals in the group. All the egos have access to similar communication routes and they are all close. In this group, communicating an intervention to one member is sufficient for communication information to all of Group A members. That is, both cohesion and equivalence predicts diffusion innovation adoption. However, notice that three members have ties with Group B and no Group A members have ties with Group C. Therefore, disseminating information in Group A and having it known in Group C requires that the information travel through Group B. Group B is the largest and has the most density.

It is important to note, however, that cohesion might predict diffusion of innovation adoption, that is, contagion, when equivalence does not. More specifically, it does not predict diffusion adoption between nonequivalent individuals. For example, notice Rahema has a connection to two individuals outside of her group. She has equivalence within her group. She also has strong ties with one individual from Group A and one individual from Group C. We do not expect her contacts in Groups A and C to see one another as significant others. Therefore, in this situation we

Hypothetical Network Sociogram

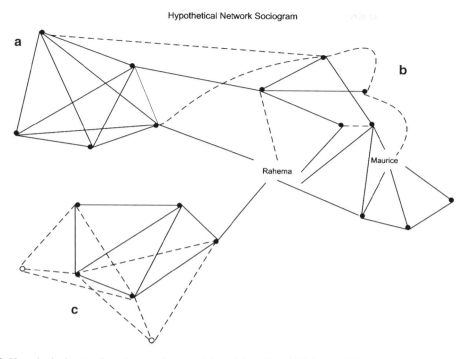

Fig. 1.2 Hypothetical network sociogram. Source: Adapted from Ronald S. Burt (1999). The social capital of opinion leaders, p. 40. Note: *Solid lines* are strong relationships. *Dashed lines* are weak relationships. *Dots* refer to individuals. *White dots* refer to satellite individuals to the group cluster

would not expect contagion. In some situations, it might also become the case where equivalence predicts contagion, and cohesion does not. For example, there is a subgroup in Group C. The white dots represent these two individuals. Notice they have no strong ties with anyone else in Group C. Furthermore, they have no direct strong or weak ties with any of the other groups. However, they are a satellite subgroup; individuals that claim a relationship with popular people but have only an indirect relationship with them. In this situation, cohesion does not predict contagion between individuals in the satellite; however, those individuals compete with one another to be attractive to individuals with whom they have strong relations. They are likely innovators that create their own rules of behavior and belief that are unique to the leading individuals in Group C (Burt, 1982, p. 245 ff; cited in, Burt, 1999, p. 43).

The following propositions that Burt presents are useful for health social and behavioral interventions:

1. Competition between strongly equivalent people can be expected to make them so aware of one another's behavior that socializing communication is superfluous to contagion between them.
2. Opinion leaders are the people whose conversations trigger contagion across the social boundaries between groups.
3. Opinion leaders…are more precisely opinion brokers who transmit information across the social boundaries between-status groups.
4. Opinion leaders are not people at the top of things so much as people on the edge of things, not leaders within groups so much as brokers between groups. (Burt, 1999, pp. 44–51).

Structural holes and weak ties. If we look at Fig. 1.2 again, we see people on the edges. For example, in Group B, Maurice occupies an edge position where he has strong ties with three individuals to the far right of the sociogram; one of them has strong ties with Rahema, another edge person.

Rahema's edge position facilitates communication with two individuals from Groups A and C. The most parsimonious use of health communication using diffusion models is to reduce redundancy. This also implies decreasing imperfect competition. For example, imagine that below the satellite in Group C, another group appears that has no ties with Group C or any of the other groups because of some social characteristic; however, they have cohesion and equivalence within their group, as does Group A. Now, imagine health workers ignored this group, not intentionally, rather because of oversight regarding their differences. In this sense, we could say that communication is not competitive. That is, there is an information barrier where some groups have access to information flow while the organization of things systematically excludes others from the flow. On the other hand, the organizational structure if saturated with the same information results in redundancy. We could imagine both redundancy by cohesion and redundancy by structural equivalence.

Redundancy by cohesion happens when a communicating alter has strong ties with everyone in the group and everyone in the group has strong ties with every other person in the group. Communicating the same message to all of them is likely inefficient. For efficiency, health promoters should maximize the number of nonredundant contacts. Redundancy by structural equivalence is alter's strong ties with several contacts who each have several ties with another group like Group A; that is, a highly cohesive and equivalent group. A structural hole is a relationship of nonredundancy. That is, a unique communicative link between network groups. Rahema's link to the one person in Group C is a structural hole. If information is flowing in Group B, Rahema is the important person for communicating that information to Group C. Notice how information might flow from Group B to Group A. Even there Rahema might play an overlapping role. However, the greatest efficiency is accomplished when one alter communicates to an ego that communicates to another tie, and so forth without redundancy. Therefore, the more network ties, the more social capital, and the greater the decrease in redundancy. The cost of the diffusion of innovation decreases with greater network diversity and an increase in structural holes (Burt, 1992, pp. 65–72).

It is also important to think about the reality that people who tend to be alike cluster together for friendship. Therefore, if information is to flow persistently, it is necessary for it to flow from one cluster to the next despite the fact that emotional strength of the ties are not great. In other words, health promoters must encourage communication flow through weak ties; weak ties are acquaintances rather than friends. Mark Granovetter analyzed how weak ties are important for information flow because it integrates otherwise disconnected social clusters into the larger society (Granovetter, 1973, 1983).

Conclusion

In the field of the elimination of health disparities, there are various groups of players. In a large-scale sense of reasoning, we might use the analogy alter ego and ego, where alters are the significant representatives for ego attitudes, beliefs, and behaviors. If we think this way, we reason a great deal of downward comparison. In this sense, the alter groups communicate parental status to subordinate child-ego groups. The major problem with such a model is that it omits the unhealthy attitudes, beliefs, and behaviors that contribute to health disparities among the parental class. Without more reflexive methodologies, research on the elimination of health disparities might compromise competitive competence.

This chapter glossed concepts used in health disparities research. It stressed that difference is not the same as disparity. It also provided commentary on two other major concepts in health disparity research, the concept of African Americans and of social and behavioral interventions. It explained theory guiding these concepts and the advancement of social and behavioral theories from empirically studying initial guiding theories. In the commentary process, the chapter suggested some operational changes for future research. The major argument is to bridge theories so that social and behavioral science could efficiently advance the elimination of health disparities. The chapter pointed out how the bioecological frame is helpful in bridging self-theory to intervention theory. In other words, self-theory is microlevel theory associated with the symbolic interaction frame. However, the chapter used structural symbolic interaction of the Stryker strand to connect identification to African American identity. There the chapter found that we might conceptualize stigma and stressors as inherent parts in African American identity. It is inextricable. However, it does not explain all social strain. From this point of view, "tribal" strain requires constant acknowledgement. Moreover, bioecology connects micro and macro elements of the human condition. By using it, we are able to bridge in practical ways accountability, instrumentality, and responsibility for action when we confront observations of health disparities. It is interesting to note that health disparities exist; we already know that. The point is to eliminate them.

When it comes to intervention, the chapter took the position that social and behavioral interventions in their various forms are reducible to social learning. However, the most important part of learning is self-knowledge from the chapter's perspective. Self-theory taught this, the symbolic interaction frame, James and Mead initially taught it; and Herbert Blumer penned its name and promoted it (Blumer, 1958, 1969, 1973, 1981). An essential element of the symbolic interaction frame is that humans make objects out of themselves; they speak to themselves when they are socially interacting. This means humans are reflexive. The chapter stressed the axiom that social scientists and other elites also use their reflexive capacity; however, when they do so in terms of health disparities, they often forget their roles as humans, giving into an impulse to see themselves as objective elites. These identities carry a great deal of baggage. For one thing, elites often forget to intervene on their class in the promotion of health disparities. They become so involved in controlling and directing others, they overlook the possibility that they might inadvertently promote classism, heterosexism, racialization, sexism, and other social strains, that is, other social disease, in their practices. To combat this elitism in social and behavioral intervention practices often results in horrible repercussions. The statuses position for battle. They downward compare health consumers to their roles and the social system holds these inequities in check. Therefore, the chapter offers ways to initiate change for the elimination of African American health disparities among the various classes with a theory of dosing contagion in competitive ecology where competition is not always perfect.

References

Albert, N. M., Trochelman, K., Meyer, K. H., & Nutter, B. (2010). Characteristics associated with racial disparities in illness beliefs of patients with heart failure. *Behavioral Medicine, 35*(4), 112–125.

Barker, D. J. P. (1998). *Mothers, babies, and health in later life* (2nd ed.). New York: Churchill Livingstone.

Bauer, R. A., & Bauer, A. H. (1942). Day to day resistance to slavery. *The Journal of Negro History, 27*(4), 388–419.

Blackwell, D. L., Hayward, M. D., & Crimmins, E. M. (2001). Does childhood health affect chronic morbidity in later life? *Social Science & Medicine, 52*(8), 1269.

Blalock, H. M., Jr. (1979). The Presidential Address: Measurement and conceptualization problems: The major obstacle to integrating theory and research. *American Sociological Review, 44*(6), 881–894.

Blumer, H. (1958). Race prejudice as a sense of group position. *Pacific Sociological Review, 1*(1), 3–7.

Blumer, H. (1969). *Symbolic interaction: Perspective and method.* Englewood Cliffs, NJ: Prentice Hall.

Blumer, H. (1973). Symbolic interactionism as a pragmatic perspective: The bias of emergent theory. *American Sociological Review, 38*(6), 797–798.

Blumer, H. (1981). George Herbert Mead: Self, language, and the world. *The American Journal of Sociology, 86*(4), 902–904.

Bonacich, E. (1975). Abolition, the extension of slavery, and the position of free Blacks: A study of split labor markets in the United States, 1830–1863. *The American Journal of Sociology, 81*(3), 601–628.

Braveman, P. A. (2005). The question is not "Is race or class more important?". *Journal of Epidemiology and Community Health, 59*(12), 1029–1029.

Braveman, P. A. (2006). Health disparities and health equity: Concepts and measurement. *Annual Review of Public Health, 27*, 167–194.

Braveman, P. A., Cubbin, C., Egerter, S., & Marchi, K. S. (2006). Use of socioeconomic status in health research. *JAMA, the Journal of the American Medical Association, 295*(15), 1770–1770.

Braveman, P. A., Cubbin, C., Marchi, K., Egerter, S., & Chavez, G. (2001). Measuring socioeconomic status/position in studies of racial/ethnic disparities: Maternal and infant health. *Public Health Reports, 116*(5), 449.

Bridges, E. (2010). Racial identity development and psychological coping strategies of African American males at a predominately White university. *Annals of the American Psychotherapy Association, 13*(1), 14–26.

Bronfenbrenner, U. (1986). Ecology of the family as a context for human development: Research perspectives. *Developmental Psychology, 22*(6), 723–742.

Bronfenbrenner, U. (2000). Ecological systems theory. In A. E. Kazdin (Ed.), *Encyclopedia of psychology* (Vol. 3, pp. 129–133). New York: Oxford University Press.

Bronfenbrenner, U. (2005a). Interacting systems in human development. Research paradigms: Present and future (1988). In *Making human beings human: Bioecological perspectives on human development* (pp. 67–93). Thousand Oaks, CA: Sage Publications Ltd.

Bronfenbrenner, U. (2005b). The social ecology of human development: A retrospective conclusion (1973). In *Making human beings human: Bioecological perspectives on human development* (pp. 27–40). Thousand Oaks, CA: Sage Publications Ltd.

Bronfenbrenner, U., Friedman, S. L., & Wachs, T. D. (1999). Environments in developmental perspective: Theoretical and operational models. In *Measuring environment across the life span: Emerging methods and concepts* (pp. 3–28). Washington, DC: American Psychological Association.

Bronfenbrenner, U., & Morris, P. A. (1998). The ecology of developmental processes. In W. Damon & R. M. Lerner (Eds.), *Handbook of child psychology: Volume 1: Theorectical models of human development* (5th ed., pp. 993–1028). Hoboken, NJ: John Wiley & Sons, Inc.

Bronfenbrenner, U., Morris, P. A., Lerner, R. M., & Damon, W. (2006). The bioecological model of human development. In *Handbook of child psychology (6th ed.): Vol 1, Theoretical models of human development*. (pp. 793–828). Hoboken, NJ: John Wiley & Sons, Inc.

Brown, T. N., Sellers, S. L., Brown, K. T., Jackson, J. S., Aneshensel, C. S., & Phelan, J. C. (1999). Race, ethnicity, and culture in the sociology of mental health. In *Handbook of sociology of mental health* (pp. 167–182). Dordrecht, Netherlands: Kluwer Academic Publishers.

Burke, P. J. (1980). The self: Measurement requirements from an interactionist perspective. *Social Psychology Quarterly, 43*(1), 18–29.

Burt, R. S. (1982). *Toward a structural theory of action: Network models of social structure, perception, and action.* New York: Academic Press.

Burt, R. S. (1990). Detecting role equivalence. *Social Networks, 12*(1), 83–97.

Burt, R. S. (1992). The social structure of competition. In N. Nohria & R. Eccles (Eds.), *Networks and organizations: Structure, form and action* (pp. 57–93). Boston: Harvard Business School Press.

Burt, R. S. (1999). The social capital of opinion leaders. *The Annals of the American Academy of Political and Social Science, 566*, 37–54.

Burt, R. S. (2000). The network structure of social capital. *Research in Organizational Behavior, 22*, 345.

Burt, R. S. (2007). Secondhand brokerage: Evidence on the importance of local structure for managers, bankers, and analysts. *Academy of Management Journal, 50*(1), 119–148.

Burt, R. S. (2010). The shadow of other people: Socialization and social comparison in marketing. In S. Wuyts, M. G. Dekimpe, E. Gijsbrechts, & R. Pieters (Eds.), *The connected customer: The changing nature of consumer and business markets* (pp. 217–256). New York: Routledge.

Burt, R. S., Bartkus, V. O., & Davis, J. H. (2009). Network duality of social capital. In *Social capital: Reaching out, reaching in* (pp. 39–65). Northampton, MA: Edward Elgar Publishing.

Burt, R. S., Jannotta, J. E., & Mahoney, J. T. (1998). Personality correlates of structural holes. *Social Networks, 20*(1), 63–87.

Burt, R. S., & Ronchi, D. (1994). Measuring a large network quickly. *Social Networks, 16*(2), 91–135.

Colley, J. R., Douglas, J. W., & Reid, D. D. (1973). Respiratory disease in young adults: Influence of early childhood lower respiratory tract illness, social class, air pollution, and smoking. *British Medical Journal, 3*(5873), 195–198.

Cross, W. E. (1991). *Shades of Black: Diversity in African American identity*. Philadelphia: Temple University Press.

Cross, W. E., Jr., Vandiver, B. J., Ponterotto, J. G., Casas, J. M., Suzuki, L. A., & Alexander, C. M. (2001). Nigrescence theory and measurement: Introducing the Cross Racial Identity Scale (CRIS). In *Handbook of multicultural counseling (2nd ed.)*. (pp. 371–393). Thousand Oaks, CA: Sage Publications, Inc.

Dallman, M. F., Akana, S. F., Laugero, K. D., Gomez, F., Manalo, S., Bell, M. E., et al. (2003). A spoonful of sugar: Feedback signals of energy stores and corticosterone regulate responses to chronic stress. *Physiology & Behavior, 79*(1), 3–12.

Dallman, M. F., Pecoraro, N., Akana, S. F., La Fleur, S. E., Gomez, F., Houshyar, H., et al. (2003). Chronic stress and obesity: A new view of "comfort food". *Proceedings of the National Academy of Sciences of the United States of America, 100*(20), 11696–11701.

Davis, J. A., Spaeth, J. L., & Huson, C. (1961). A technique for analyzing the effects of group composition. *American Sociological Review, 26*, 215–225.

Denney, J. T., Rogers, R. G., Hummer, R. A., & Pampel, F. C. (2010). Education inequality in mortality: The age and gender specific mediating effects of cigarette smoking. *Social Science Research, 39*(4), 662–673.

Duncan, G. J., Daly, M. C., McDonough, P., & Williams, D. R. (2002). Optimal Indicators of socioeconomic status for health research. *American Journal of Public Health, 92*(7), 1151–1157.

Feagin, J. R. (2004). Toward an integrated theory of systemic racism. In M. Krysan & A. E. Lewis (Eds.), *The changing terrain of race and ethnicity* (pp. 203–223). New York: Russell Sage.

Freire, P. (1983). *Pedagogy of the oppressed.* New York: Continuum.

Fry-Johnson, Y. W., Levine, R., Rowley, D., Agboto, V., & Rust, G. (2010). United States black-white infant mortality disparities are not inevitable: Identification of community resilience independent of socioeconomic status. *Ethnicity & Disease, 20*(1 Suppl 1), S1-131–135.

Fuller-Thomson, E., Nuru-Jeter, A., Minkler, M., & Guralnik, J. M. (2009). BlackWhite disparities in disability among older Americans. *Journal of Aging and Health, 22*(5), 677–698.

Fullilove, M. T. (1998). Comment: Abandoning "race" as a variable in public health research – an idea whose time has come. *American Journal of Public Health, 88*(9), 1297–1298.

Fullilove, M. T., & Fullilove, R. E., III. (1994). Post-traumatic stress disorder in women recovering from substance abuse. In S. Friedman (Ed.), *Anxiety disorders in African Americans* (pp. 89–101). New York: Springer Publishing Company.

Ginzburg, R. (1988). *100 years of lynchings.* Baltimore, MD: Black Classic Press.

Goodman, R. M., & Steckler, A. (1989). A model for the institutionalization of health promotion programs. *Family & Community Health, 11*(4), 63–78.

Grana, R. A., Black, D., Sun, P., Rohrbach, L. A., Gunning, M., & Sussman, S. (2010). School disrepair and substance use among regular and alternative high school students. *The Journal of School Health, 80*(8), 387–393.

Granovetter, M. (1973). The strength of weak ties. *The American Journal of Sociology, 78*(6), 1360–1380.

Granovetter, M. (1983). The strength of weak ties: A network theory revisited. *Sociological Theory, 1*, 201–233.

Guralnik, J. M., Butterworth, S., Wadsworth, M. E. J., & Kuh, D. (2006). Childhood socioeconomic status predicts physical functioning a half century later. *The Journals of Gerontology. Series A: Biological Sciences and Medical Sciences, 61A*(7), 694–701.

Haas, S. (2008). Trajectories of functional health: The long arm of childhood health and socioeconomic factors. *Social Science & Medicine, 66*(4), 849–861.

Haas, S., & Rohlfsen, L. (2010). Life course determinants of racial and ethnic disparities in functional health trajectories. *Social Science & Medicine, 70*(2), 240–250.

Hacker, A. (1992). *Two nations: Black and White, separate, hostile, unequal.* New York: Scribner's.

Hajat, A., Diez-Roux, A., Franklin, T. G., Seeman, T., Shrager, S., Ranjit, N., et al. (2010). Socioeconomic and race/ethnic differences in daily salivary cortisol profiles: The multi-ethnic study of atherosclerosis. *Psychoneuroendocrinology, 35*(6), 932–943.

Hertweck, S. P., Ziegler, C. H., & Logsdon, M. C. (2010). Outcome of exposure to community violence in female adolescents. *Journal of Pediatric and Adolescent Gynecology, 23*(4), 202–208.

Hull, J. G., & Levy, A. S. (1979). The organizational functions of self: An alternative to Duval and Wicklund model of self-awareness. *Journal of Personality and Social Psychology, 37*, 756–768.

Jackson, J. S., Knight, K. M., & Rafferty, J. A. (2010). Race and unhealthy behaviors: Chronic stress, the HPA axis, and physical and mental health disparities over the life course. *American Journal of Public Health, 100*(5), 933–939.

James, W. ([1892] 1968). The self. In C. Gorden & K. J. Gergen (Eds.), *The self in social interaction* (pp. 41–49). New York: John Wiley and Sons, Inc.

Jung Hoon, H., Sunderland, N., Kendall, E., Gudes, O., & Henniker, G. (2010). Professional practice and innovation: Chronic disease, geographic location and socioeconomic disadvantage as obstacles to equitable access to e-health. *Health Information Management Journal, 39*(2), 30–36.

Kamphuis, C. B. M., Mackenbach, J. P., Giskes, K., Huisman, M., Brug, J., & van Lenthe, F. J. (2010). Why do poor people perceive poor neighbourhoods? The role of objective neighbourhood features and psychosocial factors. *Health & Place, 16*(4), 744–754.

Kaner, E. F., Lock, C. A., McAvoy, B. R., Heather, N., & Gilvarry, E. (1999). A RCT of three training and support strategies to encourage implementation of screening and brief alcohol intervention by general practitioners. *The British Journal of General Practice: The Journal of The Royal College Of General Practitioners, 49*(446), 699–703.

Karlamangla, A. S., Merkin, S. S., Crimmins, E. M., & Seeman, T. E. (2010). Socioeconomic and ethnic disparities in cardiovascular risk in the United States, 2001–2006. *Annals of Epidemiology, 20*(8), 617–628.

Keith, V. M., Brown, D. R., Scheid, T. L., & Brown, T. N. (2010). African American women and mental well-being: The triangulation of race, gender, and socioeconomic status. In *A handbook for the study of mental health: Social contexts, theories, and systems* (2nd ed) (pp. 291–305). New York: Cambridge University Press.

Keller, D. S., & Galanter, M. (1999). Technology transfer of network therapy to community-based addictions counselors. *Journal of Substance Abuse Treatment, 16*(2), 183.

Kim, S., Dolecek, T. A., & Davis, F. G. (2010). Racial differences in stage at diagnosis and survival from epithelial ovarian cancer: A fundamental cause of disease approach. *Social Science & Medicine, 71*(2), 274–281.

King, C. W., & Summers, J. O. (1970). Overlap of opinion leadership across consumer product categories. *Journal of Marketing Research, 7*(1), 43–50.

Kuh, D., Bassey, J., Hardy, R., Aihie Sayer, A., Wadsworth, M., & Cooper, C. (2002). Birth weight, childhood size, and muscle strength in adult life: Evidence from a birth cohort study. *American Journal of Epidemiology, 156*(7), 627–633.

Kuh, D., Hardy, R., Butterworth, S., Okell, L., Richards, M., Wadsworth, M., et al. (2006). Developmental origins of midlife physical performance: Evidence from a British birth cohort. *American Journal of Epidemiology, 164*(2), 110–121.

Kuh, D. J., & Wadsworth, M. E. (1993). Physical health status at 36 years in a British national birth cohort (1982). *Social Science & Medicine, 37*(7), 905–916.

LaVeist, T. A. (2005). *Minority populations and health: An introduction to health disparities in the United States* (1st ed.). San Francisco: Jossey-Bass.

Lawlor, D. A., Ebrahim, S., & Smith, G. D. (2005). Adverse socioeconomic position across the life course increases coronary heart disease risk cumulatively: Findings from the British Women's Heart and Health Study. *Heart, 91*(12), 1594–1594.

Lemelle, A. J. (2007). One drop rule. In G. Ritzer (Ed.), *Blackwell encyclopedia of sociology* (pp. 3265–3266). Malden, MA: Blackwell Publishing.

Lewin, K. (1997). The background of conflict in marriage (1940). In *Resolving social conflicts and field theory in social science* (pp. 68–79). Washington, DC: American Psychological Association.

Lewin, K., Gentile, B. F., & Miller, B. O. (2009). Experiments in social space (1939). In *Foundations of psychological thought: A history of psychology* (pp. 454–467). Thousand Oaks, CA: Sage Publications, Inc.

Lewin, K., & Gold, M. (1999). The dynamics of group action. In *The complete social scientist: A Kurt Lewin reader* (pp. 285–291). Washington, DC: American Psychological Association.

Lock, C. A., & Kaner, E. F. S. (2000). Use of marketing to disseminate brief alcohol intervention to general practitioners: Promoting health care interventions to health promoters. *Journal of Evaluation in Clinical Practice, 6*(4), 345–357.

Marable, M., Steinberg, I., & Middlemass, K. (2007). *Racializing justice, disenfranchising lives: The racism, criminal justice, and law reader*. New York: Palgrave Macmillan.

Mariner, J., & Human Rights Watch. (2001). *No escape: Male rape in U.S. prisons*. New York: Human Rights Watch.

Marmot, M., Shipley, M., Brunner, E., & Hemingway, H. (2001). Relative contribution of early life and adult socioeconomic factors to adult morbidity in the Whitehall II study. *Journal of Epidemiology and Community Health, 55*(5), 301–307.

Martin, G. W., Herie, M. A., Turner, B. J., & Cunningham, J. A. (1998). A social marketing model for disseminating research-based treatments to addictions treatment providers. *Addiction, 93*(11), 1703–1715.

Marx, A. W. (1998). *Making race and nation: A comparison of South Africa, the United States, and Brazil*. New York: Cambridge University Press. 1st pbk. ed.

McWhorter, J. H. (2000). *Losing the race: Self-sabotage in Black America*. New York: Free Press.

Mead, G. H., & Morris, C. W. (1934). *Mind, self & society from the standpoint of a social behaviorist*. Chicago: The University of Chicago Press.

Mitchell, S. J., Engelman, J., Kent, C. K., Lukehart, S. A., Godornes, C., & Klausner, J. D. (2006). Azithromycin-resistant syphilis infection: San Francisco, California, 2000–2004. *Clinical Infectious Diseases, 42*(3), 337–345.

Nyswander, D. B. (2006). Public health education: Sources, growth and operational philosophy. *International Quarterly of Community Health Education, 25*(1–2), 5–18.

Nyswander, D. B., New York Department of Health, & New York Board of Education. (1942). *Solving school health problems: The Astoria Demonstration Study*. New York: Oxford University Press.

Ochs, H. L. (2006). Colorblind policy in Black and White: Racial consequences of disenfranchisement policy. *Policy Studies Journal, 34*(1), 81–93.

Pan, I. J., Daniels, J. L., & Zhu, K. (2010). Poverty and childhood cancer incidence in the United States. *Cancer Causes & Control, 21*(7), 1139–1145.

Pollack, C. E., Chideya, S., Cubbin, C., Williams, B., Dekker, M., & Braveman, P. A. (2007). Should health studies measure wealth?: A systematic review. *American Journal of Preventive Medicine, 33*(3), 250–264.

Quinn, K., Kaufman, J., Siddiqi, A., & Yeatts, K. (2010). Stress and the city: Housing stressors are associated with respiratory health among low socioeconomic status Chicago children. *Journal of Urban Health, 87*(4), 688–702.

Robinson, W. S. (1950). Ecological correlations and the behavior of individuals. *American Sociological Review, 15*(3), 351–357.

Rogers, E. M. (2002). Diffusion of preventive innovations. *Addictive Behaviors, 27*(6), 989.

Rogers, E. M. (2003). *Diffusion of innovations* (5th ed.). New York: Free Press.

Rogers, E. M. (2004). A prospective and retrospective look at the diffusion model. *Journal of Health Communication, 9*, 13–19.

Rotter, J. B. (1975). Some problems and misconceptions related to the construct of internal versus external control of reinforcement. *Journal of Consulting and Clinical Psychology, 43*(1), 56–67.

Schwartz, S., & Meyer, I. H. (2010). Mental health disparities research: The impact of within and between group analyses on tests of social stress hypotheses. *Social Science & Medicine, 70*(8), 1111–1118.

Signorello, L. B., Schlundt, D. G., Cohen, S. S., Steinwandel, M. D., Buchowski, M. S., McLaughlin, J. K., et al. (2007). Comparing diabetes prevalence between African Americans and Whites of similar socioeconomic status. *American Journal of Public Health, 97*(12), 2260–2267.

Singhal, A., & Rogers, E. M. (1999). *Entertainment-education: A communication strategy for social change.* Mahwah, NJ: L. Erlbaum Associates.

Smith, G. D., & Hart, C. (1997). Lifetime socioeconomic position and mortality: Prospective observational study. *British Medical Journal, 314*(7080), 547–552.

Sowell, T. (1981). *Ethnic America: A history.* New York: Basic Books.

Steinberg, S. (2007). *Race relations: A critique.* Stanford, CA: Stanford.

Stryker, S. (1968). Identity salience and role performance: The relevance of symbolic interaction theory for family research. *Journal of Marriage and the Family, 30*(4), 558–564.

Stryker, S. (2008). From Mead to a structural symbolic interactionism and beyond. *Annual Review of Sociology, 34*(1), 15–31.

U.S. Census Bureau. (2000). 2000 Census of population, Public law 94–171 redistricting data file. Updated every 10 years. [Electronic Version]. Retrieved July 3, 2010, from http://quickfacts.census.gov/qfd/meta/long_68176.htm

Vandiver, B. J., Cross, W. E., Jr., Worrell, F. C., & Fhagen-Smith, P. E. (2002). Validating the cross racial identity scale. *Journal of Counseling Psychology, 49*(1), 71.

Vandiver, B. J., Fhagen-smith, P. E., Cokley, K. O., Cross, W. E., Jr., & Worrell, F. C. (2001). Cross's Nigrescence model: From theory to scale to theory. *Journal of Multicultural Counseling & Development, 29*(3), 174.

Wannamethee, S. G., & Whincup, P. H. (1996). Influence of fathers' social class on cardiovascular disease in middle-aged men. *Lancet, 348*(9037), 1259.

Williams, D. R., Adler, N. E., Marmot, M., McEwen, B. S., & Stewart, J. (1999). Race, socioeconomic status, and health: The added effects of racism and discrimination. In *Socioeconomic status and health in industrial nations: Social, psychological, and biological pathways* (pp. 173–188). New York: New York Academy of Sciences.

Williams, D. R., & Collins, C. (1995). US socioeconomic and racial differences in health: Patterns and explanations. *Annual Review of Sociology, 21*, 349–386.

Williams, D. R., & Collins, C. (2004). Reparations: A viable strategy to address the enigma of African American health. *The American Behavioral Scientist, 47*(7), 977–100.

Williams, D. R., Mohammed, S. A., Leavell, J., & Collins, C. (2010). Race, socioeconomic status, and health: Complexities, ongoing challenges, and research opportunities. *Annals of the New York Academy of Sciences, 1186*, 69–101.

Wohlfeiler, D. (1998). Community organizing and community building among gay and bisexual men: The Stop AIDS Project. In M. Minkler (Ed.), *Community organizing and community building for health* (pp. 230–243). New Brunswick, NJ: Rutgers University Press.

World Health Organization, Braveman, P. A., Tarimo, E., Creese, A., Monasch, R., & Nelson, L. (1996). *Equity in health and health care: A WHO/SIDA initiative.* Geneva: World Health Organization.

Worrall, J. L., & Pratt, T. C. (2004). On the consequences of ignoring unobserved heterogeneity when estimating macro-level models of crime. *Social Science Research, 33*(1), 79.

Worrell, F. C., Cross, W. K., Jr., & Vandiver, B. J. (2001). Nigrescence theory: Current status and challenges for the future. *Journal of Multicultural Counseling & Development, 29*(3), 201.

Worrell, F. C., Vandiver, B. J., Cross, W. E., Jr., & Fhagen-Smith, P. E. (2004). Reliability and structural validity of cross racial identity scale scores in a sample of African American adults. *Journal of Black Psychology, 30*(4), 489–505.

Worrell, F. C., Vandiver, B. J., Schaefer, B. A., Cross, W. E., Jr., & Fhagen-Smith, P. E. (2006). Generalizing Nigrescence profiles: Cluster analyses of cross racial identity scale (CRIS) scores in three independent samples. *The Counseling Psychologist, 34*(4), 519–547.

Yancey, G. A. (2003). *Who is White?: Latinos, Asians, and the new Black/nonBlack divide.* Boulder: Lynne Rienner.

Ye, L., & Waite, L. J. (2005). The Impact of childhood and adult SES on physical, mental, and cognitive well-being in later life. *The Journals of Gerontology. Series B: Psychological Sciences and Social Sciences, 60B*(2), S93–S101.

Chapter 2
Ethics and Intervention Programming

Cynthia Hudley

Disparities in health outcomes, or the differential burden of health conditions for specific population groups, are a continuing problem that cuts short the lives and compromises the health and well being of African Americans in the USA. For example, the Centers for Disease Control and Prevention (2007) reported that in 2004, African Americans had the highest age-adjusted death rate for any cause of all races and ethnicities in the USA, and these elevated death rates persist throughout life, from birth through senior citizen years (Williams, 2005). Specifically, African Americans had the highest age-adjusted death rate for heart disease, cancer, diabetes, and HIV/AIDS; Black children in particular had a 200% higher prevalence rate and a 500% higher death rate from asthma, a 250% higher infant mortality rate, and a 200% higher incidence of SIDS as compared to their White peers. Relative to health compromises in daily living, roughly 40% of African American adults have some form of heart disease that can affect daily living, compared to 30% of White men and 24% of White women. African Americans are also twice as likely to suffer from diabetes, 1.7 times more likely to suffer a stroke, and 30% more likely to report serious psychological distress. African American senior citizens are half as likely to receive vaccinations for influenza and pneumonia as their White counterparts. African American children as a group have the highest rates of daily activity limitation (9%) of any child group due to chronic health, including mental health, conditions.

A common perspective on health outcomes focuses on behavior and personal choices. Although health outcomes can certainly be affected by life choices and personal behavior, physical and mental health disparities in the African American community may also be attributable to an array of social structural factors that are not directly controllable by an individual, including lack of affordable health insurance, lack of access to medical facilities and healthy food, substandard housing, environmental toxins, and environmental stressors. Limited access to health care may play some role in reported health disparities, for example, as 40% of low-income African Americans lack health insurance, and the uninsured are more than six times less likely to receive care for a chronic condition than those with health insurance (Kaiser Family Foundation, 2009). Racism, or the propensity to deny societal goods and advantages to selected racial groups, represents a constellation of stressors that may have consequences for health disparities that unduly compromise African American health. For example, higher levels of discrimination are associated with poorer mental health (Brown et al., 2000), and perceived discrimination fosters negative changes in symptoms, rather than the reverse

C. Hudley (✉)
Department of Education, Gervirtz School, University of California,
S anta Barbara, CA, USA
e-mail: hudley@education.ucsb.edu

A.J. Lemelle et al. (eds.), *Handbook of African American Health: Social and Behavioral Interventions*,
DOI 10.1007/978-1-4419-9616-9_2, © Springer Science+Business Media, LLC 2011

(Brody et al., 2006). Other prospective longitudinal data reveal that perceived discrimination predicts coronary artery disease (Lewis et al., 2006). Most importantly for our discussion, the failure to seek preventative screening such as cholesterol testing and eye examinations among diabetes is related to perceived discrimination in the health delivery system (Trivedi & Ayanian, 2006).

Thus, on the one hand, physical and mental health disparities speak to the need for more effective interventions with African Americans. On the other hand, the most likely sources of prevention and intervention services may also be implicated in poorer health outcomes for African Americans due to lack of access to or perceived discrimination in the health delivery system. This conundrum speaks directly to ethical concerns in designing intervention practices with African Americans. Ethical intervention practice is culturally competent intervention practice. Culturally competent interventions require practitioners with skills that facilitate successful interactions and intervention materials and procedures that are relevant to the population of interest. Most importantly, ethical intervention practice will prepare participants to address the institutional as well as the personal sources of health disparities. In short, ethical interventions are those that empower participants to address the health needs of their unique cultural contexts. Conversely, culturally irrelevant interventions applied in multicultural contexts may represent one of the root causes of lack of intervention efficacy and resulting unhealthy outcomes for participants. Ethically responsible intervention practitioners must consider not only adequacy of their own skill set but also the relevance of their intervention programs and the relevance of the outcomes those programs are designed to foster.

The chapter is organized into three broad sections. First, I review and discuss the meaning of culture and its significance for understanding health intervention programming. Next, I review current theorizing about the construct of cultural competence. Finally, using extant practice as a foundation, I provide a multidimensional model of cultural competence that might guide ethical practice. I conclude with a brief discussion of implications of the model for health maintenance interventions.

Culture: What and Why

Consistent with the systems view (e.g., Kitayama, 2002), I define culture as a set of variable, loosely organized systems of meanings that shape ways of living and are learned and shared by an identifiable group of people (Betancourt & López, 1993). These systems of meanings include beliefs, values, and goals that serve as foundations of social exchange in a given culture. They organize group members' associated psychological processes and behaviors, including social norms, communication styles, and rituals that allow members to successfully adapt within a particular ecocultural niche. An ecocultural niche represents the cultural and ecological contexts in which people live out their daily lives. This view of culture is particularly valuable for examining the relation between culture and health interventions, because it links culture in meaningful ways to cognitive and behavioral change as well as to social context.

This definition of culture is foundational to ethical health intervention programming. There is compelling evidence that theory and practice developed in one cultural context may not apply successfully in another context. These findings are not surprising once we understand culture as the system that organizes adaptation to a unique environment. For example, a substantial body of literature in human development has described how models of successful parenting originally developed in white middle-class contexts may not adequately capture and define successful parenting in other ecocultural contexts that present supports and challenges that may not exist in the context in which the model was developed (Baldwin, Baldwin, & Cole, 1990; Lamborn, Dornbusch, & Steinberg, 1996). Similarly, education research consistently finds that practices developed for one student group are not equally successful with all groups in a diverse society, often resulting in a significant, culturally defined "achievement gap" (Garcia, 1993; McAllister & Irvine, 2000). Finally, research on the efficacy of mental health treatment practices has shown that a cultural match between client and service provider improves client participation and persistence (Sue, 1998), perhaps due to a shared understanding of values, goals, and norms that define appropriate treatment practice and outcomes.

Practitioners should therefore anticipate that models and methods for health interventions will have a far greater chance for success if they are framed and presented in ways that are appropriate to participants' cultural systems (Roosa, Dumka, Gonzales, & Knight, 2002). Efforts to address the participants' ecocultural niche should increase the attractiveness and motivational impetus of prevention programs. The true measure of prevention programming is a capacity to effect real change that is valued in a given community. Participants and families must actually believe that intervention programming will lead to enhanced health or more effective disease management if programs are to be successful and outcomes sustainable (Roosa et al.).

Models of Cultural Competence

The construct of cultural competence has become an integral part of training and service delivery in a variety of helping professions including health and human services and mental health. Cultural competence refers to the capacity to function effectively in a given cultural/ecological niche based on knowledge of relevant social norms, roles, beliefs, and values. I will first describe the dominant theoretical models of the content and operation of cultural competence in the helping professions before presenting a model of the construct that will be of particular value for intervention programming for African Americans.

Health and Human Services

Within the last decade, the health services and mental health domains have generated a substantial literature around the construct of cultural competence (e.g., Pope-Davis & Coleman, 1997). Across these helping professions, practitioners view cultural competence as a necessary component for treating clients from diverse ethnic backgrounds. The prevalent theories of cultural competence include several themes. Self-understanding, viewed as the basis for cultural competence, provides an awareness of one's own culturally grounded assumptions and expectations about human behavior (Sue, Arredondo, & McDavis, 1992). Beyond that, the culturally competent practitioner also recognizes and appreciates the worldview of other cultural groups and displays skills appropriate to work effectively across cultures (Sue, 1998).

The focus is on the competence of the professional practitioner to effectively serve an increasingly diverse client population. Cultural competence is attained through a therapist's developmental progression from unconscious incompetence to unconscious competence (Purnell, 2002). Reviews of the cultural competence literature have acknowledged the absence of the client's perspective (Pope-Davis, Liu, Toporek, & Brittan-Powell, 2001). Nonetheless, this work continues to focus specifically on the practitioner's competence.

Cultural Competence and Education Research

Education research and practice have generated a rich and long-standing body of knowledge focused specifically on issues of culture (e.g., research in multicultural education). The education literature has introduced a variety of terms (culturally appropriate, culturally congruent, culturally compatible, culturally responsive, culturally relevant) to define particular models of cultural competence. Similar to other helping professions, all of these models posit self-knowledge, affirming attitudes toward the worldviews of other cultural groups, and the skills to successfully educate children from diverse backgrounds as foundational elements for culturally competent teachers (e.g., McAllister & Irvine, 2000).

This literature moves beyond a focus on the teacher, however, to incorporate specific instructional practices and desired student outcomes as equally necessary elements of cultural competence (Villegas & Lucas, 2002). Culturally relevant pedagogy comprises instructional practices that are responsive to and grounded in students' cultural patterns of learning and knowing and thus maximize academic learning for all students (Ladson-Billings, 1995). Cultural competence as defined from this perspective presumes that students are able to maintain the cultural knowledge and identity necessary to successfully navigate their ecocultural niche while succeeding academically (Ladson-Billings, 1995). Students' cultural competence, in turn, prepares them to become critical advocates for social justice by making visible the bias inherent in using a single cultural lens to understand a multicultural society such as ours (Villegas & Lucas).

Cultural Competence and Ethical Practice

The comprehensive model of cultural competence represented in the multicultural education literature can serve as a useful guide for the design of ethical health interventions for African Americans. Drawing on the literatures reviewed, a model of cultural competence relevant to ethical health practice comprises three elements. Cultural competence refers to

1. The requisite self-knowledge, attitudes, and skills that allow helping professionals to be effective with diverse populations. This usage is similar to the existing definition in the mental health field. I use the term *culturally effective* to refer to this specific subdomain of cultural competence that addresses practitioner competence.
2. Intervention methods and programming that are responsive to and respectful of participants' cultures and communities. Programs will present strategies for disease management and health promotion in ways that support participants' and families' cultural values and traditions (e.g., diet restrictions, appropriate exercise for women) as well as recognizing the unique demands of a given ecocultural niche (e.g., strategies for accessing care). Methods for assessment and evaluation will be similarly cognizant of the dynamics, opportunities, and constraints of participants' ecocultural niche. I use the term *culturally responsive* to refer to this specific subdomain of cultural competence that refers to programmatic adequacy and appropriateness.
3. Program goals and desired outcomes that support participants' ability to successfully navigate their own ecocultural niche. This includes cultural pride, a positive sense of self, and the critical awareness to challenge inequality in access and treatment of all kinds. I use the term *culturally engaged* to refer to this specific subdomain of cultural competence that describes desired outcomes.

The model is grounded in current thinking on positive psychology (Seligman & Csikszentmihalyi, 2000). For individuals, families, and communities to truly thrive, programs must concentrate explicitly on building positive health habits, healthy behaviors, and skills in advocacy in addition to managing disease states and navigating unhealthful environments. Lack of access to fresh, healthy food in inner city communities, for example, and unhealthful food choices in schools are two of many institutional health challenges confronted by too many African American families. It is not enough to provide listings of healthful diets or directions to supermarkets outside one's communities. Ethical practice must move beyond service delivery to include capacity building for social mobilization and advocacy with institutional and political structures. Interventions that support human thriving will provide the critical consciousness to confront institutional racism and bias in the provision of access to health care, healthful living environments, and resources to support healthful living (e.g., community green spaces, fresh groceries). Ethical intervention programming will provide the knowledge and the skills for participants to become change agents and participants in shaping the quality of health and life in their homes, their families, and their communities.

Culturally Effective Service Providers

As previously defined, the culturally effective program leader is one with a particular constellation of knowledge, attitudes, and skills. Self-knowledge, the first component of cultural effectiveness, comprises both an awareness of one's own cultural worldview and the understanding that worldview is the product of prior life history and experience. Any one worldview is not universally shared; rather there are multiple worldviews mediated by a range of factors including social class, ethnicity, language, gender, and power relations. It is important to remember that ethnic match *per se* is not definitive of matching worldviews between participant and client.

Worldview may be particularly powerful in shaping one's judgments about and reactions to individual behavior. Thus, cultural effectiveness is virtually unattainable for those who work in behavioral medicine and health intervention in the absence of self-knowledge. Self-knowledge is a precursor to comprehending how participants' cultural systems organize behavior, as it makes visible the distorting power of one's own worldview. Evidence from counselor training research supports the link between self-knowledge and efficacy; awareness of one's own cultural and personal biases has shown a positive relationship with multicultural counseling competence (Pope-Davis & Ottavi, 1994).

Prior examinations of ethical research practice have identified two critical habits of mind concerning racial categorizations that may also burden service providers and practitioners of any race and ethnicity (Stanfield, 1993). The assumption of homogeneity refers to the belief that racial labels represent homogeneous populations. In particular, the African American community is rich with ethnic variability that is glossed over or ignored by the use of a global label. The historical American understanding of race is rooted in faulty assertions of genetics and biology, due largely to European adventurers' historical attempts to rationalize colonization, slavery, and state-sanctioned racial terrorism (Cornell & Hartman, 1998). Fortunately, over time the definition of race has evolved to include an understanding of race as a social construction (Bolaffi, Bracalenti, Braham, & Gindro, 2003); however, the terms Black and African American too often ignore cultural differentiation in a population that typically represents considerable ethnic and cultural diversity. Regional distinctions, generational differences, social class differences, and immigrant populations are some of the dimensions of cultural diversity hidden beneath the labels African American and Black. Intervention practitioners must be conscious of the danger of using a gross label to inform intervention practice.

Analogous to the assumption of homogeneity, the belief in a monolithic identity similarly ignores the broad range of individual variation present in groups labeled African American or Black. Perceiving African American as a monolithic identity presumes that each person of that racial group is similar in all respects to all others of that racial group; individual characteristics, social class, or other forms of individual identity are masked within the monolithic identifier. Acknowledging the broad variation in identities in the African American population is a necessary but difficult step for the ethical practitioner because the recognition of variability refutes the stereotypical representations of African Americans that shape current thinking (Hudley & Graham, 2001). Ethical practice recognizes individual difference, not socially constructed labels that essentialize race.

The culturally effective program provider sees the culture of each participant as a valid representation of ways of living, thinking, talking, etc. that allows the participant to respond to the particular demands of his/her dynamic ecocultural niche. The culture of the dominant group (i.e., middle class Whites) is understood to enjoy high status due to institutionalized power inequality rather than an inherent superiority. Culturally effective providers in African American communities realize that participants will need to become bicultural or multicultural in order to function successfully in the existing social hierarchy. However, providers recognize that participants benefit by maintaining their own culture and therefore see change as additive and transformative rather than the replacement of an inferior culture. Such an affirming attitude is particularly relevant in health services work, as it protects both providers and participants from the toxic effects of stereotypes about particular minority groups and pathological, self-destructive behavior.

Culturally effective leaders are also committed to a safe and just future for all and thus often function as advocates for participants and their communities. For example, many children living in inner-city communities are exposed to multiple environmental risk factors (Osofsky, 1997) that can lead to serious health consequences. Early and constant exposure to community violence can lead to elevated levels of youth violence in the community, perpetuating a cycle of violence and violence exposure. Environmental toxins can lead to a range of chronic conditions including asthma due to poor air quality, learning disabilities due to early lead exposure, and childhood obesity due to insufficient fresh and healthy food choices in the community. Culturally effective practitioners understand how structural conditions present in the ecocultural niche are risk factors for poor health outcomes and work to minimize or eliminate the risks.

Culturally Responsive Materials and Methods

Culturally responsive methods and materials develop and support participants' skills in health promotion and disease management in a manner consistent with the discussion of culturally effective leaders. Such methods may be specific to particular groups or may comprise more general competence in working in multicultural settings. Effective practitioners are able to translate general interventions into strategies that are appropriate for a given cultural group. For example, participants will vary in their level of comfort with a variety of interpersonal processes (e.g., speaking in front of a group, interacting across gender boundaries, autonomous or interdependent activities). Practitioners must know how to manage these varied needs, some of which will be culturally grounded, in order to create constructive interventions.

Perhaps most important, interventions must provide capacity building experiences that develop critical analysis and social action skills that allow participants to become advocates for the health of themselves, their families, and their communities. Such capacity building activities will also help participants identify their own culturally defined worldviews in a manner similar to the awareness that is necessary for a culturally effective leader. Recall that African Americans, like members of all minority cultures, must function successfully in their ecocultural niche as well as becoming skilled at navigating the dominant culture. Ethical intervention programming will comprise deliberate efforts to strengthen health promoting behavior while developing the personal knowledge and competence necessary to advocate successfully in the mainstream culture (Hill, Soriano, Chen, & LaFromboise, 1994). Culturally responsive prevention and intervention programming can address institutional bias and racism, for example, by including training in political organizing to address issues of access to more healthful lifestyle options and health services, conducting community service projects (clean-up, beautification) to enhance the local community, or cross-age mentoring in which youth are mentored by trained, caring members of the community and in turn mentor peers and younger students in health promotion and healthy behaviors.

Methods for assessment and evaluation should be similarly cognizant of the dynamics of participants' ecocultural niche. Assessment tools should be developed and validated with samples that are sufficiently diverse to ensure cultural appropriateness and measurement equivalence for all of the cultural groups subsumed under the broad label African American. Improper measures carry the risks of inaccurate matches between need and services, meaning that participants may be inaccurately targeted for services or may not receive needed services (Hudley et al., 2001). Improper assessments can contribute to the labeling of entire social groups (e.g., "violent" African American teens) (Pumariega, 2001). Conversely, the lack of needed services may lead to a host of negative health outcomes (mental health challenges, uncontrolled chronic disease, youth violence, childhood obesity, etc.).

Culturally Engaged Participants

Cultural engagement is arguably the most important element in our model. Certainly, this component of cultural competence is difficult if not impossible to achieve in the absence of the other two components; however, the development of competence is the highest priority of prevention and intervention programming. Cultural engagement, as defined in this model, is an important competence that can support personal health promotion and disease management as well as empower participants to become socially engaged in promoting healthy lifestyles and healthy communities (Grant & Haynes, 1995).

One goal of ethical interventions with African Americans is therefore to empower participants to work against the influence of extant cultural stereotypes in their own behavior, (e.g., sexual stereotypes that promote risky sexual behavior including the rejection of condoms), the behavior of their families (e.g., negative stereotypes of Black youth including experimentation with substance abuse and antisocial behavior), and the social policies that influence their communities (e.g., stereotypes of Black communities as impoverished and uncared for that promote the disproportionate placement of environmental toxins including waste disposal facilities).

Recall that the definition of cultural engagement includes cultural pride, a positive identity, and bicultural competence, as well as the skills to challenge inequality. Cultural engagement is conceptually linked to racial/ethnic identity, as cultural attitudes are one component of many empirically validated models of ethnic (Phinney, 1990) and racial (Sellers et al., 1998) identity. Thus, culturally engaged participants will be grounded in a positive ethnic identity. By racial/ethnic identity we mean one's extent of identification with a distinguishable racial and cultural group in a given society. Individuals with a strong racial/ethnic identity have developed a knowledge of their own cultural values (a process of exploration) and integrated a positive attitude toward the sociocultural group into a coherent personal identity (arriving at commitment) (Phinney). These elements of a positive racial/ethnic identity map on to cultural pride, a key element of cultural engagement.

Knowledge of cultural values can be an important protective factor for health maintenance in the face of a potentially unhealthful proximal environment. Interdependence, communalism, and spirituality are all salient values of the traditional cultures of many African Americans in the USA that are explicitly in conflict with acquiescence to unhealthful, dangerous environments and self-destructive behaviors (Hill et al., 1994). Commitment to and pride in traditional values can also protect against the debilitating effects of racism and stereotypes, known risk factors for the development of antisocial behavior (Utsey, Chae, Brown, & Kelly, 2002) and depression and withdrawal (Belle & Doucet, 2003). From this base of an affirming ethnic identity, African Americans are better prepared to develop bicultural competence. Bicultural competence comprises skills that allow participants to successfully advocate within the mainstream opportunity structure without feeling they are compromising their identity or "selling out." This capacity to attain success in a dominant culture while maintaining a positive identity and connection within one's home culture is often labeled the "alternation model" of bicultural functioning rather than a substitution model that represents giving up the home culture in favor of mainstream culture. This kind of bicultural competence has shown a positive relationship with cognitive functioning, mental health, and self-esteem (LaFromboise, Coleman, & Gerton, 1993).

Elements of cultural engagement are subject to developmental processes (e.g., identity development); thus the construct will take on age appropriate forms as cultural knowledge, attitudes, and bicultural competence evolve with normative development. For example, children may be developing an awareness of their own racial and cultural heritage, as well as distinguishing their cultural heritage from those of other groups. Cultural engagement in health prevention programs at this age may take the form of increasing cultural knowledge and positive attitudes toward participants' own heritage as well as the heritage of groups other than their own. This form of cultural engagement should be effective in allaying or forestalling the development of negative attitudes, connecting cultural values to healthy and positive lifestyles and behaviors, and developing critical reasoning skills concerning fairness and social justice.

By adolescence, children of color in particular have typically formed a stable ethnic identity (Phinney, 1990) and have an awareness of the broader society's attitudes toward their particular sociocultural group. They will also be ready to build on a foundation of cultural awareness and critical thinking skills. Cultural engagement for this age group should take the form of involvement in cooperative activities including community improvement projects, mentoring and mediation programs, and volunteer opportunities to support social justice and equality. As youth move into adulthood, cultural engagement will include bicultural competence, a lifelong developmental process that supports individuals' capacities to increase successful functioning in the milieu of the dominant cultural group and overcome traditional risk factors for poor health outcomes, chronic disease, and self-destructive behavior, such as poverty, unemployment, lack of education, and institutional racism. At the same time, culturally engaged African Americans will remain grounded in their home culture and thus buffered by a strong sense of positive identity. Building on developmentally appropriate experience, cultural engagement will take the form of a progressively greater commitment to health promotion, disease prevention, and social justice.

This admittedly selective review discusses a model of cultural competence that underpins ethical intervention and prevention programming. Ethical interventions empower participants acting as individuals, members of families, supporters of schools, residents of communities, and contributors to society to support positive, health promoting attitudes and behaviors. Person-focused interventions, albeit important in their own right, will be insufficient to produce long term, equitable health outcomes, if used alone. Race-based health disparities are situated not only in the internal and behavioral systems of individuals but also reside equally in the external effects of a social context that continues to be dominated by racial inequality (Mays, Cochran, & Barnes, 2007). Only a concerted effort by all stakeholders working together will ensure that positive health outcomes will be enjoyed by all people.

References

Baldwin, A., Baldwin, C., & Cole, R. (1990). Stress-resistant families and stress-resistant children. In J. Rolf et al. (Eds.), *Risk and protective factors in the development of psychopathology* (pp. 257–280). New York: Cambridge University Press.

Belle, D., & Doucet, J. (2003). Poverty, inequality, and discrimination as sources of depression among U.S. women. *Psychology of Women Quarterly, 27*, 101–113.

Betancourt, H., & López, S. (1993). The study of culture, ethnicity, and race in American psychology. *The American Psychologist, 48*, 629–637.

Bolaffi, G., Bracalenti, R., Braham, P., & Gindro, S. (2003). *Dictionary of race, ethnicity, and culture*. Thousand Oaks, CA: Sage.

Brody, G., Chen, Y., Murry, V., Ge, X., Simons, R., Gibbons, F., et al. (2006). Perceived discrimination and the adjustment of African American youths: A five-year longitudinal analysis with contextual moderation effects. *Child Development, 77*(5), 1170–1189.

Brown, T., Williams, D., Jackson, J., Neighbors, H., Torres, M., Sellers, S., et al. (2000). Being black and feeling blue: The mental health consequences of racial discrimination. *Race and Society, 2*, 117–131.

Centers for Disease Control and Prevention – National Center for Health Statistics. (2007). *Health, United States, 2007*. Hyattsville, MD: Centers for Disease Control and Prevention. Retrieved Dec 1, 2010, from http://www.cdc.gov/nchs/data/hus/hus07.pdf.

Cornell, S., & Hartman, D. (1998). *Ethnicity and race: Making identities in a changing world*. Thousand Oaks, CA: Pine Forge.

Garcia, E. (1993). Language, culture, and education. *Review of Research in Education, 19*, 51–98.

Grant, D., & Haynes, D. (1995). A developmental framework for cultural competence training for children. *Social Work in Education, 17*, 171–182.

Hill, H., Soriano, F., Chen, S., & LaFromboise, T. (1994). Sociocultural factors in the etiology and prevention of violence among ethnic minority youth. In L. Eron, J. Gentry, & R. Schlegel (Eds.), *Reason to hope: A psychosocial perspective on violence and youth* (pp. 59–97). Washington, DC: American Psychological Association.

Hudley, C., & Graham, S. (2001). Stereotypes of achievement striving among early adolescents. *Social Psychology of Education: An International Journal, 5*, 201–224.

Hudley, C., Wakefield, W., Britsch, B., Cho, S., Smith, T., & DeMorat, M. (2001). Multiple perceptions of children's aggression: Differences across neighborhood, age, gender, and perceiver. *Psychology in the Schools, 38*, 45–56.

Kaiser Family Foundation. (2009). *Medicaid and the uninsured*. Washington, DC: Kaiser Family Foundation.

Kitayama, S. (2002). Culture and basic psychological processes – Toward a system view of culture: Comment on Oyserman et al. *Psychological Bulletin, 128*, 89–96.

Ladson-Billings, G. (1995). Toward a theory of culturally relevant pedagogy. *American Educational Research Journal, 32*, 465–491.

LaFromboise, T., Coleman, H., & Gerton, J. (1993). Psychological impact of biculturalism: Evidence and theory. *Psychological Bulletin, 114*, 395–412.

Lamborn, S., Dornbusch, S., & Steinberg, L. (1996). Ethnicity and community context as moderators of the relations between family decision making and adolescent adjustment. *Child Development, 67*, 283–301.

Lewis, T., Everson-Rose, S., Powell, L., Matthews, K., Brown, C., Karavolos, K., et al. (2006). Chronic exposure to everyday discrimination and coronary artery calcification in African American women: The SWAN Heart Study. *Psychosomatic Medicine, 68*, 362–368.

Mays, V., Cochran, S., & Barnes, N. (2007). Race, race-based discrimination, and health outcomes among African Americans. *Annual Review of Psychology, 58*, 201–225.

McAllister, G., & Irvine, J. (2000). Cultural competency and multicultural teacher education. *Review of Educational Research, 70*, 3–24.

Osofsky, J. (1997). *Children in a violent society*. New York: Guilford.

Phinney, J. (1990). Ethnic identity in adolescence and adults: A review of research. *Psychological Bulletin, 108*, 499–514.

Pope-Davis, D., & Coleman, H. (1997). *Multicultural counseling competencies: Assessment, education and training, and supervision*. Thousand Oaks, CA: Sage.

Pope-Davis, D., Liu, W., Toporek, R., & Brittan-Powell, C. (2001). What's missing from multicultural competency research: Review, introspection, and recommendations. *Cultural Diversity and Ethnic Minority Psychology, 7*, 121–138.

Pope-Davis, D., & Ottavi, T. (1994). The relationship between racism and racial identity among White Americans. *Journal of Counseling and Development, 72*, 293–297.

Pumariega, A. (2001). Cultural competence in treatment interventions. In H. Vance & A. Pumariega (Eds.), *Clinical assessment of child and adolescent behavior* (pp. 494–512). New York: Wiley.

Purnell, L. (2002). The Purnell model for cultural competence. *Journal of Transcultural Nursing, 13*, 193–196.

Roosa, M., Dumka, L., Gonzales, N., & Knight, G. (2002, January 15). Cultural/ethnic issues and the prevention scientist in the 21st Century. *Prevention & Treatment, 5*, Article 0005a. Retrieved January 30, 2003, from http://journals.apa.org/prevention/volume5/pre0050005a.html.

Seligman, M., & Csikszentmihalyi, M. (2000). Positive psychology: An introduction. *The American Psychologist, 55*, 5–14.

Sellers, R., Smith, M., Shelton, J., Rowley, S., & Chavous, T. (1998). Multidimensional model of racial identity: A reconceptualization of African American racial identity. *Personality and Social Psychology Review, 2*, 18–39.

Stanfield, J. (1993). Epistemological considerations. In J. Stanfield & R. Dennis (Eds.), *Race and ethnicity in research methods* (pp. 16–36). Newbury Park, CA: Sage.

Sue, S. (1998). In search of cultural competence in psychotherapy and counseling. *The American Psychologist, 53*, 440–448.

Sue, D. W., Arredondo, P., & McDavis, R. (1992). Multicultural counseling competencies and standards: A call to the profession. *Journal of Multicultural Counseling and Development, 20*, 64–88.

Trivedi, A., & Ayanian, J. (2006). Perceived discrimination and use of preventive health services. *Journal of General Internal Medicine, 21*, 553–558.

Utsey, S., Chae, M., Brown, C., & Kelly, D. (2002). Effect of ethnic group membership on ethnic identity, race-related stress and quality of life. *Cultural Diversity & Ethnic Minority Psychology, 8*, 366–377.

Villegas, A., & Lucas, T. (2002). *Educating culturally responsive teachers: A coherent approach.* Albany, NY: SUNY.

Williams, D. (2005). The health of U.S. racial and ethnic populations. *Journal of Gerontology, 2*, 53–62.

Part II
Fundamental Intervention Needs

Chapter 3
Health, Nutrition, Access to Healthy Food and Well-Being Among African Americans

Angela J. Hattery and Earl Smith

> *Today, the average American can expect to live 5 years longer than a Palestinian – unless that American is a black male, in which case he can expect to die 3 years sooner.*
>
> *National Center for Health Statistics. Health, United States, 2005 with Chartbook on Trends in the Health of Americans. Hyattsville, MD: U.S. Dept. of Health and Human Services, Centers for Disease Control and Prevention, 2005.*

Objectives

- Examine the overall state of health among African Americans with attention to health disparities with regards to chronic illnesses such as diabetes and heart disease
- Focus on the ways in which lifestyle – specifically nutrition – shapes the health outcomes of African Americans
- Examine the role that access to nutritious food plays in shaping life chances for African Americans
- Focus on the particular phenomenon of "food deserts" as they impact African American health
- Provide some suggestions for solutions and policy recommendations

Introduction

It has become more or less widely accepted as common sense that nutrition is related to health and wellness and that poor nutrition and/or unhealthy eating will lead to higher rates of obesity and higher rates of chronic diseases like diabetes, stroke, heart disease, cancer, and ultimately to death. Thus, in order to move beyond the obvious, we must consider and explore the other factors that lead to or result in poor nutrition and ultimately poor health. In this chapter, we explore the role that social class plays in shaping individual access to a healthy diet, and we consider the role that social structure, particularly social and racial housing segregation, plays in shaping the access that entire

A.J. Hattery (✉)
Women and Gender Studies, George Mason University, Fairfax, VA, USA
e-mail: ahattery@gmu.edu

A.J. Lemelle et al. (eds.), *Handbook of African American Health: Social and Behavioral Interventions*,
DOI 10.1007/978-1-4419-9616-9_3, © Springer Science+Business Media, LLC 2011

populations, e.g., African Americans in urban centers, have to healthy, nutritious food. In our case study on food deserts we also examine the role that perceptions and ideologies play in shaping food choices. We begin this chapter by arguing that hegemonic ideologies that connect racial/ethnic identity and food are very powerful in shaping individuals' food choices even in the face of common sense understandings of the importance of nutrition in leading a healthy life.

We provide two illustrations. One of the most prominent "voices" in the African American community is radio personality and morning talk show host, Tom Joyner. Listening to just a few minutes of *The Tom Joyner Morning Show* any day of the week the listener will hear numerous advertisements for McDonalds. In fact, Joyner has coined a slogan: "McDonalds: 365 Black" suggesting that African Americans can find a "food home" at McDonalds each and every day of the week. One does not need to view the documentary *Super Size Me* to know that eating at McDonalds even once a week is probably going to result in a nutritionally poor diet that will inevitably lead to diseases such as diabetes, colon cancer, and cardiovascular disease. By playing on a history of segregation and African Americans being denied a service in restaurants and seats at the lunch counter, Joyner is promoting an ideology of racial identity and linking it to food in such a way that is contributing to rates of obesity in the African American community that are higher than those found in any other racial/ethnic population.

Second, common to many racial/ethnic minorities is what can best be described as a "culture of food" that shapes the choices that individuals make both on a daily basis but perhaps especially when celebrating important events – ranging from holidays such as labor day to funerals and birthday parties. This "culture of food" is intimately connected to the racial/ethnic identity of minorities. For example, it is not uncommon to hear food described with a racial/ethnic tag: "soul food" or "Latin food." Similarly, people talk about the kinds of food that they perceive as "insiders" and others, who are identified as "outsiders" eat. These can be either positive or negative stereotypes, for example, African Americans are said to have an insatiable appetite for fried chicken and watermelon.[1] In contrast, many African Americans express concern that whites are too health conscious. For example, this summer one of the authors was listening to the radio one morning and an African American radio host was describing her experience "hanging out with white people" on the 4th of July. She regaled the audience, who are primarily African American, with tales of fresh fruit and vegetables and skinless chicken breasts, and how hungry she was after the event.

Thus, choosing foods and designing menus can be an act of reinforcing racial/ethnic identity. And, especially for minorities who have struggled to have their identities recognized and validated these expressions may trump their own understanding of the role of nutrition in shaping health and disease risks.

In this chapter, we examine and analyze the state of health in the African American community, specifically the role that lifestyle – nutrition specifically – plays in shaping the health of African Americans. Despite living in the most advanced economy in the world with the most advanced health care system in the world, many Americans live with chronic disease and health crises that are similar to citizens of developing nations. Yet even within the USA, health and illness are not distributed randomly: in fact African Americans are more likely to suffer from chronic diseases, to lack access to health care, and to die earlier than their white counterparts. In this chapter, we explore some of the ways in which nutrition and access to food shapes the disease landscape faced by African Americans. Additionally, we will include a case study: an examination of "food deserts" as they exist in rural and urban African American communities and the role they play in shaping the health outcomes of African Americans.

The health of African American women, children, and men has been chronicled for years now with varying degrees off follow-up (Du Bois, 1898, 1899; Smedley, Stith, & Nelson, 2003).

---

[1] When Tiger Woods won his first Masters, Fuzzy Zeller remarked that he supposed this meant they'd eat fried chicken and watermelon for dinner. The Masters winner chooses the clubhouse dinner for all previous Masters champions.

As recently as the mid-1990s the *New England Journal of Medicine* published many articles and editorials on the state of health among African Americans, often comparing this to health and well-being in the Third World (McCord & Freeman, 1990) In fact African American males have the shortest life span of all racial or ethnic groups in the nation – a fact that has remained unchanged for at least the past 100 years (Marmot, 2001). We begin by providing an overall summary of the state of the health of African Americans in the twenty-first Century USA.

The State of Health and Well-Being in African American Civil Society

As we look out a decade into the third millennium, the state of health of African American *citizens* living in the United States is grim indeed (Mead et al., 2008). For a variety of reasons African Americans suffer from higher rates of many of the most lethal chronic diseases: cardiovascular disease (leading to heart attacks and strokes), diabetes, as well as certain forms of cancer.[2]

Health disparities between African Americans and Americans of other racial/ethnic backgrounds have existed since these various groups began to populate – as colonists, settlers, and slaves – what is now the United States of America (Franklin, 1947). The power of lingering disparities can best be understood in the context of the United States economy and the United States system of health care. One of the reasons that the life expectancy for all Americans nearly doubled during the twentieth century was because of the changing nature of the economy. During the long period of agriculture that dominated the economies of the eighteenth, nineteenth, and early twentieth centuries, many laborers died in work-related accidents. Farming was and remains one of the most dangerous occupations (OSHA, n.d.). In fact, data from the National Safety Council still shows the dangers of farming which are surpassed as an occupational hazard in today's economy only by those associated with mining. Manufacturing occupations, such as mining and steel mills, which replaced agricultural work, were safer, but also dangerous.[3] At the close of the twentieth century, as the economy shifted to its current postindustrial service phase, occupational fatalities continue to decline. Yet, as work becomes safer, and life expectancies grow longer, African Americans, and *African American men in particular lag behind*. Thus, the probability is high that men, fathers, grandfathers, uncles, and brothers will die prematurely and be less likely to be part of their families, disrupting African American family life (Hattery & Smith, 2007a; Stewart, Dundas, Howard, Rudd, & Wolfe, 1999).[4]

---

[2] Though these diseases kill more Americans than other diseases or events (such as accidents or homicides), a matter of significant concern when considering the overall health, morbidity and mortality of African Americans are the impact of two phenomenon that rob African American communities of their young: homicide and HIV/AIDS and thus we feel it is critical to note the impact of these producers of early death on the state of African American health (LaVeist, 2005).

[3] Writing this paper we learned that 13 or 14 miners were killed in mining accidents in West Virginia. To be clear we do recognize that there has been a long history of workplace violence. Recently, in August 2010, a beer truck driver shot and killed eight co-workers in Connecticut. http://news.yahoo.com/s/ap/20100804/ap_on_re_us/us_beer_distributor_shootings A postal worker, Jennifer Sanmarco, killed eight co-workers in Oleta, California. This is the most deadly serial murders of co-workers by a woman and in 2003 Dough Williams shot 14 co-workers, killing six at a Lockheed Martin aircraft plant in Meriden, Mississippi.

[4] We note that access to health care and health insurance plays a major role in producing race and class disparities, but that is not our area of concern in this chapter. See LaVeist, http://tlaveist.blogspot.com/2009/10/are-people-in-government-health.html.

Racial Disparities in Chronic Diseases

We begin by briefly reviewing the data on the most serious and prevalent chronic diseases as they exist by race and gender groupings in the United States (all statistics on health come from the Centers for Disease Control). These data are important because they tell us something about the overall health and well-being of African Americans. Furthermore, as the data will show, a major cause of the chronic diseases that many African Americans live with and ultimately die from is poor nutrition (Table 3.1).

These data indicate that stroke death rates are substantially higher for African Americans than for whites. Stewart and colleagues note that the incident rate for first stroke is twice as high for African Americans as it is for whites even when age, gender, and social class are controlled (Stewart et al., 1999). But, as with many other diseases, our understanding of the impact of stroke must be examined through the race, class, and gender paradigm. Though stroke rates are significantly higher for African Americans, the gap between the rates for men and women is as important. In the case of stroke, there is no significant gender difference for whites, but there is a significant gender difference for African Americans; the rate for African American men is ten points higher than for African American women; a gap that has held steady for decades.

Stroke is only one of the serious cardiovascular diseases that affect men and women. The leading cause of death for Americans, regardless of race and gender, is heart disease.

Heart disease is a major cause of death for all Americans. As the data in Table 3.2 reveal, the biggest discrepancies in heart disease are actually by gender – with men of all race/ethnicities suffering significantly more heart disease than women of all racial/ethnic groups. That said, race/ethnicity also significantly shapes heart disease; African American men have the highest rates and white women have the lowest.

After cardiovascular disease, diabetes ranks as the next most significant chronic disease among Americans. Diabetes is of particular importance for both its prevalence but also for the impact it has on people's lives. Type 2, or what used to be called adult on-set diabetes, has reached epidemic proportions in the United States, affecting nearly 20 million Americans (CDC, 2007). Diabetes, if it is not controlled through diet and oral medications, afflicts many significant systems in the human body, most notably the circulatory and excretory systems. The outcomes for patients include lower body amputations (toes, feet, and legs) and kidney failure.

On average, African Americans are 1.6 times more likely to have diabetes as are whites of similar age. The rate of diabetes is important because it is related to so many other diseases. Patients with diabetes are two to four times more likely to develop heart disease, four to six times more likely to suffer a stroke, and they account for 60% of all nontrauma-related amputations (CDC, 2007) (Table 3.3).

Cancer is another serious disease that is nearly always fatal without treatment, and even with treatment, certain forms of cancer have a high rate of mortality.

Table 3.1 Death rates by stroke per 100,000 population by race and gender, 2009

Race	Males	Females
White	41.7	41.1
African American	67.1	57

Table 3.2 Death rates by heart disease per 100,000 population by race, 2009

Race	Males	Females
White	245.2	158.6
African American	320.6	212.5

Table 3.3 Total prevalence of diabetes by race among people aged 20 years or older, United States, 2005

Whites	13.1 million
	8.1% of all whites aged 20 years or older have diabetes
African Americans	3.2 million
	13.4% of all blacks aged 20 years or older have diabetes

In a study by Jessup, Stewart, and Greene (2005), using the National Cancer Data Base between 1990 and 2002, we are told that the incidences for colon cancer are high for African Americans. And, while the study does not spend time with the causes of colon cancer, we find that several easily understood causes have been demonstrated to contribute to the causes of colon cancer among African Americans.

According to the American Cancer Society (2006), variables such as age over 50; diabetes; consumption of foods high in cholesterol (especially from animal sources) and saturated fats; race, ethnicity, social class, and family history are associated with higher rates of colon cancer. While researchers disagree on the impact of these variables, it is clear to us that most of these show up in other leading causes of illness for African Americans such as diabetes. We know for sure that poor diet and imbalance in nutrition are critical in terms of who contracts colon cancer. (We address this last issue when we turn to "food deserts.") (Editorial, 2010, February 9th).

Troubling, though, is the focus of the Jessup, Stewart and Greene (2005) research in the use of adjuvant chemotherapy to treat colon cancer – that even though we know who is susceptible for colon cancer, the level of treatment is minimal. They put it thus:

> Potosky et al. examined the use of adjuvant therapy in colon and rectal cancer in different Surveillance, Epidemiology, and End Results registries and found that in addition to disparities in the administration of adjuvant chemotherapy in stage III colon cancer for elderly patients there were similar disparities based on racial differences with blacks receiving it less often… However, use of adjuvant chemotherapy differed considerably by race/ethnicity, age group, and sex. Its usage was significantly less in blacks (pp. 2706 and 2710).

Leading Causes of Death

Another way to examine health and well-being is to examine causes of death as these are determined by the physician signing the death certificate. These statistics are not free of problems either; however, they are often a more consistent source of data. The problems with this source of data are primarily related to the situation in which the medical examiner may not have access to all of the information. For example, a person who has been receiving chemotherapy for colon cancer but dies of an upper respiratory infection that is a result of a suppressed immune system will have listed as the cause of death "upper respiratory failure" not colon cancer. In fact, the medical examiner may not be aware of the colon cancer unless he or she has access to the medical records or a reliable friend or family member of the deceased. However, unlike diagnoses which require a person to go to see a doctor, because the death certificate is required by law and must be signed by the medical examiner, there will be a record, no matter how imperfect, for every person who dies. Thus, "causes of death" is a more standardized measure.

Another reason it is important to examine causes of death is because they tell us something about how various individuals and groups cope with illnesses. For example, if 8% of whites have diabetes, but few die of the illness (or related complications) then we can assume that they have the support (financial resources, access to medical care, access to a nutritious diet) needed to control the disease. Thus, causes of death tell us something more about health and well-being among different groups of Americans. And, the data on causes of death reveal that though the top causes of death for all Americans are heart disease and stroke, African Americans are more likely to die of chronic diseases like diabetes and homicide, where as Whites, and White women in particular, are more likely to die of "old age."

Infant Mortality

One measure of health and well-being is the Infant Mortality Rate which refers to the probability that a child will die before his/her first birthday. The rate represents the number of children/infants who die before their first birthday per 1,000 live births. Thus, an infant mortality rate of 7.1 (the US average) means that of every 1,000 babies born alive, 7 will die in their first year of life.

The infant mortality rate is considered by researchers to be a good measure of poverty and access to health care because of what it represents as well as the fact that it is (1) a clear measure and (2) it is comparable across geographic region. What do we mean by "clear measure"? We mean that unlike many other measures of poverty such as literacy or malnourishment, it is clear whether an infant has lived or died by his/her first birthday. Second, unlike measures of income that are difficult to standardize because of variance in cost of living and other factors, infant mortality, the death or life of an infant, has the same meaning across all geographic regions and all cultures and societies on the planet.

Finally, though some infants die accidentally or because of genetic birth defects, or sadly, some are murdered by their parent, the majority of infants die because of preventable causes such as infections that go untreated, birth defects that are preventable through prenatal care and a healthy diet for both mother – pregnant or nursing – and the young child (Table 3.4).

Internationally, infant mortality rates vary from a low of 2.28 deaths/1,000 in Singapore to a high of 192.5 deaths/1,000 in Angola. To put the infant mortality rate in perspective, the United States ranks 36 of the 208 countries for which there are infant mortality data. We are outranked by all of the western European countries as well as many countries in Asia such as Singapore, Japan, and Hong Kong. Our infant mortality rate is slightly higher than those in the countries of the former Soviet block and slightly lower than many Caribbean nations. Thus, an African American child born in the United States is as likely to die before his or her first birthday as a child born in the developing economies of the Caribbean and more likely to die before his or her first birthday than children born in former Soviet block countries such as Latvia and Estonia.

As with many other phenomena, infant mortality rates are not uniform across the United States. Not only are African American babies twice as likely to die in their first year as white babies, infant mortality rates for African Americans are also significantly higher in segregated, poor, southern counties (Hattery & Smith, 2007b).[5] *In fact, an African American infant born in parts of the Deep South is more likely to die before its first birthday than one born in many developing nations.* At the extreme,

Table 3.4 Infant mortality rates by race, 1999

US population	African American	White
7.1	14.6	5.8

[5]The results of an analysis of census data for counties in the Deep South indicate that counties in which African Americans are disproportionately represented (greater than 40% of the county population) have infant mortality rates that are many times greater than the rate for counties in which African Americans are not disproportionately represented. Furthermore, in many cases, the infant mortality rates of these counties are more similar to those of countries in the developing world than to the rate in the USA.

only four *countries* in the Western Hemisphere have infant mortality rates *higher* than Tippah County, Mississippi: Dominican Republic (41); Guyana (45.2); Bolivia (66); and Haiti (88.9).

As noted, infant mortality is affected primarily by poverty and access to health care. The role that poverty plays in infant mortality is related to at least two key factors: maternal diet and infant diet. Women who do not have adequate nutrition during pregnancy are more likely to deliver low-birth weight babies as well as babies with particular birth defects (mostly related to the consumption of folic acid). These low-birth weight babies are more likely to die in their first year of life. Second, new mothers who do not have adequate nutrition during the period of lactation will be unable to produce enough nutrition-rich breast milk to nurture their infant. Third, mothers who are unable to produce enough nutrient-rich milk may need to rely on formula. If they cannot afford formula or do not have access to a clean water supply their infants will be at serious risk for death during the first year.[6]

Outcomes of Poor Health: Premature Death

We have already discussed the primary outcome of poor health in the African American community and that is death. Because we will all die some day what becomes important, as noted above, are the causes of death that (1) are preventable and (2) result in premature death.

One of the standardized measures of health and well-being is life expectancy. Life expectancy is a statistic that represents the *average* number of years remaining for a person of a given age to live. Life expectancies are calculated for each new cohort. Thus, the life expectancy for a child born in 2006 is significantly longer than the life expectancy of a person born in 1940.

Many scholars talk about the cumulative stress associated with racism[7] (Shapiro, 2003; Williams, 1999). One outcome of that accumulated stress as well as of poverty (lack of access to health care, poor nutrition, etc.) is a lower life expectancy. This relationship between race, poverty, and health is nowhere more clear than in life expectancy data. For Americans born in 2002, whites can expect to live longer as can women. White women have the longest life expectancy and African American men have the shortest, in fact African American men can expect to live nearly 12 years less than white women. What is also interesting about Table 3.5 is the interaction effect of race and gender. We see, for example, that the gap between African American and white women is narrower (white women can expect to live 5 years longer than their African American counterparts) than it is for

Table 3.5 Life expectancy by selected race, 2002

	White	African American
Male	75.1	68.8
Female	80.3	75.6

Source: Arias, E. (2002). "United States Life Tables, 2002." *National Vital Statistics Reports,* Atlanta, GA: Centers for Disease Control and Prevention. http://www.cdc.gov/nchs/data/nvsr53/nvsr53_06.pdf

---

[6] Access to health care, both pre- and postnatal, is also significantly linked to infant mortality. Mothers who receive prenatal care are more likely to deliver healthy babies of normal birth weight. Similarly, when mothers and their babies receive health care, check ups, and vaccinations in the first year of life, the babies are far less likely to die in the first year. Finally, mother's age is also a significant predictor of low-birth weight and ultimately of infant mortality. Babies born to teenage mothers are at significantly higher risk for low birth weight and infant mortality. Because teen childbearing is significantly more likely among African Americans than whites, this stands as another factor in the racial disparities in infant mortality.

[7] We highly recommend Kai Wright's essay on his father's early death at age 57. His father, a surgeon, suffered from many of the hidden costs of being African American that Shapiro describes (Wright, 2006).

African American and white men. Thus, African American women, for example, share some of the protections that all women have relative to men, but they suffer some of the negative health outcomes that we associate with racism and poverty.

There are a variety of causes of poor health and death for all Americans. Many experts argue that obesity is the number one health problem of all Americans. Today 65% of Americans are overweight or obese, a 16% increase over the rate just a decade ago (Flegal, Ogden, & Johnson, 2002). African American women have the highest rate of obesity of all race/gender groups: 77.1% are overweight and they are 20% more likely to be overweight than white women (57.2%). Men, both African American and white, fall between these two extremes, with white men being somewhat more likely to be overweight (69.4%) than African American men (62.6%). Overweight and obese individuals are at increased risk for many diseases and health conditions, including hypertension, type 2 diabetes, coronary heart disease, stroke, and some cancers (endometrial, breast, and colon).

Comparing the health conditions associated with being overweight or obese and the leading causes of death for Americans, it is clear that one of the major causes of poor health (and even death) in the United States is lifestyle: eating too much, eating an unhealthy diet, and not getting enough exercise. Though this is less of a problem for African American men, it is a serious problem for African American women.

Poverty and Lifestyle[8]

The relationship between lifestyle causes of poor health and illness and race is confounded by social class. In order to disentangle this set of relationships we will begin with a brief discussion of the relationship between social class and lifestyle. The relationship is complex and occurs at both the individual level and the societal level.

At the societal level, America is the land of wealth and abundance. Americans eat more meat, for example, than people in most other nations: both developed and developing. Fewer and fewer Americans have jobs that require much if any physical activity, and as the literal land of the automobile, except for those Americans living in major cities (New York, Chicago, Washington, D.C.) few Americans walk anywhere. Thus, compared to citizens in other countries, both developed and developing, Americans eat more, especially calorie rich foods, and get less physical activity.

Like most everything else, however, even this is shaped by social class. The affluent, for example, are the least likely to have jobs that are physically demanding, but they are the most likely to own memberships to exclusive gyms and country clubs where they can exercise, play golf, and so forth. Similarly, though the affluent have the resources to purchase more meat and "rich" foods, it is the poor who find it difficult to afford or even find healthy food such as fresh fruits and vegetables, leaner cuts of meat and fish, and lower fat dairy products. Thus, in this land of plenty, social class shapes lifestyle, in particular access to healthy food and exercise.

Because African Americans are disproportionately likely to be poor, they are less likely to eat healthfully and exercise and more likely to suffer diseases such as stroke, diabetes, and heart disease. The rates especially of diabetes bear this out. Thus, Americans almost never die of the diseases the world's poor die of malaria and cholera for example, they die instead of diseases of

---

[8] There is ample scientific evidence to conclude that at least two other factors contribute to higher rates of chronic disease and death among African Americans and the poor: (1) lack of health insurance and lack of access to medical care and (2) racial disparities that produce delays in diagnosis. Again, for a lengthy discussion of these issues as they related to the health of African Americans see: (Hattery & Smith, 2007a).

over consumption such as diabetes and heart disease. And, just as the poor in other parts of the world are more vulnerable to diseases like malaria and cholera, the poor, and increasingly African Americans, are more vulnerable to the diseases associated with an unhealthy lifestyle.

Case Study: Food Deserts

Food deserts are a relatively recent concept that describes the variability in accessibility of healthy, high quality food in urban and rural areas. A food desert refers to an area in either a rural or urban community in which several conditions exist either independently or simultaneously: (1) a lack of grocery stores that stock healthy, nutritional food; (2) a high rate of "fast food" stores; (3) a high rate of convenience or other types of "grocery" stores that stock food that is cheap but not high in nutritional value; and (4) the ratio of availability of healthy food to unhealthy food is low.

Scholarly attention on food deserts began when urban researchers observed that one consequence – most likely unintended of white flight (Wilson, 1996) and "ghettoization" – was the flight of chain supermarkets that offered a variety of food choices to local residents. Of course, the variety was not always of the best quality, as news exposes such as the 20–20 investigative program that showcased Food Lion demonstrated, nevertheless, chain supermarkets had at a minimum provided some access to produce, fresh meat and dairy products, even if the quality and nutritional value was somewhat diminished relative to these same supermarkets in the upscale wealthier neighborhoods and suburbs. For the most part, access to any "grocery" has been replaced by convenience stores and "bodegas" which in some cases may carry some produce and dairy products but for the most part carry only packaged and prepared food items that are both more expensive and less nutritionally complete. Along with the demise of the supermarket in urban "ghettos" is the rise of fast-food restaurants, ranging at the "high" end with McDonald's which in its attempt to stay competitive has added "healthy" options to its menu to the "low" end which includes Church's and other similar stores that specialize in selling grizzle at low prices.

This is illustrated in Fig. 3.1 which demonstrates that in Chicago, compared to all other racial/ethnic groups, African Americans had about equal access to fast food, but their access to stores that sold healthy food was significantly reduced by the barrier of distance. Whereas, most whites lived within one-third of a mile to a supermarket, African Americans lived nearly twice as far.

What is the impact of living in a food desert? Based on the research done in Chicago (Gallagher, 2006) and reflected in Fig. 3.2, living in a food desert contributed significantly to higher rates of "diet related death." Yet, as with everything we have discussed in this chapter, the impact varies by race/ethnicity.

Fig. 3.1 Food access in Chicago. Source: Gallagher, M. (2006). *Examining the Impact of Food Deserts on Public Health in Chicago*

Food Access by Avg. Distance in Miles by City of Chicago Block				
Majority Race	Chain Grocers	Small Grocers	All Grocers	Fast Food
White	.57	.54	.39	.35
Afr.-Am.	.77	.86	.59	.34
Latino	.62	.42	.36	.34
Diverse	.52	.53	.36	.30
Chicago	.65	.62	.45	.34

Fig. 3.2 Food deserts and
diet-related deaths in
Chicago. Source: Gallagher, M.
(2006). *Examining the Impact
of Food Deserts on Public
Health in Chicago*

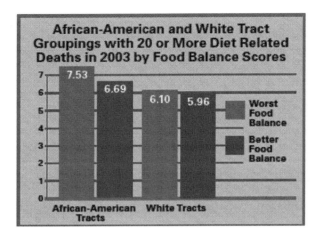

There is no significant difference between the rates of diet related deaths among Whites regardless of whether they live in a food desert or not. In contrast, African Americans who live in food deserts are significantly more likely to suffer from diet-related deaths than those who live in neighborhoods with regular access to food.

This finding is important because it underscores and reinforces our research that documented the impact of racial housing segregation on African Americans and whites in the rural Deep South. We found that whites who lived in majority "black" counties did not differ significantly in terms of overall well-being (educational attainment, employment, wealth, and infant mortality) than those who lived in majority "white" counties. In contrast, for African Americans the impact of living in a majority "black" county were devastating on all measures of well-being; the previous discussion of infant mortality is a case in point (Hattery & Smith, 2007b).

We argue that part of the reason for this similarity is the fact that food deserts exist in rural, farming communities as well, especially across the Deep South where the majority of African Americans continue to live and where rates of obesity and diet-related diseases are the highest in the nation. For example, the Delta counties of rural Mississippi and the Black Belt counties of Alabama are referred to by public health scientists as constituting the "stroke belt" (Glymour, Avendaño, & Berkman, 2007).

Anecdotally we can confirm, after spending many weeks each summer driving through and living in the Mississippi Delta, that these are indeed profound food deserts. Even moderately sized cities such as Clarksdale, Mississippi offer only one supermarket for the entire city. And, with no public transportation, it is out of reach for most of the African American population, that instead rely on a series of "7–11" style convenience stores and local take out restaurants that boast "meat boxes" and every conceivable fried food to meet all of their nutritional needs. In the rural communities that dot the Delta between the moderate cities it is difficult even to find a "healthier" fast food option such as Subway or McDonalds. The vastness of rural food deserts is incomprehensible to those who have not witnessed them. And, the impact on health is clear; these counties, many of which have not a single stop light in the whole county, "boast" the highest rate of obesity, diet-related diseases, and infant mortality. And, because a substantial portion of the US African American population lives in these communities, the impact on African American health is devastating.

What is so surprising about rural food deserts is that they exist in one of the most agriculturally rich areas of the planet. Based on research that we conducted in the Delta in the summer of 2010 we learned that one of the major barriers to growing local food is the history of the slave plantation and share cropper systems that were in place until relatively recently in this hidden part of the

United States. Folks who were interviewed in the Delta indicated that they were not interested in growing their own food because they interpreted this as a step backward, a step back toward the oppressive lives their parents and grandparents lived as former slaves or sharecroppers. Additionally, because the land has always been cultivated with commercial crops – cotton and now soybeans – there is very little collective history or experience with growing food that one can consume or sell at a local farmer's market. Lastly, though many of the larger communities, like Clarksdale, offer weekly farmers' markets rich with healthy and nutritional food, access is limited for many because of a lack of public transportation and barriers such as the inability for them to accept "food stamps" inhibiting access of poor African Americans to the bounty grown in their own "backyards."[9]

Conclusion

In this chapter, we have provided an overview of issues related to health and well-being in the African American community. Unfortunately, on nearly every front, the story is dismal. African Americans are more likely to suffer from many diet-related chronic diseases such as cardiovascular disease and diabetes. They are more likely to be among the uninsured, and when they are insured, they are often relegated to the rolls of Medicaid rather than having private, employer-based health insurance. This situation seriously limits their access to all kinds of health care, but especially the kinds of preventative and on-going care that would reduce the incidence and severity of chronic diseases.

African Americans die earlier than white Americans. And, for different reasons. Whereas 90% of the leading causes of death for whites are diseases of lifestyle and age, 20% of the leading causes of death for African Americans are preventable and premature: HIV/AIDS for both African American men and women and homicide for African American men. Furthermore, African Americans are significantly more likely to die prematurely of diet-related diseases such as diabetes and heart disease because they lack the resources for proper care, they experience discrimination in treatment and delays in diagnosis, and because they lack the resources to control the diseases through diet and exercise.

The African American community is being devastated by illness and premature death. And the effects on African American families are extraordinary. Because African Americans are more likely to face health crises and live with chronic diseases, the burdens on family members are tremendous. These burdens include both financial and emotional strain as well as the burn-out associated with long-term care giving. But, clearly the greatest impact is the disruption that premature death causes in families. Children grow up without parents and grandparents, partners are widowed and live out their lives alone. It is impossible to measure the impact of this on African American families.

In this chapter, we have also explored the utility of the race, class and gender paradigm in understanding health and disease among African Americans (Farmer, 2005). As demonstrated repeatedly, many diseases include both a race and gender component and the data from the Chicago Food desert study (Gallagher) – as well as our small project in the Mississippi Delta – reveal the importance of class, as well. Though it is critical to point out that with regards to diet-related illness, race trumps class. This is largely explained by our research (Hattery & Smith, 2007b), which demonstrates that high degrees of racial housing segregation force even middle income African Americans to live in low-income neighborhoods that are often characterized as "food deserts." Additionally, because of significant racial disparities in wealth accumulation (Conley, 1999; Shapiro, 2003) even middle class African Americans may face additional financial barriers to housing and food security as well

---

[9]For a podcast dealing directly with food deserts in rural Mississippi see: http://www.youtube.com/user/msussrc#p/a/u/0/i5ZnNMU72Sk.

as the history and traditions around "food" shape their risk for diet-related diseases. Kai Wright, an essayist, poignantly demonstrates, through the premature death of his father, at 57, from complications of diabetes, the impact of race, class, and gender on the health and well-being of individual African Americans and their families.

> This theory holds that black folks carry a legacy of disease that isn't genetic but that nonetheless is transferred from one generation to the next – and eventually catches up even with those who clamber up the socioeconomic ladder. Dad died, according to this theory, from the side effects of racism (Wright, 2006).

Solutions

We argue that access to nutritionally healthy food is a human right that must be expanded in the United States. In the "land of plenty" where much food is discarded every year before it gets to market, where fields are left fallow as part of price support programs, and where the legacy of slavery has created ideologies around food that negatively impact African Americans, especially those living in the rural south, the issue is clearly not the amount of food grown but the access and distribution of that food to segments of our population. Reconstituting access to healthy food as a human right would be one step in shaping food policies in ways that would reduce the impact of diet-related illness among all Americans and African Americans in particular.

Practically speaking, we recommend the following:

- Rendering illegal the practice of supermarket chains that as part of their delivery cycle remove rotting and nearly expired food from upscale neighborhood stores and restocking it in their stores in low-income neighborhoods.
- Creating zoning laws that restrict the number of fast-food restaurants based on geography and population density.
- Creating zoning laws that require supermarkets or local food markets be built or retained based on geography and population density.
- Creating incentives for local food producers and farmers' markets to sell in low-income neighborhoods; e.g., accept food stamps, provide transportation, etc.
- Require health courses – and provide the staff to teach them – in all public schools.
- Adjust the requirements of school lunch programs to restrict access to unhealthy food and increase the healthy food offerings…this is especially critical given the percentage of African American students who qualify for and receive free and/or reduced lunch.

A bright spot: We conclude our chapter by highlighting the initiative in Clarksdale, Mississippi. With the help of several programs, including Delta Initiatives and the placement of a HealthCorps staff, a garden program has been developed at the local high school. During the school year, students participate in an afterschool program and during the summer they are paid, to raise food in the high school garden. During the spring, summer and fall, the students sell the food at the local farmer's market. This produces income for the program, provides employment for a few students, teaches skills ranging from farming practices to business practices, and improves the eating habits of the young men. The early indications are that this program is successful, and perhaps can stand as a model for both rural and urban communities in efforts to improve health, changing ideologies, and increasing access to healthy food.

Finally, we began this chapter by arguing that hegemonic ideologies of identity and food create a context or landscape in which people make food choices – on a daily basis perhaps but especially for special events and holidays – based on their racial/ethnic identity and their understanding of what kinds of food "their people" eat. These powerful ideologies, broadcast over the radio station and in popular culture, reinforce the notion that in order to "be black" one must eat certain kinds of foods and not others. When this is coupled with a landscape of accessible and cheap food that is unhealthy and a veritable desert of healthy food, the food choices people make, even when they defy common sense, are understandable and may actually seem to be based on common sense for the individual purchasing the food. Thus, in order to address issues of nutrition and health in the African American community, interventions must be designed that take into consideration hegemonic ideologies that merge racial/ethnic identities and food as well as the practicality of locating and affording healthy food on a daily basis for those people living on very low incomes or in food deserts. Health care providers and nutrition counselors must move beyond the common sense of nutrition and health and think like sociologists in order to address the practical aspects of individuals' lives that shape their food choices and ultimately their risk for chronic disease and premature death.

References

American Cancer Society. (2006, March 15). *Overview: Colon and rectum cancer: What Causes Colorectal Cancer*. Retrieved August 2, 2010, from http://www.cancer.org/docroot/CRI/contentCRI_2_2_2X_What_causes_colorectal_cancer.asp?sitearea=

CDC. (2007). *Diabetes fact sheet*. Retrieved July 25, 2007, from http://www.cdc.gov/diabetes/pubs/pdf/ndfs_2007.pdf

Conley, D. (1999). *Being black, living in the red: Race, wealth, and social policy in America*. Berkeley: University of California Press.

Du Bois, W. E. B. (1898). The negroes of Farmville, Virginia: A social study. *Bulletin of the Department of Labor, 14*, 1–38.

Du Bois, W. E. B. (1899). *The Philadelphia negro*. New York: Lippincott.

Editorial. (2010, February 9). Hungry in America. *New York Times* [electronic version]. Retrieved July 25, 2010, from http://www.nytimes.com/2010/02/10/opinion/10wed4.html?th&emc=th

Farmer, P. (2005). Rethinking health and human rights: Time for a paradigm shift. In P. Farmer (Ed.), *Pathologies of power* (pp. 213–246). Berekeley: University of California Press.

Flegal, K. M., Ogden, C. L., & Johnson, C. L. (2002). Prevalence and trends in obesity among US adults, 1999–2000. *Journal of the American Medical Association, 288*, 1723–1727.

Franklin, J. H. (1947). *From slavery to freedom: A history of African Americans*. New York City: Knopf.

Gallagher, M. (2006). *Examining the Impact of Food Deserts on Public Health in Chicago*. Retrieved July 10, 2010, from http://marigallagher.com/projects/14/4

Glymour, M., Avendaño, M., & Berkman, L. (2007). Is the 'Stroke Belt' worn from childhood?: Risk of first stroke and state of residence in childhood and adulthood. *Stroke, 38*, 2415–2421.

Hattery, A. J., & Smith, E. (2007a). *African American families*. Thousand Oaks, CA: Sage Publishers.

Hattery, A. J., & Smith, E. (2007b). Social stratification in the New/Old South: The Influences of racial segregation on social class in the Deep South. *Journal of Poverty Research, 11*, 55–81.

Jessup, M., Stewart, A., & Greene, F. (2005). Adjuvant chemotherapy for stage III colon cancer: Implications of race/ethnicity, age, and differentiation. *Journal of the American Medical Association, 294*(21), 2703–2711.

LaVeist, T. (2005). *Minority populations and health: An introduction to health disparities in the U.S.*. New York: Jossey-Bass.

Marmot, M. (2001). Inequalities in health. *The New England Journal of Medicine, 345*, 134–136.

McCord, C., & Freeman, H. (1990). Excess mortality in Harlem. *The New England Journal of Medicine, 322*, 173–177.

Mead, H., Cartwright-Smith, L., Jones, K., Ramos, C., Woods, K., & Siegel, B. (2008). *Racial and ethnic disparities in U.S. health care: A chartbook*. New York: Commonwealth Fund.

OSHA. (n.d.). *Farm safety*. Retrieved May 13, 2010, from http://www.osha.gov/OshDoc/data_General_Facts/FarmFactS2.pdf

Shapiro, T. (2003). *The hidden cost of being African American: How wealth perpetuates inequality*. New York: Oxford University Press.

Smedley, B., Stith, A., & Nelson, A. (Eds.). (2003). *Unequal treatment: Confronting racial and ethnic disparities in health care*. Washington, DC: National Academy of Science.

Stewart, J., Dundas, R., Howard, R., Rudd, A. G., & Wolfe, C. D. (1999). Ethnic differences in incidence of stroke: Prospective study with stroke register. *British Medical Journal, 318*, 967–971.

Williams, D. (1999). Race, socioeconomic status, and health: The added effects of racism and discrimination. *Annals of the New York Academy of Science, 896*, 173–188.

Wilson, W. J. (1996). *When work disappears: The world of the new urban poor*. New York: Knopf.

Wright, K. (2006, May/June). Upward Mortality [Electronic version]. *Mother Jones*. Retrieved July 10, 2010, from http://motherjones.com/politics/2006/05/upward-mortality

Chapter 4
Promoting Physical Activity in Black Children and Adolescents: Intervention Strategies Health Practitioners Have Put into Play

Raegan A. Tuff and Billy Hawkins

Introduction and Overview

Physical activity (PA) provides benefits to physical health, psychological well-being, and overall quality of life. Many of the protective effects of physical activity are related to its positive impact on hypertension, diabetes mellitus, and overweight and obesity (Agurs-Collins, Kumanyika, Ten Have, & Adams-Campbell, 1997; Kesaniemi et al., 2001). Physical activity also has a positive impact on psychological health as it decreases symptoms of anxiety, poor self-esteem, and depression (Irwin, 2006; Kesaniemi et al., 2001; Wolin et al., 2007). To achieve the benefits of physical activity, federal experts recommend that healthy youth between the ages of 6 and 17 participate in 60 min of age appropriate moderate aerobic activity each day and/or vigorous-intensity aerobic activity at least three times a week. As part of their 60 or more minutes of daily physical activity, youth should include 3 days of muscle-strengthening activities such as playing on playground equipment, climbing trees, and playing tug-of-war, and 3 days of bone strengthening activities like running, jumping rope, basketball, tennis, or hopscotch (US Department of Health and Human Services [USDHHS], 2008).

Despite the abundance of information documenting the role of physical activity in health and quality of life, this information alone has been insufficient in promoting active lifestyles in some groups of the US population, particularly youth. Youth are believed to be sedentary or physically active at levels below the threshold to reap substantial health benefits. Youth is recognized as a time of physical, psychosocial, cognitive, and emotional changes within varied social cultural contexts. Changes in each context influences participation in physical activity. Furthermore, youth is a critical time when many future heath behaviors begin and provides an opportunity for interventions that encourage physical activity participation (Clemmens & Haymen, 2004). Healthy People 2020 objectives include increasing the proportion of adolescent who meet current Federal physical activity guidelines for aerobic and muscle-strengthening physical activities (objectives PA-3). Even though attention has grown toward designing and implementing health interventions that address obesity-related risk factors (e.g., nutrition) in the general population of adolescents, intervention approaches designed to increase physical activity among African American youth who suffer most from physical activity disparities has been limited. The purpose of this paper is to review interventions that have been developed and implemented for Black children and adolescents with the goal of helping public health practitioners identify approaches to improve physical activity in this population.

B. Hawkins (✉)
Department of Kinesiology, University of Georgia, Athens, GA, USA
e-mail: bhawk@uga.edu

A.J. Lemelle et al. (eds.), *Handbook of African American Health: Social and Behavioral Interventions*,
DOI 10.1007/978-1-4419-9616-9_4, © Springer Science+Business Media, LLC 2011

Over the past decade, several studies have investigated physical activity correlates specific to African Americans or other ethnically diverse youth (Barr-Anderson et al., 2007; Dishman, Saunders, Motl, Dowda, & Pate, 2009). These studies are generally helpful for determining necessary intervention components and have identified personal and parental positive outcome expectations about physical activity, and self-esteem, as correlates to physical activity participation and adherence. In other correlate studies, factors such as "parental involvement, enjoyment of physical education or physical activity, self-efficacy, access, and quality and location of physical activity-related resources, regardless of participant characteristics (e.g., race/ethnicity, gender)," have also been identified (Whitt-Glover et al., 2009, p. S323) and may be considered when developing interventions for African American youth.

In a systematic review of physical activity interventions published between 1985 and 2006, Whitt-Glover and Kumanyika (2009) identified 43 studies that reported physical activity or fitness changes in African American participants. Of these, 14 interventions included African American children and youth between the ages of 7 and 17 years. Interventions including children and youth were generally controlled trials conducted in "schools community centers, a church, a housing development, a combined summer camp and an internet program, a neighborhood clinic, and a medical center" (p. S35). Interventions were also conducted in after-school programs. Interventions incorporated behavioral, cognitive, and cultural components but had limited success in helping participants sustain physical activity over time due to lack of long-term post-intervention follow-up. Wilson (2009) reviewed intervention approaches that targeted obesity-related behavior in minority adolescents. The chapter highlighted home, school, and community environments as key settings for supporting healthy diet and physical activity. Intervention approaches that integrated culturally targeted and tailored approaches showed the most potential for improving health behavior.

Previous research demonstrates that school-based intervention approaches may be effective in increasing physical activity since it is where children spend a large portion of their day (Jago & Baranowski, 2004; Sallis et al., 2003; Stone, McKenzie, Welk, & Booth, 1998). Furthermore, school settings reach youth across various ethnic and socioeconomic strata (Naylor & McKay, 2009). Such interventions have been implemented to change existing physical education curricula and other classroom educational approaches. The Centers for Disease Control and Prevention (CDC) supports school-based approaches and encourages schools to require and ensure that children and adolescents (1) participate in PE classes each day, (2) participate in moderate to vigorous physical activity for at least half of the time spent in PE classes, (3) are provided with opportunities to participate in PA programs after school, and (4) spend limited amounts of time watching televisions and using computers in licensed child care facilities (Kettle Kahn et al., 2009).

Policy and systems change approaches in schools and after school programs in communities will allow these types of recommendations to be effectively implemented. However, there is limited understanding for how these approaches work with African American populations and minority groups. As a result, it is imperative to design, implement, and evaluate programs for this population (Klebnoff & Muramatus, 2002). The purpose of this chapter is to provide a narrative review of school and after-school-based physical activity interventions for African American children and adolescents. This chapter is divided into three sections. "Prevalence and Consequences of Physical Inactivity" describes the prevalence and consequences of physical inactivity. "Methods" describes the selected interventions. The final section provides recommendations and implications for public health researchers and practitioners working with African American adolescents and underserved populations.

Prevelance and Consequences of Physical Inactivity

To examine the prevalence of priority health risk behavior such as physical inactivity, the CDC conducts the Youth Risk Behavior Surveillance System (YRBSS). As illustrated in Fig. 4.1, results

Fig. 4.1 Percentage of high school students who met recommended levels of physical activity, by sex and race/ethnicity, 2007 (CDC, 2008)

Fig. 4.2 Percentage of high school students who did not participate in 60 or more minutes of physical activity on any day, by sex and race/ethnicity, 2007 (CDC, 2008)

Fig. 4.3 Percentage of female high school students who did not participate in 60 or more minutes of physical activity on any day, by race/ethnicity and grade, 2007 (CDC, 2008)

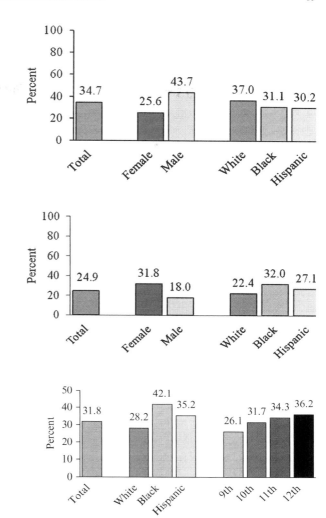

from the 2007 YRBSS indicate that African American youth in grades 9–12 had a lower prevalence of meeting the physical activity recommendations than other adolescent groups. The recommended levels include any kind of physical activity that increased their heart rate and made them breathe hard some of the time for a total of at least 60 min/day on 5 or more days during the past 7 days before the survey. Other studies have found similar results among African American youth. In a study of Chicago inner city youth, only 26% of African American adolescents engaged in more than 20 min of moderate to vigorous physical activity each day, while 71% spent four or more hours each day watching TV, using the computer, or playing video games.

Figure 4.2 demonstrates that nationwide the largest disparities in meeting the physical activity recommendation in 2007 were observed by gender, which has been previously documented (Whitt-Glover et al., 2009).

Furthermore, the prevalence of not meeting physical activity recommendations increased as participants aged regardless of race or ethnicity (Fig. 4.3).

Similar results were noted in the longitudinal National Heart, Lung, and Blood Institute (NHLBI) Growth and Health Study in which 2,400 Black and White girls were prospectively followed for 10 years to determine how their physical activity participation changed over time (Kimm et al., 2002). For both groups physical activity declined significantly between the ages of 13 and 17. However, the decline for Black girls was much steeper than the decline for White girls. Even as activity participation rose slightly by the age of 18 years for White participants, Black participants remained steadily inactive (Kimm et al., 2002). The dramatic decrease in physical activity during adolescence is cause for concern because it is associated with increased morbidity and the development of obesity, other chronic diseases, and type 2 diabetes (Epstein, Paluch, Gordy, & Dorn, 2000; Webber et al., 1996).

Physical inactivity and unhealthy eating habits have contributed to an unprecedented epidemic of overweight that is currently plaguing children and adolescents. Results from the 2007 National Survey of Children's Health (NSCH) revealed that approximately 32% of children aged 10–17 years are overweight or obese – nationwide defined as having a body mass index (BMI) greater than the 85th percentile BMI for an age group (Trust for America's Health, 2009). Eight of the ten states with the highest prevalence of overweight and obese 10- to 17-year-old children are in the south – Mississippi (44.4%), Arkansas (37.5%), Georgia (37.3%), Kentucky (37.1%), Tennessee (36.5%), Alabama (36.1%), Louisiana (35.9%), and West Virginia (35.5%) (Trust for America's Health, 2009). African American children as well as those of lower socioeconomic status have been disproportionately affected by the obesity epidemic (Richmond, Field, & Rich, 2007). The same data show that approximately 41% of African American children and adolescents aged 10–17 years are disproportionately affected by overweight and obesity when compared to the general population.

The prevalence of overweight African American youth is contributing to an increase in the diseases that were mainly seen in adult populations. Studies have shown that as many as 80% of overweight or obese adolescents will become obese adults predisposing this population to a range of health and medical conditions including cardiovascular disease (CVD), high cholesterol levels, high blood pressure, gallbladder disease, and abnormal glucose tolerance (Cruz et al., 2005). Research has shown that children as young as 4 years of age have been diagnosed with type II diabetes, with the average age of onset being 13 years (Nwobu & Johnson, 2007).

The most immediate consequence of overweight, as perceived by children themselves, is social discrimination. In a society that values thinness, overweight children and adolescents are often targets of early and systematic social discrimination. Neumark-Sztainer, Story, and Faibisch (1998) explored the issue of weight-related stigmatization among 55 overweight African American and Caucasian adolescent girls and found that, regardless of ethnicity, girls endured teasing, joking, and name calling in home, school, and peer contexts due to their overweight status.

Stern et al. (2006) studied 39 African American adolescent girls who were participating in an obesity treatment program and found high rates of self-reported stigmatization and poor overall psychosocial functioning, which interfered with their quality of life. Some researchers have found that teachers have low expectations for success for overweight students and view overweight students as untidy, more emotional, less likely to succeed on homework, and more likely to have family problems (Neumark-Sztainer, Story, & Harris, 1999; O'Brien, Hunter, & Banks, 2007). The psychological stress of social stigmatization can cause low self-confidence and may consequently impede academic success and social interaction (Schwartz & Puhl, 2003). Judge and Jahns (2007) found that overweight children in the third and fourth grade had lower reading and math assessment scores, lower interpersonal skills, and more instances of problem behavior than normal weight children in the same grade.

Methods

To identify after school and school-based approaches for increasing physical activity in African American youth, a literature search was conducted for studies that were published in the English language between 2000 and 2009. This search included computerized searches of online databases such as PubMed, the Cochrane Database of Systematic Reviews, Psychnet, and SportsDiscuss.

Keywords for the search included Black, African American, teenage, child, adolescent, intervention, program, project, school, after-school, recreation physical activity, physical education, training, physical fitness, exercise, and sports. Additional studies of interest were located though bibliographic searches of key articles and the authors knowledge of the literature. Studies included in the review (a) targeted a large group of African American children or adolescents (≥47%), (b) engaged participants between the ages of 6 and 17 years old, (c) measured physical activity as a main outcome or as an intervention component, (d) used either objective or self-report assessments of physical activity, and (e) measured physical activity before and after the intervention. Since there is likely limited literature on PA interventions in African American children we also included interventions that focused on increasing energy expenditure, physical fitness, or leisure time physical activity. As any increase in the amount of these components in which children and adolescents engaged is likely to result in health benefits, this review included studies that assessed the effect of the intervention on either physical activity or energy expenditure at the intervention location or in habitual activity. Unpublished works such as dissertation and theses were not included in the review. Further, studies were not included in the review if the demographics of the target population or the effect of the PA intervention were not described.

Results

Summaries of the intervention studies that met the inclusion criteria are shown in Table 4.1. The table includes the study author, publication date, outcome measures, setting, participant description, intervention method, and overall findings. In addition to physical activity and fitness, some studies measure multiple health outcomes (BMI, fast glucose, etc.). Since this study is primarily focused on the effects of physical activity in interventions only, the results of the PA component of the intervention are reported in the table.

Study Characteristics

The interventions reviewed fell into four general categories: instructional, policy, environmental, and multicomponent. These categories are similar to those found in previous reviews of school-based physical activity interventions (Naylor & McKay, 2009). The instructional interventions in the review provided informational classes and education to improve physical activity knowledge, behavior, and attitudes. Policy interventions are those in which implementation of physical activity was guided by some written or unwritten standard or professional practice (Schmid, Pratt, & Witmer, 2006). The environmental approaches in the review changed the physical environment such as by changing playground markings, providing playground equipment, or improving park appearance. Finally, multicomponent interventions employed a systems approach to impacted several layers of the child environment simultaneously such as the physical education classroom, family, physical educational class, and the playground (Naylor & McKay).

Fifteen studies were controlled trials, and thirteen of these were randomized controlled trials. Seven studies measured physical activity as a primary outcome in terms of estimated daily expenditure or time (h/week) spent in moderate to vigorous physical activity (Barbeau et al., 2007; Gutin, Yin, Johnson, & Barbeau, 2008; Pate et al., 2003; Pate et al., 2005; Rohm Young, Phillips, Yu, & Haythornthwaite, 2006; Story et al., 2003; Wilson et al., 2005). Eight studies measured physical activity or cardiovascular fitness as one of several target outcomes (Baranowski et al., 2003; Beech et al., 2003; Fitzgibbon et al., 2005; Foster et al., 2008; Neumark-Sztainer et al., 2009; Shaw-Perry et al., 2007; Yin et al., 2005).

Table 4.1 Summary of intervention studies

Study	Design	Outcome measures	Setting	Participants	Intervention method	Overall findings
Pate et al. (2005) LEAP	Random control trials (RCT)	Primary: % of girls who reported participating in VPA during ≥1, 30-min blocks/day Secondary: ≥2, 30-min blocks/ day of MVPA (≥3 METs) 3-day physical activity recall (3DPAR)	Schools, USA	Grade: 8th Age: 13.6 years (SD 0.6) N=2,744 Black: 48.7% Gender: Girls only	Theory: Social ecological model Timeframe: 1 year Context: Multicomponent; focused on changing PE and health education instruction and creating a supportive school environment Instruction: Changed PE content to enhance self-efficacy and enjoyment, teach girls physical and behavioral skills, and use of 50% of PE time for MVPA Environment target: Activities that enhanced role modeling by faculty and staff, increased communication about physical activity, and provided opportunities for family and community involvement Control group: No intervention	Prevalence of regular VPA intervention schools>control schools (P=0.05) After baseline adjustments 45% of girls in intervention schools and 36% of girls in control schools had reported participating in VPA during ≥1, 30 min blocks/day during the 3-day recall period
Rohm Young et al. (2006)	RCT	Primary: Estimated daily energy expenditure 7-day physical activity recall	School, USA	Grade: 9th N=221 Black: 83% Gender: Girls only	Theory: Social action theory Timeframe: 8 months Context: Conducted to maximize PA during PE classes Less sedentary games (e.g., soccer vs. softball). One semester of individual sports and team sports each on 5 days/week Included small group activities such as skits to enhance goal setting and problem solving Family support component: Monthly newsletters, family workshops Control group: Standard physical education class	No significant between-treatment group differences for mean daily energy expenditure (P=0.93), moderate-intensity energy expenditure (P=0.77), or hard to very hard energy expenditure (P=0.69). Intervention classes spent 46.9% of physical education class time in moderate to vigorous activity compared with 30.5% of time for control classes (P=0.001)

Study	Design	Measures	Sample	Intervention	Results
Robinson et al. (2003) Stanford GEMS	RCT	Computer sciences and applications (CSA) accelerometer GEMS activity questionnaire (GAQ)	Age: 9.5 (SD 0.8) N=61 Black: 100% Gender: Girls (and their guardians/parents) Community health centers, USA	Theory: Social cognitive Timeframe: 12 weeks Context: 45–60 min of MVPA, 5 days/week structured around hip hop, African, and step dance classes Family support component: Five home lessons with a behavior change partner/role model on reducing TV time and AA history. Five newsletters mailed to parents/guardians to reinforce lessons Active control group: Monthly community health lectures, health newsletter updates on obesity, heart disease, and stroke	At follow-up girls in intervention group showed trends towards increased physical activity (although not as much as predicted) Both the average counts per minute of PA as measured by CSA and minutes of MVPA between 12 and 6 PM increased by 7% relative to control group (p. 53) no significant differences
Story et al. (2003) "Girlfriends for KEEPS": Minnesota GEMS	RCT	Computer sciences and applications (CSA) accelerometer GEMS activity questionnaire (GAQ)	Girls N=54 Age: 9.3 (SD 0.9) Black: 83% Gender: Girls Community after-school program, USA	Theory: Social cognitive Timeframe: 12 weeks Context: Club meeting format. "Members" met 1 h 2x/week after-school Environmental targets: Peer support and role modeling; as well as personal and behavioral factors such as knowledge, self-efficacy, goal setting, and social reinforcement Increased MVPA by allowing girls to choose among physical activity options (e.g., ethnic dancing, Double Dutch, jump rope tag, and step aerobics) Incentives built into the program Family support component: Families received take home packets of information; participated in activities such as family night events, and received encouragement telephone calls Active control group: Created memory books, attended arts and crafts meetings and workshop on African percussion	Consistently, higher physical activity levels in the intervention group than in the control group; CSA counts per minute, minutes of MVPA, and self-report of PA although not statistically significant

(continued)

Table 4.1 (continued)

Study	Design	Setting	Outcome measures	Participants	Intervention method	Overall findings
Wilson et al. (2005)	Quasi-experimental	Schools, USA	Primary: Time spent in MVPA over five consecutive days Accelerometer Secondary: Enjoyment of PA scale	Age = 11 ± 0.6 Intervention n = 28 Control n = 20 Gender: Intervention 61% female, 39% male Control: 85% female, 15% male Black: 85% Free/reduced lunch: 89% BMI = 21 ± 4	Theory: Social cognitive theory, Self-motivation theory Time: Context: 3 days/week 2-h after school. Intervention included strategic self-presentation videotape sessions and three components (1) homework/snack, (2) 60 min of student selected MVPA (e.g., basketball, hip-hop dance, step, double Dutch), and (3) behavioral and motivational skills training to increase PA with friends and family at home Control:	Participants in the intervention demonstrated a significantly larger increase in time spent in MVPA than those in the comparison group. No significant differences in accelerometer estimates of MPA levels on program versus non-program days
Yin et al. (2005) Fit Kid Project	RCT	School/after-school, USA	Primary: %Body fat (DXA) Secondary: Cardiovascular fitness Submaximal 3-step bench test	Age = 8.7 ± 0.5 N = 601 (Intervention N = 312; Control N = 28) Boys: 48% Girls: 52% Black: 61%	Theory: Timeframe: 8 months Context: Supportive after-school environment for PA that included a 40-min homework period and a 70-min physical activity period. 20 min warm-up skills instruction 40 min of continuous MVPA (6 MET) 10 min of stretching and cool down	Average attendance rate: 69% 92% retention rate over 1 year Compared to control group intervention group participants with 40%+ attendance showed significantly great gains in BMD and CVF
Wilson et al. (2002)	RCT	School	Primary: Increase in aerobic activity to 30–60 min/day for 7 days a week by the end of the program Computer sciences and applications (CSA) accelerometer	N = 53 Black: 100% Boys: 58.4% Girls: 41.5% Age: 11–15 years Weight status: Within 30% of ideal weight	Theory: Social cognitive Timeframe: 12 weeks Context: Students randomized into SCT + motivational interviewing, SCT only, or education only group for increasing FV intake and PA. Used strategic self-presentation videotape sessions Control group: Given information material about general health issues	Within group: NA No significant effects found for any of the PA measures between intervention and comparison group

Barbeau et al. (2007)	RCT	Schools, USA	$N=201$ (Intervention $n=118$; Control $n=83$) Gender: Girls Black: 100% weighing less 300 lbs	Theory: Timeframe: 10 months 5 days/week focus on decreasing accumulation of fatty tissue through PA. Sessions were 110 min divided into 30 min for HW/snack and 25 skill development 35 MVPA. Implemented by classroom teachers and teacher assistants. Transportation provided after each session Control: No intervention
Gutin et al. (2008)	RCT	Schools, USA	Intervention: $n=42$ Age: 3rd grade Boys: 46% Girls: 54% Black: 67% Control: $n=168$ Gender: 47% Male; 53% female Black: 59%	Theory: Timeframe: 3 school years Context: 5 days/week focus on increasing aerobic fitness. 2-h sessions combined 40 min of academic time and snack followed by 80 min of PA Environment: Designed as a mastery oriented climate with 40 min allocated for VPA. Sessions supervised by physical education teachers and classroom teachers from schools Control: Not discussed

(continued)

Table 4.1 (continued)

Study	Design	Outcome measures	Setting	Participants	Intervention method	Overall findings
Beech et al. (2003) Memphis GEMS	RCT	Primary: %Body fat-dual energy X-ray absorptiometry (DEXA) Secondary: Average daily counts per minute and number of minutes of MVPA occurring between 12 and 6 PM Computer science applications (CSA) accelerometer. The GEMS activity questionnaire (GAQ), a modification of the self-administered physical activity checklist (SAPAC)	Community health center, USA	$N=60$ (21 in child intervention, 21 in parent intervention, 18 in control group) Black: 100% Gender: Girls Age: 8.9 (0.8) BMI 23.7 (6.3)	Theory: Social cognitive Timeframe: 12 weeks Context: 90-min weekly session – child targeted: 30 min of hip-hop dance and lessons on reducing sedentary activity. Parents: 25 min 70/80 s music dance sessions and learn current dance moves from their daughters. Nutrition lessons through cooking demonstrations	In relation to the comparison group girls in both the child-targeted and parent-targeted interventions when averaged increased their level of MVPA by 11.7%
Baranowski et al. (2003) The Fun Food and Fitness Project (FFFP): Baylor GEMS	RCT	Primary: Body mass index (BMI)-dual energy X-ray absorptiometry (DEXA) Secondary: MVPA computer science applications (CSA) accelerometer. GEMS activity questionnaire (GAQ), a modification of the self-administered physical activity checklist (SAPAC)	Summer day camp, Homes	$N=35$ (Intervention $n=19$; Control $n=16$) Black: 100% Gender: Girls Age: 8.3 (0.3) BMI: Intervention: 21.1 (4.4); Control: 26.6 (7.9)	Theory: Social cognitive theory Timeframe: 12 weeks Context: Girls in the intervention group attended a special 4-week summer day camp, followed by a special 8-week home Internet intervention for the girls and their parents Control group girls attended a different 4-week summer day camp, followed by a monthly home Internet intervention, neither of which components included the GEMS-FFFP enhancements	Intervention group had more 24-h CSA counts per minute and MET adjusted minutes of activity based on the GEMS questionnaire than the comparison group although not statistically significant. The intervention group also had fewer DCSA MVPA counts per minute than the control group

Study	Design	Setting	Measures	Sample	Intervention	Results
Resnicow et al. (2000) Go Girls!	UCT	Public housing development	Primary: Increased FV intake, decreased fat intake, decreased fast food intake, decreased TV viewing, and increased PA		Context: 30–60 min of PA including aerobics, toning, walking, jumping rope, and outdoor games, visits to local health clubs	No significant differences in physical activity variables between intervention and comparison group
Pate et al. (2003) Active Winners	Quasi-experimental	Rural communities	Primary: Physical activity during after school hours. Previous day physical activity recall (PDPAR)	Total $N=436$ (Intervention $n=175$, Comparison $n=129$) Age: 10–12 years Gender: Male 49%, female 51% Black: Intervention=87.4%, Comparison=59.4%	An after school and summer physical activity program: Students entered the program the summer after 5th grade (Summer I) and continued the summer after 6th grade (Fall I–Summer II). Transition program fall of 7th grade (Fall II). Sessions ranged between 2 and 15 weeks and covered topics on fitness, physical activity, social skills, and academic skills	
Shaw-Perry et al. (2007) NEEMA	Quasi-experimental	Schools low income	Glucose (FCG) Body composition: %Body fat Anthropometric BMI Fitness laps completed	$N=58$ Black: 42% Age: $10.54+0.74$ Female: 55.9 Male: 44.1% Overweight students (BMI>95th): 22.1%	Theory: Timeframe: 14 weeks Context: Diabetes prevention pilot study. Based on Bienestar. Organized health programming transmitted to students through four NEEMA social network components: Health and physical education class – 13 sessions on nutrition, PA self-esteem and self-control Health club – 18 sessions to promote leisure time PA. Parents encouraged to attend. Student participation voluntary. Includes aerobics, dancing, and singing Family fun fair – parent manual and parent handouts to promote healthy nutrition and exercise choices School food service program – Seven cafeteria lesson plans designed to improve nutrition knowledge of food service staff and encourage students to eat healthy F&V	From baseline to follow-up fitness laps increased from 16.40 (SD=9.98) to 23.72 (SD=14.79) ($P<0.000$)

(continued)

Table 4.1 (continued)

Study	Design	Outcome measures	Setting	Participants	Intervention method	Overall findings
Neumark-Sztainer et al. (2009) Ready Set Action	RCT	BMI Dietary Intake Physical activity (h/day after school) – Past day physical activity recall TV viewing Self-efficacy for healthy eating and physical activity Enjoyment of FV Enjoyment of PA	Schools/after school low income	N=96 children and their parents Age: 10.3 (1.1) BMI>95th percentile: 23 (41%) 41% overweight Black: 54%	Theory: Social cognitive 14.2-h after school theatre sessions to discuss behavioral changes, prepare healthy snacks, and engage in PA (dancing/walking). Included theatrical activities – intervention messages transformed into play scenes. Eight weekly booster sessions. Family component to enhance home support through parent participation in PA and health eating practices	Self-efficacy to be physically active showed a statistically significant difference between intervention and control 13 out of 21 outcomes were in the hypothesized positive direction but there were no meaningful differences between intervention and control groups for these outcomes at follow-up

Measurement of physical activity was mostly carried out with self-reported questionnaire or recall instruments in six studies (Baranowski et al., 2003; Beech et al., 2003; Pate et al., 2005, Robinson et al., 2003; Rohm Young et al., 2006; Story et al., 2003). Four studies relied on objective measures such as the computer sciences applications accelerometer, physical fitness tests, or activity monitors (Baranowski et al.; Beech et al.; Robinson et al.; Shaw-Perry et al., 2007; Story et al.; Wilson et al., 2005). Sample sizes ranged from 35 to more than 2,500 for studies included in the review. The timeframe for most interventions was short, lasting between 12 weeks and 10 months. One study described results that occurred after 3 years (Gutin et al., 2008). Most studies recruited only girls and girls comprised most of the participants in other studies. Four studies included both boys and girls (Gutin et al., 2008; Yin et al., 2005; Wilson et al., 2002, 2005). The effect of intervention strategies on adult family members or caregivers was also included in several studies. The age of the participants in the study ranged from 6 to 15 years of age.

Ten studies included healthy participants. Six studies selected or included participants based on the overweight or obese weight status of the participant or their parents (Robinson, Barbeau, Baranowski, Resnicow, Neumark-Sztainer, Shaw-Perry.) Other special populations included obese children at risk for diabetes (Shaw-Perry et al., 2007).

While several of the studies reported a positive intervention effect, only three achieved a statistically significant increase in physical activity between intervention and comparison groups (Pate et al., 2005; Shaw-Perry et al., 2007; Wilson et al., 2005). One study reported a significant difference in physical inactivity so that children in the interventions' schools reported less television watching (Foster et al., 2008). Since only four studies reported a significant result, it is difficult to stratify the intervention elements that caused the most impact. However, it appears that family participation and role modeling from school staff may be critical elements to increasing physical activity. This is consistent with previous research that shows that family is the primary and most essential socializing agent for physical activity during childhood. Additionally, studies using objective previously validated instruments also reported significant positive results on physical activity and sedentary behavior.

Conclusion

This chapter provided a summary of school and after-school-based physical activity interventions for African American children and adolescents. It described the prevalence and consequences of physical inactivity, the selected interventions, and implications for public health researchers and practitioners working with African American adolescents and underserved populations.

Dramatic declines in physical activity among Black youth require the development of programs that aim to increase physical activity to subsequently improve other obesity-related health outcomes. Evidence in published literature indicates that policy and multicomponent physical activity approaches that enhance family participation and take place in schools and after school programs are likely to be successful among Black youth and should be promoted.

The results of this review must be considered in light of its limitations. First, we only included studies that had been published in the scientific literature, potentially omitting publications (e.g. dissertations, thesis, or unpublished works) that might have relevance to African American children and adolescents in schools and communities. Second, since current physical activity guidelines focus on children and adolescents between the ages of 6 and 17, our review only focused on studies that included this age group. Therefore, we are unable to comment on the effectiveness of the reviewed interventions for groups outside this age range; such as, preschool children. Future research should build upon the gaps that emerged in this review. There is currently a lack of studies among African American youth that employ environmental and policy approaches in school and after school settings. Future research should aim to increase the evidence in this area. Research should also aim to increase the time of follow-up to determine maintenance of physical activity postintervention.

References

Agurs-Collins, T. D., Kumanyika, S. K., Have Ten, T. R., & Adams-Campbell, L. L. (1997). A randomized controlled trial of weight reduction and exercise for diabetes management in older African American subjects. *Diabetes Care, 20,* 1503–1511.

Barbeau, P., Johnson, M. H., Howe, C. A., Allsion, J., Davis, C. L., Gutin, B., et al. (2007). Ten months of exercise improves general and visceral adiposity, bone, and fitness in black girls. *Obesity, 15,* 2077–2082.

Barr-Anderson, D. J., Young, D. R., Sallis, J. F., Newmark-Sztainer, D. R., Gittelsohn, J., Webber, L., et al. (2007). Structured physical activity and psychosocial correlates in middle school girls. *Preventive Medicine, 44,* 404–409.

Baranowski, T., Baranowski, J. C., Cullen, K. W., Thompson, D. I., Nicklas, T., Zakeri, I., et al. (2003). The fun, food, and fitness project (FFFP): The Baylor GEMS pilot study. *Ethnicity & Disease, 13,* S1-30–S1-39.

Beech, B., Klesges, R. C., Kumanyika, S. K., Murray, D. M., Klesges, L., McClanahan, B., et al. (2003). Child- and parent-targeted interventions: The Memphis GEMS pilot study. *Ethnicity & Disease, 13,* S1-40–S1-53.

CDC. (2008). Youth risk behavior surveillance – United States, 2007. *Morbidity and Mortality Weekly Report, 57,* 1–131.

Clemmens, D., & Haymen, L. L. (2004). Increasing activity to reduce obesity in adolescent girls: A research review. *Journal of Obstetric, Gynecologic, and Neonatal Nursing, 33,* 801–808.

Cruz, M. L., Shaibi, G. Q., Weigensberg, M. J., Spruijt-Metz, D., Ball, G. D., & Goran, M. I. (2005). Pediatric obesity and insulin resistance: Chronic disease risk and implications for treatment and prevention beyond body weight modification. *Annual Review of Nutrition, 25,* 435–468.

Dishman, R. K., Saunders, R. P., Motl, R. W., Dowda, M., & Pate, R. R. (2009). Self efficacy moderates the relation between declines in physical activity and perceived social support in high school girls. *Journal of Pediatric Psychology, 34,* 441–451.

Epstein, L. H., Paluch, R. A., Gordy, C. C., & Dorn, J. (2000). Decreasing sedentary behaviors in treating pediatric obesity. *Archives of Pediatrics & Adolescent Medicine, 154,* 220–226.

Fitzgibbon, M. L., Stolley, M. R., Schiffer, L., Van Horn, L., KauferChristoffel, K., Dyer, A. (2005). Two-year follow-up results for Hip-Hop to Health Jr.: A randomized controlled trial for overweight prevention in preschool minority children. *Journal of Pediatrics, 146,* 618–625.

Foster, G. D., Sherman, S., Borradaile, K. E., Grundy, K. M., Vander Veur, S. S., Nachmani, J., et al. (2008). A policy based school intervention to prevent overweight and obesity. *Pediatrics, 121,* e794–e802.

Gutin, B., Yin, Z., Johnson, M., & Barbeau, P. (2008). Preliminary findings of the effect of a 3-year after-school physical activity intervention on fitness and body fat: The Medical College of Georgia Fitkid Project. *International Journal of Pediatric Obesity, 3,* S1-3–S1-9.

Irwin, M. L. (2006). Randomized controlled trials of physical activity and breast cancer prevention. *Exercise and Sport Sciences Reviews, 34,* 182–193.

Jago, R., & Baranowski, T. (2004). Non-curricular approaches for increasing physical activity in youth: A review. *Preventive Medicine, 39,* 157–163.

Kimm, S. Y., Glynn, N. W., Kriska, A. M., Barton, B. A., Kronsberg, S. S., Daniels, S. R., et al. (2002). Decline in physical activity in black girls and white girls during adolescence. *The New England Journal of Medicine, 347,* 709–715.

Klebanoff, R., & Muramatsu, N. (2002). A community-based physical education and activity intervention for African American preadolescent girls: A strategy to reduce racial disparities in health. *Health Promotion Practice, 3,* 276–285.

Judge, S., & Jahns, L. (2007). Association of overweight with academic performance and social and behavioral problems: An update from the early childhood longitudinal study. *The Journal of School Health, 77,* 672–678.

Kesaniemi, Y. K., Danforth, E., Jr., Jensen, M. D., Kopelman, P. G., Lefebvre, P., & Reeder, B. A. (2001). Dose-response issues concerning physical activity and health: An evidence-based symposium. *Medicine and Science in Sports and Exercise, 33,* S351–S358.

Kettle Kahn, L., Sobush, K., Keener, D., Goodman, K., Lowry, A., Kakietek, J., et al. (2009). Recommended community strategies and measurements to prevent obesity in the United States. *Morbidity and Mortality Weekly Report, 58,* 1–26.

McKay, H. A., & Naylor, P.-J. (2009). Prevention in the first place: Schools a setting for action on physical activity. *British Journal of Sports Medicine, 43,* 10–13.

Neumark-Sztainer, D., Story, M., & Harris, T. (1999). Beliefs and attitudes about obesity among teachers and school health care providers working with adolescents. *Journal of Nutrition Education, 31,* 3–9.

Neumark-Sztainer, D., Story, M., & Faibisch, E. (1998). Perceived stigmatization among overweight African American and Caucasian adolescent girls. *The Journal of Adolescent Health, 23,* 264–270.

Neumark-Sztainer, D., Haines, J., Robinson-O-Brien, R., Hannan, P. J., Robins, M., Morris, B., et al. (2009). 'Ready. Set. Action!' A theatre-based obesity prevention program for children: A feasibility study. *Health Education Research, 24*, 407–420.

Nwobu, C. O., & Johnson, C. C. (2007). Targeting obesity to reduce the risk for type 2 diabetes and other co-morbidities in African American youth: A review of the literature and recommendations for prevention. *Diabetes & Vascular Disease Research, 4*, 311–319.

O'Brien, K. S., Hunter, J. A., & Banks, M. (2007). Implicit anti-fat bias in physical educators: Physical attributes, ideology, and socialization. *International Journal of Obesity, 31*, 308–314.

Pate, R. R., Ward, D. S., Saunders, R. P., Felton, G., Dishman, R. K., & Dowda, M. (2005). Promotion of physical activity among high school girls: A randomized controlled trial. *American Journal of Public Health, 95*, 1582–1587.

Pate, R. R., Ward, D. S., Saunders, R. P., Ward, D. S., Felton, G., Trost, S. G., et al. (2003). Evaluation of a community based intervention to promote physical activity in youth: Lessons from active winners. *American Journal of Health Promotion, 17*, 171–182.

Resnicow, K., Yaroch, A. L., Davis, A., Wang, D. T., Carter, S., Slaughter, L., et al. (2000). GO GIRLS!: Results from a nutrition and physical activity program for low-income, overweight African American adolescent females. *Health Education & Behavior, 27*, 616–629.

Richmond, T. K., Field, A. E., & Rich, M. (2007). Can neighborhoods explain racial/ethnic differences in adolescent inactivity? *International Journal of Pediatric Obesity, 2*, 202–210.

Robinson, T. N., Killen, J. D., Kramer, H. C., Wilson, D. M., Matheson, D. M., Haskell, W. L., et al. (2003). Dance and reducing television viewing to prevent weight gain in African American girls: The Stanford GEMS pilot study. *Ethnicity & Disease, 13*, S1-65–S1-77.

Rohm Young, D., Phillips, J. A., Yu, T., & Haythornthwaite, J. A. (2006). Effects of life skills intervention for increasing physical activity in adolescent girls. *Archives of Pediatrics & Adolescent Medicine, 160*, 155–1261.

Sallis, J. F., McKenzie, T. L., Conway, T. L., Elder, J. P., Prochaska, J. J., Brown, M., et al. (2003). Environmental interventions for eating and physical activity: A randomized controlled trial in middle schools. *American Journal of Preventive Medicine, 24*, 209–217.

Schmid, T. L., Pratt, M., & Witmer, L. (2006). A framework for physical activity policy research. *Journal of Physical Activity and Health, 3*, S20–S29.

Schwartz, M. B., & Puhl, R. (2003). Childhood obesity: A societal problem to solve. *Obesity Review, 4*, 57–71.

Shaw-Perry, M., Horner, C., Trevina, R., Sasa, E. T., Hernandez, I., & Phardwaj, A. (2007). NEEMA: A school-based diabetes risk prevention program designed for African American children. *Journal of the National Medical Association, 99*, 368–375.

Stern, M., Mazzeo, S. E., Porter, J., Gerke, C., Daphne, B., & Joseph, L. (2006). Self-esteem, teasing and quality of life: African American adolescent girls participating in a family-based pediatric overweight intervention. *Journal of Clinical Psychology in Medical Settings, 13*, 217–228.

Stone, E. J., McKenzie, T. L., Welk, G. J., & Booth, M. L. (1998). Effects of physical activity interventions in youth, review and synthesis. *American Journal of Preventive Medicine, 15*, 298–315.

Story, M., Sherwood, N. E., Himes, J. H., Davis, M., Jacobs, D. R., Jr., Cartwright, Y., et al. (2003). An after school obesity prevention program for African American girls: The Minnesota GEMS pilot study. *Ethnicity & Disease, 13*, S1-54–S1-63.

Trust for America's Health. (2009). How obesity policies are failing America. Retrieved October 6, 2010, from http://healthyamericans.org/reports/obesity2009/

US Department of Health and Human Services (HHS), Office of Disease Prevention and Health Promotion (2008). Physical activity guidelines for Americans. Washington: HHS.

Webber, L. S., Osganian, S. K., Feldman, H. A., Wu, M., McKenzie, T. L., Nichaman, M., et al. (1996). Cardiovascular risk factors among children after a 2 1/2-year intervention-The CATCH Study. *Preventive Medicine, 25*, 432–441.

Whitt-Glover, M. C., Taylor, W. C., Floyd, M. F., Yore, M. M., Yancey, A. K., & Matthews, C. E. (2009). Disparities in physical activity and sedentary behaviors among US children and adolescents: Prevalence, correlates, and intervention implications. *Journal of Public Health Policy, 30*, S309–S334.

Whitt-Glover, M. C., & Kumanyika, S. K. (2009). Systematic review of interventions to increase physical activity and physical fitness in African Americans. *American Journal of Health Promotion, 23*, S33–S55.

Wilson, D. K. (2009). New perspectives on health disparities and obesity interventions in youth. *Journal of Pediatric Psychology, 34*, 231–244.

Wilson, D. K., Evans, A. E., Williams, J., Mixon, G., Sirard, J. R., & Pate, R. (2005). A preliminary test of student-centered intervention on increasing physical activity in underserved adolescents. *Annals of Behavioral Medicine, 30*, 119–124.

Wilson, D. K., Friend, R., Teasley, N., Green, S., Reaves, I. L., & Sica, D. A. (2002). Motivational versus social cognitive interventions for promoting fruit and vegetable intake and physical activity in African American adolescents. *Annals of Behavioral Medicine, 24,* 310–319.

Wolin, K. Y., Lee, I. M., Colditz, G. A., Glynn, R. J., Fuchs, C., & Giovannucci, E. (2007). Leisure-time physical activity patterns and risk of colon cancer in women. *International Journal of Cancer, 121,* 2776–2781.

Yin, Z., Gutin, B., Johnson, M. H., Hones, J., Moore, J. B., Cavnar, M., et al. (2005). An environmental approach to obesity prevention in children: Medical College of Georgia FitKid Project year 1 results. *Obesity Research, 13,* 2153–2161.

Part III
Major Lifestyle Intervention Considerations

Chapter 5
Reducing Tobacco-Related Health Disparities: Using Mass Media Campaigns to Prevent Smoking and Increase Cessation in Underserved Populations

Jane A. Allen, Donna M. Vallone, and Amanda K. Richardson

Introduction

Mass media campaigns can be effectively used to reduce youth smoking prevalence and promote adult cessation within the general population, particularly when combined with other tobacco control efforts (CDC, 2007; National Cancer Institute, 2008). As a result, mass media campaigns are one of the CDC's recommended "best practices" for tobacco control (CDC, 2007). However, there is less evidence about the effectiveness of mass media campaigns to prevent or reduce smoking among socioeconomically disadvantaged or racial and ethnic minority populations. In general, evaluations of youth prevention campaigns have not included analyses by socioeconomic status (SES). Analyses by race/ethnicity have been conducted inconsistently – even by evaluators of "model" youth campaigns – and some studies have used such crude measures of race and ethnicity that it is difficult to interpret the findings. A recent review of the studies evaluating adult smoking cessation campaigns finds that they are often less effective among low SES smokers as compared with high SES smokers (Fagan, 2008; Niederdeppe, Fiore, Baker, & Smith, 2008; Niederdeppe, Kuang, Crock, & Skelton, 2008). Even among those campaigns that are specifically designed to reach low SES audiences, there are mixed or inconclusive results (Niederdeppe, Kuang, et al., 2008). Like youth campaigns, adult smoking cessation campaigns are not routinely evaluated by race/ethnicity; those that have been yield mixed results in terms of campaign effectiveness (Bala, Strzeszynski, & Cahill, 2008).

There are many factors that may be related to differential campaign effects among low SES and racial/ethnic minority groups. Tobacco use patterns and prevalence differ by SES and race/ethnicity (CDC, 2008, 2009a; Wallace et al., 2009). Product preferences, including cigarette brand and type, are strongly associated with race/ethnicity, and can impact the rate of progression to established smoking and the likelihood of successful cessation (CDC, 2009b; Clark, Gautam, & Gerson, 1996; Gandhi, Foulds, Steinberg, Lu, & Williams, 2009; Gundersen, Delnevo, & Wackowski, 2009). Cultural and socioeconomic factors can influence cessation processes and outcomes, as well as health-care seeking, and ultimately, rates of morbidity and mortality (Adams, Lucas, & Barnes, 2008; Albano et al., 2007; Cokkinides, Halpern, Barbeau, Ward, & Thun, 2008; Devesa & Diamond, 1983; Fagan, Shavers, Lawrence, Gibson, & Ponder, 2007; Giovino, 2002; Hymowitz, Jackson, Carter, & Eckholdt, 1996; Lawlor, Sterne, Tynelius, Davey Smith, & Rasmussen, 2006; Levinson, Perez-Stable, Espinoza, Flores, & Byers, 2004; Marmot & McDowall, 1986 Aug 2; Pleis &

J.A. Allen (✉)
American Legacy Foundation, Washington, DC, USA
e-mail: jallen@legacyforhealth.org

A.J. Lemelle et al. (eds.), *Handbook of African American Health: Social and Behavioral Interventions*, DOI 10.1007/978-1-4419-9616-9_5, © Springer Science+Business Media, LLC 2011

Lethbridge-Cejku, 2007; U.S. Department of Health and Human Services, 1989; U.S. Public Health Service, 1964; Wong, Shapiro, Boscardin, & Ettner, 2002; Yerger, Wertz, McGruder, Froelicher, & Malone, 2008). For example, studies suggest that racial prejudice can reduce the likelihood that an African American smoker will receive advice to quit smoking from a physician (Cokkinides et al.; Fiore, Bailey, Cohen, & al., 2000; Hymowitz et al.; Levinson et al.). In addition, patterns of media use differ by SES and race/ethnicity, including amount of exposure to media, preferred media channels and programming, and times of day in which media use takes place (Bureau, 2010; Lee & Zhou, 2009; Viswanath & Kreuter, 2007). Whether a public health advertisement resonates with a specific audience, and whether it is likely to motivate them to take action may be influenced by numerous contextual factors. To date, there has been very little research examining under what conditions, to what degree, and how these and other factors may combine to influence campaign outcomes in specific populations.

This chapter highlights this important area of research, by (1) describing the current evidence regarding use of mass media campaigns to influence tobacco use cognitions and behavior among low SES and minority populations; (2) presenting data from two mass media campaigns, one specifically designed to promote smoking cessation among low SES smokers, and the other designed to prevent smoking among youth of diverse racial/ethnic backgrounds; (3) outlining the challenges to developing a body of knowledge about the effects of mass media campaigns by SES and race/ethnicity, and; (4) making recommendations about how mass media campaigns for low SES and racial/ethnic minority populations can be optimized in the future.

Evidence Regarding the Use of Mass Media Campaigns to Influence Tobacco Use Cognitions and Behavior Among Underserved Populations

Evidence from Youth Campaigns

Four mass media campaigns can be considered "model campaigns" for youth because they have been rigorously evaluated and linked with declines in youth smoking. One of these – the national truth campaign – will be discussed at length in section on "Evidence from Legacy Mass Media Campaigns" of this chapter. The others – the state campaigns of Florida, California, and Massachusetts – preceded and provided the evidence base for the national truth campaign (Allen, Vallone, Vargyas, & Healton, 2009).

The Florida Campaign

The Florida "Truth" campaign served as a blueprint for the national campaign of the same name (Allen et al., 2009; Farrelly et al., 2002). Campaign advertisements aired within the context of a comprehensive, statewide antitobacco effort. The advertisements were considered intensive and novel; the primary message strategy was to highlight the deceptive behavior of the tobacco industry in an effort to help teens reject smoking (Bauer, Johnson, Hopkins, & Brooks, 2000; Goldman & Glantz, 1998; Sly, Heald, & Ray, 2001; Sly, Hopkins, Trapido, & Ray, 2001; Sly, Trapido, & Ray, 2002; Zucker et al., 2000).

A series of cross-sectional studies documented that over a 2-year period from 1998 to 2000, current smoking (having smoked within the past 30 days) and frequent smoking (smoked on 20 of the past 30 days), declined significantly among middle and high school students overall (Bauer et al., 2000). When the data were analyzed by race/ethnicity, however, there were no significant declines in current smoking among African American high school students, and no significant declines in frequent smoking among Hispanic high school students or African American students in middle or high school (Bauer et al.). These results were presented in tables but not addressed in the text of the study. While other longitudinal studies show that the campaign lowered the risk of smoking initiation and the likelihood of progressing to "established smoking" among students overall, results were not presented by race/ethnicity (Sly et al., 2002; Sly, Hopkins, Trapido, & Ray, 2001).

The California Campaign

The California Tobacco Control Program is a comprehensive, antitobacco program implemented in 1989 and funded by a voter-enacted cigarette surtax (Traynor & Glantz, 1996). It is the largest state tobacco-control program ever undertaken, combining tax increases and smoke-free policies with community-based programs and an aggressive media campaign (Fichtenberg & Glantz, 2000; Goldman & Glantz, 1998). The campaign was designed primarily to influence adult smoking behavior, but youth were considered a secondary audience (Fichtenberg & Glantz). Among several messaging strategies used in the media campaign is an anti-industry approach, which has been shown to be effective in reducing smoking initiation among youth (Goldman & Glantz).

The campaign has been credited with reductions in per capita cigarette consumption, smoking prevalence, and mortality from heart disease among adults (Fichtenberg & Glantz, 2000; Pierce, Choi, Gilpin, Farkas, & Berry, 1998). Among youth ages 12–17, there were statistically significant increases in the proportion of "committed never smokers" from 1990 to 1999 (Chen, Li, Unger, Liu, & Johnson, 2003). An analysis by race/ethnicity indicated that these results held true, not only among white youth, but also among African American and Hispanic youth (Gilpin et al., 2001). However, there was no increase in the proportion of "committed never smokers" among Asian youth (Gilpin et al.). The same study showed a significant decrease in the proportion of "established smokers" among all youth ages 15–17; however, an analysis by race/ethnicity indicated that the finding persisted only for white youth (Gilpin et al.).

While the most recent data from the California Department of Public Health shows overall declines in youth smoking from 2000 through 2006, data on smoking rates by race/ethnicity or SES is not reported (Health, 2009). In fact, a recent study examining population-level changes in smoking initiation from 1990 to 2005 in California did not include non-white youth in their sample (Messer & Pierce, 2010). We are therefore unable to draw any conclusions about the effectiveness of the California Tobacco Control Program in changing the age trajectories of smoking experimentation among youth other than white youth. The rationale for this exclusion was the documented evidence of differences in smoking initiation and prevalence among racial/ethnic groups (Trinidad et al., 2007; Trinidad, Gilpin, Messer, White, & Pierce, 2006). Such differences present difficulties since any change in smoking behavior over time may be at least partially related to shifts in the racial/ethnic composition of the population. Accounting for these differences can introduce analytic challenges and, for this reason, investigators may choose not to analyze program effects among racial/ethnic subgroups. However, it is critical to develop analytic approaches which account for the varying trajectories of tobacco use to help document program effects across race/ethnicity.

The Massachusetts Campaign

The Massachusetts antismoking media campaign arose out of a 1992 ballot initiative approved by Massachusetts voters that increased the cigarette excise tax and established a comprehensive antismoking tobacco control program (Siegel & Biener, 2000). The media campaign was initiated in

October 1993, and was conducted primarily through advertisements on television, radio, newspaper, and billboards (Siegel & Biener, 1997). Messages focused on countering tobacco use by highlighting tobacco industry practices and the health effects of tobacco use. The tone was considered emotionally arousing and fairly intense (L. Biener, personal communication, 2006; Siegel & Biener, 2000).

A longitudinal survey of adolescents aged 12 and 13 years was conducted in 1993, at the beginning of the campaign, and again 4 years later. A large proportion of youth reported exposure to the campaign at baseline: 71% reported exposure to television advertising, 57% to billboard advertising, and 33% to radio advertising (Siegel & Biener, 2000). While the evaluation found no differences by race in the proportion of youth who reported campaign exposure within each media channel, the race categories were crude, consisting only of white and "other" race (Siegel & Biener). It is possible that a more refined examination of campaign exposure by race and ethnicity may have revealed different results.

Within the overall sample, the 12- and 13-year-old youth who reported exposure to the television campaign in 1993 were 50% less likely to progress to "established smoking" over the next 4 years (Siegel & Biener, 2000). There was no significant difference in the likelihood of progression to "established smoking" by race (Siegel & Biener). In a separate analysis of youth ages 14 through 17, conducted in 1999, there were no significant differences by race/ethnicity in the perceived effectiveness of several antismoking advertisements aired as part of the Massachusetts campaign (Biener, 2002).

Summary of the Evidence from Youth Campaigns

Findings from the Florida, California, and Massachusetts campaigns provide mixed evidence about the effectiveness of youth counter-marketing campaigns across racial/ethnic subgroups. Furthermore, to our knowledge, there are no studies that evaluate these campaigns by SES. While SES has been repeatedly linked with higher rates of smoking, lower rates of successful cessation and greater tobacco-related morbidity and mortality among adults, (Adams et al., 2008; Albano et al., 2007; CDC, 2009a; Cokkinides et al., 2008; Devesa & Diamond, 1983; Fagan et al., 2007; Giovino, 2002; Hymowitz et al., 1996; Lawlor et al., 2006; Levinson et al., 2004; Marmot & McDowall, 1986 Aug 2; Pleis & Lethbridge-Cejku, 2007; U.S. Department of Health and Human Services, 1989; U.S. Public Health Service, 1964; Wong et al., 2002; Yerger et al., 2008) the relationship among youth is less well documented. One recent study showed that lower SES was associated with a greater likelihood of smoking among adolescent girls, but that this relationship was stronger within some racial/ethnic subgroups (i.e., white) as compared with others (i.e., African American or Hispanic) (Wallace et al., 2009).

Although evidence suggests that the Florida campaign was less effective among African American and Hispanic youth as compared with white youth, the majority of the studies evaluating the campaign do not report findings by race/ethnicity. Early evidence suggests that the California campaign was equally effective among African American, Hispanic, and white youth. However, subsequent studies examining the effects of the campaign did not include non-white youth in their analysis, making it unclear as to whether this finding held true over time. Finally, major evaluations of the Massachusetts campaign made use of a limited race variable, which may have obscured differences in smoking and media use behavior among youth of different racial/ethnic backgrounds.

Taken together, this body of information suggests the need for greater adherence to the CDC's *Best Practices for Comprehensive Tobacco Control Programs* recommendation for campaigns to be evaluated by race/ethnicity (CDC, 2007), not only to address health disparities, but also to create standardized measures so results can be interpreted and compared in meaningful ways.

Adult Campaigns

Two excellent reviews of the literature, both published in 2008, provide evidence about the effectiveness of mass media campaigns to promote smoking cessation among low SES and minority smokers (Bala et al., 2008; Niederdeppe, Kuang, et al., 2008). The first of these, conducted by Niederdeppe et al., synthesized findings from published evaluations of mass media campaigns designed to promote smoking cessation among adults, ages 18 years and over (Niederdeppe, Kuang, et al.). Each of the campaign evaluation studies examined effects by SES. Twenty-nine studies described 18 media campaigns, which were designed to influence the smoking behavior of a general audience, and 21 described 13 campaigns designed specifically to influence low SES populations. The review concluded that, among the 18 campaigns designed for a general audience, nine were less effective, six were equally effective, and three were more effective among lower SES individuals as compared with higher SES individuals. Among the 13 campaigns that specifically targeted low SES individuals, eight generated mixed or inconclusive results, and five were less effective among low SES individuals. Three of the campaigns targeted low income African Americans; none had a detectable community-level effect (Niederdeppe, Kuang, et al.).

The second review, conducted by Bala et al., sought to evaluate the effectiveness of media campaigns to increase cessation among adult smokers, ages 25 years and over (Bala et al., 2008). The primary goal of this review was to assess the effectiveness of media campaigns to increase cessation in general, and to shed light on the relative effectiveness of various types of campaigns and campaign components. Bala found 11 campaigns appropriate for inclusion in the review, of which eight "showed some positive effects on smoking behavior." However, race/ethnicity data were only collected in relation to five of the campaigns. Two of the campaigns were targeted to Vietnamese American men, and the evaluations showed a positive effect on smoking behavior (Jenkins et al., 1997; McPhee et al., 1995). Another campaign used race/ethnicity only as a control variable and did not present its effect in the published results. The campaign evaluations that examined effects by race/ethnicity included the state campaigns of California and Massachusetts. In California, from 1989 to 2005, smoking prevalence declined equally across race/ethnicity among men, while among women, declines were greater among Hispanic and white women as compared with African American women. In terms of education, the greatest decline in male smoking prevalence was among college graduates, while the greatest decline in female smoking prevalence was among those who did not complete high school. In Massachusetts, smoking prevalence declined from 1990 through 2000 overall, but further analysis showed that the decline was statistically significant only among men. The decline was more pronounced among white individuals as compared with those of other races or ethnicities (Bala et al.).

Summary of the Evidence from Adult Campaigns

These reviews underscore the need for a greater emphasis on examining the effects of adult mass media campaigns by SES and race/ethnicity. Evidence indicates that the impact of many campaigns was reduced among low SES and minority individuals – even when campaigns were specifically designed to reach and influence these individuals.

Unfortunately, it is these populations, the most vulnerable to the burden of tobacco use and tobacco-related illness, which need to benefit most from these public education efforts.

While discouraging, these findings highlight the gaps in our knowledge about how best to use mass media campaigns to increase smoking cessation among adults. As smoking becomes increasingly concentrated among those with the least resources, understanding how best to reach low SES and minority smokers can serve to improve our efforts to reach *all* smokers. Each study that links a specific campaign type, component, message, or other campaign characteristic with cognitive or behavioral effects (or lack thereof) among low SES and minority smokers can be used to help improve future public health education efforts.

Evidence from Legacy Mass Media Campaigns

The Truth Campaign

The truth campaign (truth) is a branded, national youth smoking prevention campaign launched in 2000. The campaign is designed to reach and influence those youth at greatest risk of smoking. A trait called "sensation seeking" has been used to develop, deliver, and evaluate truth advertisements. Sensation-seeking has been linked repeatedly to a variety of youth risk behaviors, including cigarette smoking (Martin et al., 2002; Slater, 2003; Zuckerman, Ball, & Black, 1990). The campaign is characterized by edgy advertisements with an antitobacco industry theme (Farrelly et al., 2002; Farrelly, Davis, Haviland, Messeri, & Healton, 2005). Campaign advertisements present facts about the addictiveness of smoking, the number of deaths and amount of disease attributed to smoking, the ingredients in cigarettes, and the marketing practices of the tobacco industry. The primary audience for the campaign is at-risk youth, ages 12–17 years, with young adults ages 18–24 composing an important secondary audience. The television component of the campaign is supplemented by radio ads, a robust and growing presence on the Internet, and an annual, grass roots "truth tour." The truth tour employs young adult "crew members" to travel across the USA in an orange "truth" truck following popular summer music venues such as the Vans Warped Tour to engage youth in a dynamic setting.

The truth campaign was based in part on the now defunct Florida truth campaign, which effectively reduced rates of youth tobacco use in Florida (Bauer et al., 2000). Both the Florida truth campaign and Legacy's national truth campaign have intellectual roots in the work of a panel of youth marketing experts convened in 1996 by the Columbia School of Public Health and funded by the CDC (Columbia University School of Public Health, 1996; McKenna, Gutierrez, & McCall, 2000). The Columbia expert panel identified three critical elements for a successful youth tobacco prevention media campaign. First, noting teens' extreme brand-consciousness and the pervasiveness of tobacco brands, it called for the creation of a teen-focused nonsmoking – or "counter" tobacco – brand. Second, it recognized that a teen-focused campaign must talk to teens in their own voice and not patronize them. Third, the panel recommended that the counter brand highlight the actions of the tobacco industry in marketing cigarettes, including its failures to be truthful about the addictiveness and health effects of tobacco (Columbia University School of Public Health; McKenna, Gutierrez, & McCall). These became key elements of Legacy's national truth campaign.

Multicomponent Evaluation

Legacy designed a multicomponent evaluation to assess the effects of the truth campaign, necessary given its national scope and lack of a true control condition. The evaluation consists of qualitative data collection, including ethnographies and focus groups; extensive market research; telephone and online quantitative surveys; a biochemical validation (cotinine) study; and use of established surveillance resources, such as Monitoring the Future (MTF) data. We focus on the media monitoring tools in the following section.

The Legacy Media Tracking Survey

The Legacy Media Tracking Survey (LMTS) is a nationally representative, random-digit-dial (RDD), cross-sectional telephone survey of youth and young adults ages 12–24 years (Thrasher et al., 2004). It was developed to track awareness of, and receptivity to, Legacy's truth campaign, and also measures tobacco-related beliefs, attitudes and behaviors, sensation seeking, openness to smoking among youth who are not current smokers, exposure to secondhand smoke, and exposure to pro- and antitobacco influences in the home, the school, and the mass media.

Eight waves of LMTS data (including a baseline wave) were collected from December 1999 through January 2004. African American, Hispanic, and Asian youth were oversampled in each survey wave to ensure that sample sizes would be large enough to produce accurate estimates for these populations. Response rates ranged from 60% in 2001 to 30% in 2004 (Vallone, Allen, & Xiao, 2009). The decline in response rates for telephone surveys reflects a pattern that has been observed throughout the field in recent years, possibly because of the increase in the numbers of sales and survey calls (Curtin, Presser, & Singer, 2000). In 2005, Legacy shifted to an online media tracking survey called Legacy Media Tracking Online (LMTO) (Wunderink et al., 2007).

Legacy Media Tracking Online

The LMTO is a cross-sectional, nationally representative online survey of US youth, ages 13–18. It was developed to take the place of the LMTS, with the primary goal being to measure youth awareness of, and reactions to, truth advertising. The survey also measures youth tobacco use behavior, beliefs and attitudes, and other pro- and antitobacco media messages. To ensure sufficient sample size for subgroup analyses, oversamples of African American and Hispanic youth are obtained.

The LMTO was launched in 2005, a time when telephone response rates were declining, the cost of telephone surveys was increasing, and the benefits of online data collection were becoming impossible to ignore, including lower cost, far greater flexibility in the timing of a survey, and a much shorter data collection period. LMTO is administered by Harris Interactive, Inc. to youth members of their Harris Poll Online (HPOL) database. Members of the HPOL are recruited through a variety of strategies, and receive incentives to take periodic online surveys. Youth who agree to participate in the LMTO receive a unique web link that allows them to enter the survey, ensuring that each respondent completes the survey only once. The LMTO has been administered approximately twice a year since 2005, yielding nine waves of data. The survey is fielded following the launch of new truth advertising.

Overall Effects of the Truth Campaign

Awareness and Receptivity

A 2002 study based on LMTS data showed that in the first 9 months of the campaign, 75% of all 12- to 17-year olds nationwide could accurately describe at least one truth advertisement (Farrelly et al., 2002). This finding was based on a conservative measure of awareness called confirmed awareness. Confirmed awareness is documented in the following way. The interviewer asks the respondent if they are aware of any truth ads. If the respondent reports awareness, the interviewer then describe the beginning of a truth ad currently or recently on the air. If the youth can accurately describe the end of the ad in question, they are categorized as having confirmed awareness. This conservative measure of awareness reduces the likelihood of false awareness.

The same 2002 study showed that during the first 9 months of the campaign, truth influenced key youth attitudes toward tobacco in the expected direction and was associated with lower intention to smoke (OR = 1.66), though this latter finding was marginally statistically significant at $p = 0.09$ (Farrelly et al., 2002). Interestingly, this study also examined the association between confirmed awareness of Philip Morris' "Think. Don't Smoke" (TDS) campaign and youths' intention to smoke in the coming year. Confirmed awareness of TDS was associated with an *increase* in the odds of intending to smoking in the coming year (OR = 0.64, $p < 0.05$). A dose–response analysis, which included information about the number of TDS advertisements a youth could accurately describe, was robust ($p < 0.02$), suggesting that increased exposure to the Philip Morris campaign placed youth at greater risk of smoking in the future (Farrelly et al.).

Behavioral Change

A 2005 study used MTF and media delivery data (gross ratings points, or GRPs) to demonstrate a dose–response relationship between campaign exposure and smoking prevalence among youth in grades 8 through 12. Results showed that youth with greater exposure to the campaign were less likely to be current smokers. The study concluded that the truth campaign was responsible for an estimated 22% of the nationwide decline in youth smoking from 1999 to 2002 (Farrelly et al., 2005). A more recent longitudinal study, based on data collected during annual interviews with a cohort of youth from 1997 through 2004 indicated that exposure to the truth campaign was associated with a decreased risk of smoking initiation (relative risk = 0.80, $p = 0.001$). Based on these data, the authors estimate that 450,000 youth were prevented from smoking between 2000 and 2004 as a result of the truth campaign (Farrelly, Nonnemaker, Davis, & Hussin, 2009).

Cost Effectiveness

Using methods established by the U.S. Panel on Cost-effectiveness in Health and Medicine, a recent analysis found that the truth campaign was economically efficient. The authors estimated that the campaign recovered its costs, and saved between $1.9 billion and $5.4 billion in medical costs for society (Holtgrave, Wunderink, Vallone, & Healton, 2009). Additional models, which accounted for longer life expectancy and its associated additional medical costs for those who never smoke or who quit smoking, found a saving of $4,302 per Quality Adjusted Life Year (QALY) (Holtgrave et al.).

Effects of the Truth Campaign by SES and Race/Ethnicity

Awareness of and Receptivity to the Campaign

A 2002 study used LMTS data to measure youth awareness of several antismoking media campaigns, including the truth campaign, by gender and race/ethnicity. The study showed that African American youth (ages 12–17) and young adults (ages 18–24) had statistically significantly lower levels of unaided awareness of "any" antismoking campaign as compared with their white peers (Farrelly et al., 2003). However, there were no differences by race/ethnicity in confirmed awareness of the truth campaign. Overall, 75% of youth and 68% of young adults demonstrated confirmed awareness of the truth campaign (Farrelly et al.).

This study also examined confirmed awareness of Philip Morris' Think Don't Smoke (TDS) campaign. Confirmed awareness of TDS was lower in both age groups (66% among 12–17 year olds and 53%

among 18–24 year olds) as compared with truth awareness (Farrelly et al., 2003). Also, there were statistically significant differences in confirmed awareness of TDS by race/ethnicity, in both age groups. A higher proportion of African American youth (73%) had confirmed awareness of TDS as compared with white youth (62%). Among young adults, 65% of African Americans had confirmed awareness of TDS as compared with white (51%) and Hispanic (54%) young adults (Farrelly et al.). The authors of the study speculate that the higher levels of awareness among African Americans may have been due to a single Philip Morris advertisement, "Boy on the Bus," which featured an African American teenager. It is worth noting that awareness in both age groups was statistically significantly higher among males as compared with females.

The degree to which an advertisement is relevant or salient among the target audience (receptivity) is as important as its level of exposure as measured by the size of the audience reached and the number of times the ad airs. This study evaluated receptivity to truth and TDS advertisements using a measure consisting of four survey items which asked youth whether the advertisements were convincing, grabbed their attention, and gave good reasons not to smoke, and whether they talked with friends about the advertisement. Youth of all races and ethnicities were equally receptive to truth campaign advertisements. There were no differences by gender (Farrelly et al., 2003). Overall, among youth ages 12–17, receptivity to truth advertisements was higher than to TDS ads. However, an analysis by racial/ethnic subgroups indicates that, among African American youth, there were no campaign differences in receptivity. Among those youth who were aware of the TDS campaign, African American youth had statistically significantly higher receptivity to the advertisements as compared with white, Hispanic, and Asian American youth (Farrelly et al.), perhaps due to the "Boy on the Bus" advertisement.

The first study to explore awareness of and receptivity to the truth campaign by SES was published in 2009 (Vallone et al., 2009). This study was based on seven waves of LMTS data, collected from September 2000 through January 2004 ($n=30$, 512). Because the LMTS did not include a measure of SES, LMTS data were geocoded with zip code-level median household income and median household education variables to serve as proxy measures of individual SES. The zip code data were purchased separately from a data collection company. Zip code data have been shown to be nonhomogenous as compared to other geographical measures of SES, such as census tract areas; however, because use of zip code data tends to "attenuate estimates of socioeconomic gradients in health"(Krieger et al. 2002) the expectation of the authors was that any bias resulting from use of them would likely be toward null findings for the study. Youth who lived in lower education zip codes were less likely to have confirmed awareness of the truth campaign as compared with those in higher education zip codes (Vallone et al., 2009). Zip code level median household income was not associated with confirmed awareness. Receptivity to the campaign was not associated with either zip code level median household income or education. As previously observed, females had lower levels of confirmed awareness of the truth campaign as compared with males (Vallone et al.). The findings from this study suggest that the effectiveness of the truth campaign could be enhanced by developing strategies to increase campaign awareness among youth from lower education zip codes and females. Increased campaign exposure within these populations could result in lower smoking rates and, ultimately, lower rates of tobacco-related disease.

Belief and Attitude Change, and Intention to Smoke

Another study using LMTS data analyzed racial/ethnic differences in the association between exposure to truth and youth's beliefs and attitudes about cigarette companies, as well as their intention to smoke (Cowell, Farrelly, Chou, & Vallone, 2009). Beliefs and attitudes were analyzed separately. Beliefs comprised the following items: "Cigarette companies lie"; "Cigarette companies deny that cigarettes cause cancer and other harmful disease"; and "Cigarette companies deny that cigarettes are addictive." Attitudes comprised the following items: "I would like to see cigarette companies go out of business"; "I would not work for a cigarette company"; and "On a scale from 1 to 5, how do you feel about cigarette companies." Results showed that exposure to truth was positively associated with increased antitobacco beliefs and attitudes among youth overall (Cowell et al.). Analysis by race/ethnicity, however, showed a statistically significant association between exposure to truth and the composite score on the belief and attitude indices only for whites and African American youth, not for Hispanics or Asians (Cowell et al.).

When the individual belief and attitude items that composed the measurement indices are analyzed separately, different patterns of associations emerged. For example, exposure to truth among whites was associated with statistically significant increases in each individual belief item. However, among African Americans, exposure to truth was associated only with the beliefs "Cigarette companies lie" and "Cigarette companies deny that cigarettes are addictive" (Cowell et al., 2009).

Regarding intention to smoke, exposure to the truth campaign was statistically significantly associated with intention not to smoke in the future among youth who had never smoked (OR = 2.02, p = 0.001). However, when analyzed by race/ethnicity, the results were more robust among African American youth (OR = 5.39, p = 0.001) as compared with white (OR = 1.76, p = 0.062) or Hispanic youth (OR = 2.00, p = 0.064) (Cowell et al., 2009). Among youth noncurrent "ever" smokers, the association was strong and statistically significant among youth overall, as well as within every racial/ethnic group (Cowell et al.).

Assessing Audience Segmentation Measures Across Racial/Ethnic Subgroups

Sensation-seeking has been repeatedly linked with risk-taking behavior including tobacco use among teens (Martin et al., 2002; Slater, 2003; Zuckerman et al., 1990). For this reason, the measure has been used by a number of media campaigns, including the National Youth Anti-drug Media Campaign of the Office of National Drug Control Policy (ONDCP) to assess campaign effects by audience segments (Palmgreen, Donohew, Lorch, Hoyle, & Stephenson, 2001; Palmgreen, Lorch, Stephenson, Hoyle, & Donohew, 2007; Zimmerman et al., 2007). The Brief Sensation Seeking Scale-4, or BSSS-4, is a four-item scale that measures four factors of sensation-seeking, including thrill and adventure seeking, experience seeking, disinhibition, and susceptibility to boredom (Stephenson, Hoyle, Palmgreen, & Slater, 2003). The BSSS-4 was useful in segmenting the target audience to tailor advertising for those most at risk of smoking initiation. However, the BSSS-4 was based on the eight-item Brief Sensation Seeking Scale (BSSS), in which mean sensation seeking scores were found to be significantly lower for African American youth as compared with white youth (Hoyle, Stephenson, Palmgreen, Lorch, & Donohew, 2002).

Using LMTS data, a study was conducted in 2007 to assess whether the BSSS-4 showed similar discrepancies in scores across racial/ethnic subpopulations (Vallone, Allen, Clayton, & Xiao, 2007). The study pooled six waves of LMTS data for an overall sample size of 25,560. Overall, and among youth who had experimented with cigarettes or were open to smoking, African Americans were found to have statistically significantly lower mean sensation-seeking scores than white and Hispanic youth (p < 0.001) (Vallone et al.). The internal consistency of the sensation-seeking scale, as measured by coefficient alpha, was 0.65 for the sample overall, with an average corrected item-total correlation of 0.43. Coefficient alpha was found to be statistically significantly lower among African American youth (α = 0.55) than among white (α = 0.66, p < 0.001), Hispanic (α = 0.63, p < 0.001), and Asian youth (α = 0.66, p < 0.001) (Vallone et al.). An examination by race/ethnicity and gender showed lower mean sensation-seeking scores among females as compared with males in every racial/ethnic subgroup with the exception of African Americans. The scale appeared to be least internally consistent among African American females as compared with other youth, including African American males. When scores were examined by both race/ethnicity and age, mean sensation-seeking scores were found to be highest at age 15 among African American youth as compared with age 17 among other youth. Analysis of the individual items of the BSSS-4 suggests that there is no single item or subset of items that perform especially poorly among African American youth; instead, the scale as a whole seems to resonate less well among African American youth as compared with other youth (Vallone et al.).

It is possible that the BSSS-4 may not accurately measure the latent construct of sensation-seeking among African American youth. While at least one published study suggests that a variant of the BSSS-4 does not perform equally well for African American youth (Hoyle et al., 2002), other studies have not reported on the internal consistency of the scale among racial/ethnic groups (Stephenson et al., 2003). The authors urge researchers who are measuring sensation-seeking to explore whether the scale they use is less internally consistent among African American youth and, if so, to explore what factors might contribute to this. If flawed measures of sensation-seeking are used to develop and deliver public health campaigns, the impact of these efforts could be significantly reduced, particularly among African American youth.

Summary

Studies have shown that the truth campaign was responsible for an estimated 22% of the nationwide decline in youth smoking from 1999 to 2002 (Farrelly et al., 2002), and was associated with a decreased risk of smoking initiation from 1997 to 2004 (relative risk = 0.80, $p = 0.001$) (Farrelly et al., 2009). There were no differences in campaign awareness or receptivity to the campaign by race/ethnicity. Exposure to the truth campaign was statistically significantly associated with intention not to smoke in the future among youth who had never smoked, however, the results were more robust among African American youth as compared with white or Hispanic youth. Among youth noncurrent "ever" smokers, the association was strong and statistically significant among youth overall, and within every racial/ethnic group. Research is still needed to further understand these outcomes among youth of color. Given the heavy burden of tobacco use and related illness in minority and disadvantaged populations, it is essential to understand how media messages and media dose influence awareness and shift cognitive and behavioral variables in those most vulnerable.

Future Analyses

The ability of different types and levels of media delivery to prompt changes in tobacco use behavior among racial/ethnic subgroups requires further analyses. A study conducted in 2005 using MTF data demonstrated a dose–response relationship between campaign exposure and smoking prevalence among youth in grades 8 through 12 such that youth with greater exposure to the campaign were less likely to be current smokers (Farrelly et al., 2005). Analyses are currently underway to examine whether this same relationship holds across racial/ethnic boundaries. Findings may inform our understanding of whether media dose can be considered equivalent across racial/ethnic subgroups. It may be that racial/ethnic subgroups have different dosage thresholds to achieve awareness or a cognitive or behavioral response. Similarly, there might be different points at which there is a plateau effect of dose, such that increasing dose no longer has marked effects on response. Understanding whether media dose corresponds to behavioral change across racial/ethnic subgroups is critical if we hope to tailor interventions specifically to at-risk and minority populations.

The EX Campaign

Introduction

The EX Campaign is a branded mass media campaign designed to promote cessation among lower income and blue collar smokers of diverse race/ethnicity, ages 25–49, who are interested in quitting (McCausland et al., 2009). Similar to the truth campaign, EX is based on behavior change theory, evidence about effective mass media campaigns, and extensive formative research with the target audience. Forty focus groups ($n = 300$), over 45 individual in-depth interviews, and an online survey with over 1,000 respondents were conducted to understand the smoker's perspective, develop the message strategy, and test initial reactions to the concepts (McCausland et al.). This research, conducted from 2003 through the launch of the EX pilot campaign in 2006, provided input for each stage of development, from the formulation of the EX brand through the decision making about which advertisements to produce and air.

Based on the formative research, messages were developed to reflect an empathic tone, which encourages smokers to "re-learn" life without cigarettes (McCausland et al., 2009). Personal smoking triggers – such as drinking coffee or driving a car – are showcased in messages to highlight the importance of disassociating smoking from these daily activities. For example, one advertisement tells smokers, "When you're used to always doing something with a cigarette, it can be hard doing it without one. But if you can learn how to drink coffee without cigarettes, then you can learn to do anything without cigarettes." The "re-learn" message concept resonated well with a diverse group of smokers and some remarked that the concept of "re-learning" left them feeling hopeful and optimistic about the quitting process. Smokers indicated that learning to overcome a single smoking cue was a first step, which made them feel that the process of quitting would be manageable.

EX messages are delivered via television, radio, the Internet, and other channels. Television advertising was specifically placed during programming popular with smokers such as particular day-parts (morning drive time and late night) to help ensure exposure among shift workers, who comprise a large segment of our target audience. Advertising also aired on ESPN, ESPN2, NASCAR, and NFL programming to match the high interest of smokers in sporting events. Radio advertisements were aired also on African American and Hispanic radio programs, as well as on country and classic rock stations (McCausland et al., 2009).

Evaluation Tools and Effects of the EX Campaign Overall

A comprehensive evaluation plan was established to assess both short- and longer term effects of the EX campaign. The brand, key message concepts, and advertising executions were pretested with the target audience prior to campaign launch. Data collection included both cross-sectional and longitudinal telephone surveys, some designed to measure campaign awareness and receptivity among African Americans and Hispanics, and others designed to demonstrate campaign effects, such as changes in cognition and tobacco use behavior.

The Pilot Phase of the EX Campaign: Awareness and Receptivity Study

Three cross-sectional telephone surveys were conducted in 2006 to measure awareness and receptivity to the pilot phase of the EX campaign, with a particular focus on whether the campaign would resonate equally well across race/ethnicity (McCausland et al., 2009). All adults aged 18 and over who had smoked at least 100 cigarettes in their lifetime and were current smokers were eligible to participate in the surveys. Market-lists of potential smokers were used to draw a sample of approximately 300 adult African American smokers from Baltimore, Maryland, and 300 adult Hispanic/Latino smokers from San Antonio, Texas. In a third location, Grand Rapids, Michigan, the awareness and receptivity survey was embedded within a larger evaluation effort, and differed from the other surveys in its sampling framework (Vallone et al., 2010). Over 400 smokers completed interviews in Grand Rapids. All adults aged 18 and over who had smoked at least 100 cigarettes in their lifetime and were current smokers were eligible to participate in the surveys. Interviews were conducted using computer-assisted telephone interviews. In San Antonio, bilingual interviewers were used for respondents whose primary language was Spanish (Vallone et al., 2010).

Awareness of EX varied by the average weekly level of advertising, as measured by the average number of GRP's per week in the three markets. The majority of respondents in all three markets reported that EX was a trusted, empathetic brand (McCausland et al., 2009). There were similar levels of receptivity among all demographic subgroups examined across the three samples; EX brand receptivity did not differ by education, employment status, age, or level of media exposure. Females were slightly more receptive than males. In addition, smokers who were thinking of quitting were more receptive to the EX brand than smokers not thinking about quitting. Similarly, receptivity was increased among respondents with a higher motivation to quit as compared with those who were not motivated to quit (McCausland et al., 2009).

The Pilot Phase of the EX Campaign: Cognitive and Behavioral Outcomes

This study was based on longitudinal data collected among adult smokers in Grand Rapids in 2006 and 2007 (Vallone et al., 2010). At baseline, telephone numbers were randomly selected from a list-assisted, stratified, RDD sampling frame. Of the 448 baseline smokers who agreed to participate in the follow-up survey approximately 6 months after the campaign launch, 212 completed it, resulting in a response rate of 62.1%. Outcome variables include cognitions about quitting smoking, confidence in quitting smoking, and quit attempts. The primary independent variable in this study is exposure to the EX campaign, as measured by confirmed awareness of individual EX advertisements. Variables assessed at baseline were used to control for potential factors that may be associated with the outcomes, including age, gender, education, employment status, recent quit attempts, nicotine dependence, motivation to quit, awareness of other cessation media messages, and media use (Vallone et al., 2010). Race/ethnicity could not be included as a covariate due to lack of heterogeneity in the Grand Rapids sample.

Findings demonstrated that the EX campaign generated a high level of awareness of EX, with 62% of the sample demonstrating confirmed awareness and 79% reporting aided awareness. Six months after the campaign launched, awareness of EX was associated with significant change in two of five campaign-related cognitions in this largely white sample. However, awareness was not associated with confidence in quitting or having made a quit attempt (Vallone et al., 2010).

The National Campaign: Cognitive and Behavioral Outcomes

The evaluation study of the national campaign was based on longitudinal data collected from a sample of 18–49-year-old current smokers, from eight U.S. Designated Market Areas (DMAs or "media markets") (Vallone, Duke, Cullen, McCausland, & Allen, 2011). A DMA is the standard geographic unit of measurement for mass media. The DMAs were selected to ensure cross-market variation with respect to key factors thought to potentially influence cessation outcomes: geographic location, racial/ethnic composition, strength of tobacco control policy efforts (clean indoor air legislation, state tobacco control expenditures, cigarette price), and smoking prevalence.

The baseline survey was conducted from February 5 through April 15, 2008, prior to the national launch of the EX media campaign (Vallone et al., 2011a). A list-assisted, RDD method was used to select a single stage, unclustered sample of telephone numbers across the eight DMAs. For each household contacted, up to two smokers were randomly selected and administered the survey in either English or Spanish. In this way, 8,489 eligible respondents were identified. A total of 5,616 of those eligible (66%) completed the baseline interview. All baseline survey respondents were invited to participate in a follow-up survey conducted approximately 6 months after the campaign launch; August 23 through October 19, 2008. Among baseline respondents, 4,067 successfully completed the follow-up survey, of whom 74% were non-Hispanic white, 12% non-Hispanic black, and 7% Hispanic (Vallone et al., 2011a).

Six months after the launch of the national campaign, findings indicate that respondents who demonstrated confirmed awareness of EX were significantly more likely to increase their level of agreement on a cessation-related cognitions index from baseline to follow-up (OR = 1.6, p = 0.046) (Vallone et al., 2011a). Individuals with confirmed campaign awareness had a 24% greater chance of making a quit attempt between baseline and follow-up interviews, as compared with those who were not aware (OR = 1.24, p = 0.048) (Vallone et al.).

Effects of the EX Campaign by SES and Race/Ethnicity

Awareness and Receptivity

Using three random samples of smokers drawn from each of the pilot market areas, survey results indicate that the EX brand was well received among smokers with varying levels of educational attainment, and across race/ethnicity (McCausland et al., 2009). While it is not possible to statistically compare receptivity by race/ethnicity given the sampling strategy, levels of receptivity were similar across the three racial/ethnic groups. The majority of respondents in all three markets reported that EX was a trusted, empathetic brand. For example, there was high agreement that EX provided helpful information that could be used in a future quit attempt within the African American (80%), Hispanic/Latino (65%), and white (68%) samples. The majority of smokers among the African American, Hispanic/Latino, and white samples reported that the EX brand made them feel as if there was help out there for smokers like themselves (83, 67, and 74%, respectively) (McCausland et al.).

Cognitive and Behavioral Outcomes

Following the study of the overall impact of the national EX campaign among smokers, a second analysis examined the impact of EX stratified by SES and race/ethnicity (Vallone et al., 2011b). This study provides evidence that, among smokers with less than a high school education, the national EX campaign increased favorable cessation-related cognitions and quit attempts during the first 6 months of the campaign (OR = 2.6, p = 0.037) (Vallone et al.,). The campaign also markedly increased favorable cognitions about smoking cessation among Hispanics (OR = 4.3, p = 0.028), and quit attempts among African Americans (OR = 3.3, p = 0.0005) (Vallone et al.,). These results suggest that EX – which was specifically designed to influence lower SES/blue collar smokers and smokers from diverse racial/ethnic backgrounds – can effectively serve populations, which experience a disproportionate burden of the tobacco epidemic.

Summary

Studies conducted to date indicate that the EX campaign holds promise in terms of promoting smoking cessation among adults overall (Vallone et al., 2010; Vallone et al. 2011a). Perhaps more important, results indicate that EX resonates with smokers across race/ethnicity (McCausland et al., 2009); is associated with changes in key cessation-related cognitions among low SES smokers and Hispanics; and is associated with increased quit attempts among African Americans (Vallone et al. 2011b). The positive campaign impact likely results from the extensive formative research with the target audience conducted during campaign development, as well as its strategic implementation, which was carefully designed to leverage the media preferences of the target audience. These findings represent an important contribution to the literature, particularly since a review of similar efforts shows that mass media campaigns to promote smoking cessation are often less effective among individuals of lower SES (Niederdeppe, Kuang, et al., 2008), and a second review shows that the majority of evaluators never investigate effectiveness among vulnerable populations at all (Bala et al., 2008).

Future Analyses

The current studies evaluating the EX campaign were based upon data collected approximately 6 months after campaign launch. To understand the long-term impact of this campaign, data collected 18 months after campaign launch will be analyzed. Areas of interest will include the overall impact of the campaign, and the impact of EX across SES and racial/ethnic subgroups. An additional area of study will be to identify the influence of components or characteristics of the EX campaign as well as whether and to what extent policy, social, and environmental factors contribute to the campaign effect within specific populations, which will inform the development and implementation of future campaigns.

Challenges to Developing a Body of Knowledge About the Effects of Mass Media Campaigns by SES or Race/Ethnicity

The lack of evidence related to the effects of mass media campaigns with respect to SES or race/ethnicity is often due to funding constraints, which make it difficult to conduct appropriate formative research and often results in insufficient sample sizes for racial/ethnic subgroups. This issue is compounded by inconsistent evaluation measures and analytic approaches, which hinder comparison across those studies that are conducted. Each of these issues is discussed in greater detail below.

Costs Associated with Conducting Formative Research

Developing and implementing a campaign requires extensive planning, dedicated staff time, and establishment of relationships with vendors, contractors, media, and creative agencies, all of which can be costly. Consider the case of an agency that has obtained funding to air a local or statewide mass media campaign at a fairly low level of GRPs for an undetermined length of time. Such an agency may not feel they have the resources – financial or otherwise – to conduct formative research with several segments of the target audience. Formative research would entail, at the very least, conducting focus groups of individuals recruited from these populations to generate concepts for the campaign, the brand, and the messaging. After a subsequent period of creative development, the campaign concept and messages should be pretested with the audience. A third round of testing would ideally be conducted to assess the advertising executions prior to their airing publicly.

Organizations that feel they do not have the resources to conduct formative research will often make decisions about the messaging based on existing research or on their own intuition. Unfortunately, what has worked well in one set of circumstances may not necessarily translate to another setting, and messages that are developed without input from the target audience may not be well received, or may have unintended effects. The best advertising campaigns are designed and executed with substantive input from the specific target audience.

Costs Associated with Evaluation

To determine whether a campaign has impacted the awareness, cognitions, or behavior of a group of individuals, one must have a sufficient sample size with which to conduct the analysis. This is referred to as "power." Since the expected overall effects of mass media campaigns are relatively small, larger sample sizes are generally needed in order to have an adequately powered sample. If a sample is "underpowered," it is possible to statistically calculate a null effect even if the campaign is producing "true" effects in a population (the problem of a false negative). Unfortunately, because many evaluation initiatives are limited by funding constraints, they often do not achieve an adequate sample size to determine whether there was a campaign effect within racial/ ethnic or other subgroups.

Telephone surveys have become increasingly expensive over the past decade as a result of lower respondent participation (Curtin et al., 2000). Furthermore, while RDD surveys – those in which the sample of phone numbers is randomly generated – are the gold standard, random samples often yield insufficient numbers of minority respondents to evaluate a campaign within those populations. A technique called "oversampling" can be used to supplement the RDD sample with listed numbers; for example, lists of phone numbers from geographic areas which are predominantly low SES or African American or lists of those in the phone directory with Hispanic surnames. However, oversampling does incur additional costs which may act as a barrier for obtaining sufficient samples for underrepresented populations. Online surveys are becoming more common, in large part because they are highly cost-efficient. Some online surveys utilize an RDD sampling frame followed by online data collection, which reduces costs and results in nationally representative data. One technique used to reduce SES bias in online samples is to provide a computer and internet access free of cost to respondents who agree to participate in an online panel.

Lack of Methodological Continuity

Among those who have evaluated campaign effects by SES or race/ethnicity, there is often a lack of continuity across measures and analytic approaches. SES is often categorized using a variety of variables including (1) income, education, employment; (2) mother's, father's, or parents' education; and (3) geographic measures of neighborhood SES. Unfortunately, there are limitations to each of these measures. Income data tend to have high rates of missingness in surveys, and thus, are often replaced with other variables with better response rates. In addition, the level of aggregation for geographic variables, such as census block-group or zip code, varies substantially in their ability to validly serve as a proxy for individual-level SES (Krieger et al., 2002). Challenges also occur when establishing categories of "low" versus "high" SES. Definitions often vary and are typically tailored to a specific hypothesis; however, this often prevents comparability across studies. Measurement of behavioral outcomes also varies substantially. Although there are accepted definitions of current and heavy smoking established by the Centers for Disease Control, there is less standardization in relation to measurement of cessation behavior. For example, successful cessation is often defined in relation to a particular study's project period rather than an established measure related to sustained abstinence from smoking. While measures of race/ethnicity are fairly standard, some studies combine racial and ethnic minority groups into larger categories, or even a single category representing all individuals who are non-white. This practice obscures starkly different patterns of smoking and cessation across race/ethnicity, and contributes little to our body of knowledge on campaign impact among minority populations. Analytic approaches are likewise tailored to individual campaigns and their hypothesized effects occurring within a specific time frame and target audience. While the variety of study designs is beneficial in that it provides a nuanced and multifaceted view of the effects of mass media campaigns, it also makes it difficult to compare and contrast findings to establish guidelines for future campaign development.

The Future: Optimizing the Use of Mass Media Campaigns to Prevent or Reduce Smoking Among Low SES and Minority Populations

In an effort to improve the effectiveness of mass media campaigns to prevent or reduce smoking among low SES and minority smokers, campaign developers need to be mindful of several key elements. First, and foremost, *conducting formative research with the target audience* helps ensure that the brand, message strategy, and the advertising executions will have a greater likelihood of success. Ideally, formative research should occur sequentially to: (1) understand the needs of the target audience; (2) identify message concepts and media channels; and (3) test advertising executions prior to campaign launch. Although public health agencies may not have the resources for extensive formative research, some level of formative research should be considered essential. Studies show that some well-intentioned campaigns have been ineffective or even counterproductive as a result of their lack of formative research. While formative research cannot ensure that a campaign will be effective, it does increase the likelihood of a relevant and effective campaign.

It is also essential that *every campaign evaluation includes findings by SES and race/ethnicity* to help advance our knowledge of this type of intervention among underserved communities. Reviewers of peer-reviewed manuscripts should insist that investigators address the issue of SES and race/ethnicity within the text of a study, even if it is only to explain why it was not possible to conduct subgroup analyses, why the subgroup analyses are not robust, or that the subgroup analyses will be presented in a separate study. Readers should not be left to wonder why investigators have presented SES or race/ethnicity data only in tables or as control variables. The characteristics of the study population should be described in such a way that readers can understand why an author chose to combine all racial and ethnic subgroups. This will enable us to generate the body of knowledge needed to most effectively reach and influence these populations. We urge the editors of respected, scientific peer-review journals to include an assessment of effects by SES and race/ethnicity in the standard guidance for reviewers of scientific manuscripts. Those designing, implementing, and evaluating media campaigns will expect this scrutiny of their work upon peer-review, and will make every effort to include SES and race/ethnicity. When campaign effects by SES or race/ethnicity are not included, this should be acknowledged as a limitation in the text of peer-reviewed studies. For better or for worse, substantive program effects are going unmeasured, unconsidered, and unreported.

Finally, we will improve the effectiveness of media campaigns among low SES and minority communities if we *develop and use standardized measures*. In developing surveys, we urge investigators to use established measures from national, federally funded surveys such as the National Health Interview Survey (NHIS), the Youth Risk Behavior Survey (YRBS) and the National Youth Tobacco Survey (NYTS), and the MTF Survey. The measures in these surveys have been validated, and using them helps to ensure comparability over time and across studies. Investigators should use study designs that replicate, as much as possible, those of studies that have been published in a respected peer-reviewed journals, with a preference for those that have been classified in reviews of the literature as "rigorous designs." Replication of design and methodology and use of standardized measures are necessary to ensure adequate comparability across studies.

Conclusion

Mass media campaigns are a powerful tool that can be used to reduce tobacco-related health disparities. However, many evaluations of mass media campaigns have not included an analysis of effects by SES or race/ethnicity. Among those that have published findings, results have been mixed, demonstrating that campaigns are often ineffectual or counterproductive among low SES or racial/ethnic minority populations. Given that underserved populations bear a disproportionate burden of tobacco-related disease and death, federal, state and private funding agencies should require campaign evaluations to include an SES and racial/ethnic component. We urge the public health community to help integrate the analysis of findings by SES and racial/ethnic minority populations in studies evaluating public education campaigns. In this way, each study will represent a substantive contribution to what is known about reducing the impact of tobacco use and other health threats among our most vulnerable populations.

References

Adams, P. F., Lucas, J. W., & Barnes, P. M. (2008). Summary health statistics for the U.S. population: National Health Interview Survey, 2006. *Vital Health Statistics, 10*(236), 1–104.

Albano, J. D., Ward, E., Jemal, A., Anderson, R., Cokkinides, V. E., Murray, T., et al. (2007). Cancer mortality in the United States by education level and race. *Journal of the National Cancer Institute, 99*(18), 1384–1394.

Allen, J. A., Vallone, D., Vargyas, E., & Healton, C. G. (2009). The truth campaign: Using counter marketing to reduce youth smoking. In B. Healy & R. Zimmerman (Eds.), *The new world of health promotion, New program development, implementation and evaluation* (pp. 195–215). Sudbury, MA: Jones and Bartlett.

Bala, M., Strzeszynski, L., & Cahill, K. (2008). Mass media interventions for smoking cessation in adults. *Cochrane Database of Systematic Reviews, 23*(1), CD004704.

Bauer, U. E., Johnson, T. M., Hopkins, R. S., & Brooks, R. G. (2000). Changes in youth cigarette use and intentions following implementation of a tobacco control program: Findings from the Florida Youth Tobacco Survey, 1998–2000. *Journal of the American Medical Association, 284*(6), 723–728.

Biener, L. (2002). Anti-tobacco advertisements by Massachusetts and Philip Morris: What teenagers think. *Tobacco Control, 11*(Suppl 2), ii43–ii46.

Bureau, U. S. C. (2010). Multimedia Audiences-Summary: 2008; The 2010 Statistical Abstract.

CDC. (2007). *Best Practices for Comprehensive Tobacco Control Programs – 2007*. Atlanta, GA: U.S. Department of Health and Human Services, Centers for Disease Control and Prevention, National Center for Chronic Disease Prevention and Health Promotion, Office on Smoking and Health.

CDC. (2009a). Cigarette Smoking Among Adults and Trends in Smoking Cessation – United States, 2008. *Morbidity and Mortality Weekly Report, 1358*(44), 1227–1232.

Chen, X., Li, G., Unger, J. B., Liu, X., & Johnson, C. A. (2003). Secular trends in adolescent never smoking from 1990 to 1999 in California: An age-period-cohort analysis. *American Journal of Public Health, 93*(12), 2099–2104.

Clark, P. I., Gautam, S., & Gerson, L. W. (1996). Effect of menthol cigarettes on biochemical markers of smoke exposure among black and white smokers. *Chest, 110*(5), 1194–1198.

CDC. (2009b). Cigarette brand preference among middle and high school students who are established smokers – United States, 2004 and 2006. *Morbidity and Mortality Weekly Report, 58*(5), 112–115.

CDC. (2008). Cigarette use among high school students – United States, 1991–2007. *Morbidity and Mortality Weekly Report, 57*(25), 686–688.

Cokkinides, V., Halpern, M. T., Barbeau, E., Ward, A., & Thun, M. (2008). Racial and ethnic disparities in smoking-cessation interventions: Analysis of the 2005 National Health Interview Survey. *American Journal of Preventive Medicine, 34*(5), 404–412.

Columbia University School of Public, H. (1996). *Experts panel meeting on the effect of tobacco marketing and counter-marketing on youth tobacco behavior 1996–1997*, New York.

Cowell, A. J., Farrelly, M. C., Chou, R., & Vallone, D. M. (2009). Assessing the impact of the national "truth" antismoking campaign on beliefs, attitudes, and intent to smoke by race/ethnicity. *Ethnicity & Health, 14*(1), 75–91.

Curtin, R., Presser, S., & Singer, E. (2000). The effects of response rate changes on the index of consumer sentiment. *Public Opinion Quarterly, 64*(4), 413–428.

Devesa, S. S., & Diamond, E. L. (1983). Socioeconomic and racial differences in lung cancer incidence. *American Journal of Epidemiology, 118*(6), 818–831.

Fagan, P. (2008). Examining the evidence base of mass media campaigns for socially disadvantaged populations: What do we know, what do we need to learn, and what should we do now? A commentary on Niederdeppe's article. *Social Science & Medicine, 67*(9), 1356–1358.

Fagan, P., Shavers, V., Lawrence, D., Gibson, J. T., & Ponder, P. (2007). Cigarette smoking and quitting behaviors among unemployed adults in the United States. *Nicotine & Tobacco Research, 9*(2), 241–248.

Farrelly, M., Nonnemaker, J., Davis, K., & Hussin, A. (2009). The Influence of the National truth Campaign on Smoking Initiation. *American Journal of Preventive Medicine, 36*(5), 379–384.

Farrelly, M. C., Davis, K. C., Haviland, M. L., Messeri, P., & Healton, C. G. (2005). Evidence of a dose-response relationship between "truth" antismoking ads and youth smoking prevalence. *American Journal of Public Health, 95*(3), 425–431.

Farrelly, M. C., Davis, K. C., Yarsevich, J., Haviland, M. L., Hersey, J. C., Girlando, M., et al. (2003). *Getting to the Truth: Assessing Youths' Reactions to the truthsm and "Think. Don't Smoke" Tobacco Countermarketing Campaigns*. Washington DC: American Legacy Foundation.

Farrelly, M. C., Healton, C. G., Davis, K. C., Messeri, P., Hersey, J. C., & Haviland, M. L. (2002). Getting to the truth: Evaluating national tobacco countermarketing campaigns. *American Journal of Public Health, 92*(6), 901–907.

Fichtenberg, C. M., & Glantz, S. A. (2000). Association of the California Tobacco Control Program with declines in cigarette consumption and mortality from heart disease. *The New England Journal of Medicine, 343*(24), 1772–1777.

Fiore, M. C., Bailey, W. C., Cohen, S. J., Dorfman, S. F., Fox, B. J., & Goldstein, M. G. (2000). *Treating tobacco Use and dependence. Clinical practice guideline*. Rockville, MD: U.S. Department of Health and Human Services.

Gandhi, K. K., Foulds, J., Steinberg, M. B., Lu, S. E., & Williams, J. M. (2009). Lower quit rates among African American and Latino menthol cigarette smokers at a tobacco treatment clinic. *International Journal of Clinical Practice, 63*(3), 360–367.

Gilpin, E. A., Emery, S. L., Farkas, A. J., Distefan, J. M., White, M. M., & Pierce, J. P. (2001). *The California tobacco control program: A decade of progress, results from the California tobacco surveys, 1990–1998*. San Diego: California Department of Health Services, Tobacco Control Section.

Giovino, G. A. (2002). Epidemiology of tobacco use in the United States. *Oncogene, 21*(48), 7326–7340.

Goldman, L. K., & Glantz, S. A. (1998). Evaluation of antismoking advertising campaigns. *Journal of the American Medical Association, 279*(10), 772–777.

Gundersen, D. A., Delnevo, C. D., & Wackowski, O. (2009). Exploring the relationship between race/ethnicity, menthol smoking, and cessation, in a nationally representative sample of adults. *Preventive Medicine, 49*(6), 553–557.

Health, C. D. o. P. (2009). *California Tobacco Control Update 2009: 20 Years of Tobacco Control in California*. Sacramento, CA: California Department of Public Health.

Holtgrave, D. R., Wunderink, K. A., Vallone, D. M., & Healton, C. G. (2009). Cost-utility analysis of the national truth campaign to prevent youth smoking. *American Journal of Preventive Medicine, 36*(5), 385–388.

Hoyle, R., Stephenson, M., Palmgreen, P., Lorch, E., & Donohew, R. (2002). Reliability and validity of a brief measure of sensation seeking. *Personality and Individual Differences, 32*, 401–414.

Hymowitz, N., Jackson, J., Carter, R., & Eckholdt, H. (1996). Past quit smoking assistance and doctors' advice for white and African American smokers. *Journal of the National Medical Association, 88*(4), 249–252.

Jenkins, C. N., McPhee, S. J., Le, A., Pham, G. Q., Ha, N. T., & Stewart, S. (1997). The effectiveness of a media-led intervention to reduce smoking among Vietnamese-American men. *American Journal of Public Health, 87*(6), 1031–1034.

Krieger, N., Waterman, P., Chen, J. T., Soobader, M., Subramanian, S. V., & Carson, R. (2002). Zip code caveat: Bias Due to spatiotemporal mismatches between Zip codes and US census-defined geographical areas-the public health disparities geocoding project. *American Journal of Public Health, 92*(7), 1100–1102.

Lawlor, D. A., Sterne, J. A., Tynelius, P., Davey Smith, G., & Rasmussen, F. (2006). Association of childhood socioeconomic position with cause-specific mortality in a prospective record linkage study of 1,839,384 individuals. *American Journal of Epidemiology, 164*(9), 907–915.

Lee, D., & Zhou, L. (2009). "An Empirical Test of SES and Media Use: Modeling the Knowledge Gap Hypothesis in the TV versus Newspaper Context". Paper presented at the annual meeting of the International Communication Association, New Orleans Sheraton, New Orleans, LA.

Levinson, A. H., Perez-Stable, E. J., Espinoza, P., Flores, E. T., & Byers, T. E. (2004). Latinos report less use of pharmaceutical aids when trying to quit smoking. *American Journal of Preventive Medicine, 26*(2), 105–111.

Marmot, M. G., & McDowall, M. E. (1986). Mortality decline and widening social inequalities. *Lancet, 2*(8501), 274–276.

Martin, C. A., Kelly, T. H., Rayens, M. K., Brogli, B. R., Brenzel, A., Smith, W. J., et al. (2002). Sensation seeking, puberty, and nicotine, alcohol, and marijuana use in adolescence. *Journal of the American Academy of Child and Adolescent Psychiatry, 41*(12), 1495–1502.

McCausland, K. L., Allen, J. A., Duke, J. C., Xiao, H., Asche, E. T., Costantino, J. C., et al. (2009). Piloting EX, a social marketing campaign to prompt smoking cessation. *Social Marketing Quarterly, 15*(Suppl 1), 81–101.

McKenna, J., Gutierrez, K., & McCall, K. (2000). Strategies for an effective youth counter-marketing program: Recommendations from commercial marketing experts. *Journal of public health management and practice, 6*(3), 7–13.

McPhee, S. J., Jenkins, C. N. H., Wong, C., Fordham, D., Lau, D. Q., Bird, J. A., et al. (1995). Smoking cessation intervention among Vietnamese Americans: A controlled trial. *Tobacco Control, 4*, S16–S24.

Messer, K., & Pierce, J. P. (2010). Changes in age trajectories of smoking experimentation during the California Tobacco Control Program. *American Journal of Public Health, 100*(7), 1298–1306.

National Cancer Institute. (2008). *The role of the media in promoting and reducing tobacco Use (manuscript)*. Bethesda, MD: U.S. Department of Health and Human Services, National Institutes of Health, National Cancer Institute.

Niederdeppe, J., Fiore, M. C., Baker, T. B., & Smith, S. S. (2008). Smoking-cessation media campaigns and their effectiveness among socioeconomically advantaged and disadvantaged populations. *American Journal of Public Health, 98*(5), 916–924.

Niederdeppe, J., Kuang, X., Crock, B., & Skelton, A. (2008). Media campaigns to promote smoking cessation among socioeconomically disadvantaged populations: What do we know, what do we need to learn, and what should we do now? *Social Science & Medicine, 67*(9), 1343–1355.

Palmgreen, P., Donohew, L., Lorch, E. P., Hoyle, R. H., & Stephenson, M. T. (2001). Television campaigns and adolescent marijuana use: Tests of sensation seeking targeting. *American Journal of Public Health, 91*(2), 292–296.

Palmgreen, P., Lorch, E. P., Stephenson, M. T., Hoyle, R. H., & Donohew, L. (2007). Effects of the Office of National Drug Control Policy's Marijuana Initiative Campaign on high-sensation-seeking adolescents. *American Journal of Public Health, 97*(9), 1644–1649.

Pierce, J. P., Choi, W. S., Gilpin, E. A., Farkas, A. J., & Berry, C. C. (1998). Tobacco industry promotion of cigarettes and adolescent smoking. *Journal of the American Medical Association, 279*(7), 511–515.

Pleis, J. R., & Lethbridge-Cejku, M. (2007). Summary health statistics for U.S. adults: National Health Interview Survey, 2006. *Vital and health statistics, 10*(235), 1–153.

Siegel, M., & Biener, L. (1997). Evaluating the impact of statewide anti-tobacco campaigns: The Massachusetts and California tobacco control programs. *Journal of Social Issues, 53*, 147–168.

Siegel, M., & Biener, L. (2000). The impact of an antismoking media campaign on progression to established smoking: Results of a longitudinal youth study. *American Journal of Public Health, 90*(3), 380–386.

Slater, M. D. (2003). Sensation-seeking as a moderator of the effects of peer influences, consistency with personal aspirations, and perceived harm on marijuana and cigarette use among younger adolescents. *Substance Use & Misuse, 38*(7), 865–880.

Sly, D. F., Heald, G. R., & Ray, S. (2001). The Florida "truth" anti-tobacco media evaluation: Design, first year results, and implications for planning future state media evaluations. *Tobacco Control, 10*(1), 9–15.

Sly, D. F., Hopkins, R. S., Trapido, E., & Ray, S. (2001). Influence of a counteradvertising media campaign on initiation of smoking: The Florida "truth" campaign. *American Journal of Public Health, 91*(2), 233–238.

Sly, D. F., Trapido, E., & Ray, S. (2002). Evidence of the dose effects of an antitobacco counteradvertising campaign. *Preventive Medicine, 35*(5), 511–518.

Stephenson, M. T., Hoyle, R. H., Palmgreen, P., & Slater, M. D. (2003). Brief measures of sensation seeking for screening and large-scale surveys. *Drug and Alcohol Dependence, 72*(3), 279–286.

Thrasher, J. F., Niederdeppe, J., Farrelly, M. C., Davis, K. C., Ribisl, K. M., & Haviland, M. L. (2004). The impact of anti-tobacco industry prevention messages in tobacco producing regions: Evidence from the US truth campaign. *Tobacco Control, 13*(3), 283–288.

Traynor, M. P., & Glantz, S. A. (1996). California's tobacco tax initiative: The development and passage of proposition 99. *Journal of Health Politics, Policy and Law, 21*(3), 543–585.

Trinidad, D. R., Gilpin, E. A., Messer, K., White, M. M., & Pierce, J. P. (2006). Trends in smoking among Hispanic women in California: Relationship to English language use. *American Journal of Preventive Medicine, 31*(3), 257–260.

Trinidad, D. R., Messer, K., Gilpin, E. A., Al-Delaimy, W. K., White, M. M., & Pierce, J. P. (2007). The California Tobacco Control Program's effect on adult smokers: (3) Similar effects for African Americans across states. *Tobacco Control, 16*(2), 96–100.

U.S. Department of Health and Human Services. (1989). *Reducing the health consequences of smoking: 25 years of progress. A Report of the Surgeon General*: U.S. Department of Health and Human Services, Public Health Service, Centers for Disease Control, Center for Chronic Disease Prevention and Health Promotion, Office on Smoking and Health. DHHS Publication No. (CDC) 89–8411.

U.S. Public Health Service. *Smoking and Health. Report of the Advisory Committee to the Surgeon General of the Public Health Service*. Washington, D.C.: U.S. Department of Health, Education, and Welfare, Public Health Service Publication No. 1, 103, January 1964.

Vallone, D., Allen, J. A., Clayton, R. R., & Xiao, H. (2007). How reliable and valid is the Brief Sensation Scale (BSSS-4) for youths of various racial/ethnic groups? *Addiction, 102*(Suppl 2), 71–78.

Vallone, D., Allen, J. A., & Xiao, H. (2009). Is socioeconomic status associated with awareness of and receptivity to the truth campaign among girls and young women? *Drug and Alcohol Dependence, 104*(Suppl 1), S115–S120.

Vallone, D. M., Duke, J. C., Mowery, P. D., McCausland, K. L., Xiao, H., Costantino, J. C., et al. (2010). The impact of "EX": Results from a pilot smoking-cessation media campaign. *American Journal of Preventive Medicine, 38*(3 Suppl), S312–S318.

Vallone, D., Duke, J., Cullen, J., McCausland, K., & Allen, J. (2011a). Evaluation of EX®: A national mass media smoking cessation campaign. *American Journal of Public Health, 101*(2), 302–309.

Vallone, D. M., Niederdeppe, J., Richardson, A. K., Patwardhan, P., Niaura, R., & Cullen, J. (2011b). A national mass media smoking cessation campaign: Effects by race/ethnicity and education. *American Journal of Health Promotion, May–June 2011, 25*(Suppl 5), S38–S50.

Viswanath, K., & Kreuter, M. W. (2007). Health disparities, communication inequalities and eHealth. *American Journal of Preventive Medicine, 32*(Suppl 5), S131–S133.

Wallace, J. M., Jr., Vaughn, M. G., Bachman, J. G., O'Malley, P. M., Johnston, L. D., & Schulenberg, J. E. (2009). Race/ethnicity, socioeconomic factors, and smoking among early adolescent girls in the United States. *Drug and Alcohol Dependence, 104*(Suppl 1), S42–S49.

Wong, M. D., Shapiro, M. F., Boscardin, W. J., & Ettner, S. L. (2002). Contribution of major diseases to disparities in mortality. *The New England Journal of Medicine, 347*(20), 1585–1592.

Wunderink, K. A., Allen, J. A., Xiao, H., Duke, J., Green, M., & Vallone, D. (2007). *American Legacy First Look Report 17. Cigarette preferences among youth: Results from the 2006 Legacy Media Tracking Online (LMTO)*. Washington: American Legacy Foundation.

Yerger, V. B., Wertz, M., McGruder, C., Froelicher, E., & Malone, R. (2008). Nicotine replacement therapy: Perceptions of African American smokers seeking to quit. *Journal of the National Medical Association, 100*(2), 230–236.

Zimmerman, R. S., Palmgreen, P. M., Noar, S. M., Lustria, M. L., Lu, H. Y., & Lee Horosewski, M. (2007). Effects of a televised two-city safer sex mass media campaign targeting high-sensation-seeking and impulsive-decision-making young adults. *Health Education & Behavior, 34*(5), 810–826.

Zucker, D., Hopkins, R. S., Sly, D. F., Urich, J., Kershaw, J. M., & Solari, S. (2000). Florida's "truth" campaign: A counter-marketing, anti-tobacco media campaign. *Journal of public health management and practice, 6*(3), 1–6.

Zuckerman, M., Ball, S., & Black, J. (1990). Influences of sensation seeking, gender, risk appraisal, and situational motivation on smoking. *Addictive Behaviors, 15*(3), 209–220.

Part IV
Important Interventions for Children

Chapter 6
Preventing Childhood Lead Poisoning

Wornie Reed

Preventing Childhood Lead Poisoning

Lead poisoning is a serious but preventable childhood disease, caused by exposure to lead, which is found primarily in paint, soil, and household dust. Children come in contact with these sources of lead during normal indoor and outdoor play. Lead is especially dangerous to children under 7 years of age because this is a critical phase in the development of their neurological system. The implications of lead poisoning are vast, as the neurological damage it causes can lead to such problems as learning disabilities and emotional disturbances. Lead poisoning can damage a young child's developing brain and nervous system, leading to reduced IQ and behavioral disabilities. Consequently, lead poisoning is associated with poor school performance and delinquent behavior.

Lead poisoning is the number one environmental health threat to children. Lead present in paint, dust, and soil is possibly our most significant toxic waste problem in terms of the seriousness and the extent of human health effects. It is more dangerous than some forms of cancer – yet it is virtually ignored by the American public. Lead poisoning among children has changed over the past three to four decades. Previously, it was a disease often presented as encephalopathy associated with children ingesting peels of lead paint. Now lead poisoning has become known as a largely asymptomatic condition characterized by an elevated blood lead level linked with many sources of exposure and affecting a broad range of children. Recent research has demonstrated that even low levels of blood lead produce permanent damage to the central nervous system's functions of preschool-age children.

Lead poisoning is of special significance for African Americans as they are much more likely than white children to have elevated levels of lead in their blood. Since some of the principal sources of lead in the environment are flaking paint from old houses, auto emissions, and industrial sources, inner-city neighborhoods have higher rates of child lead poisoning than rural or suburban areas. Because African Americans tend to be the primary inner-city dwellers they are more at risk for lead poisoning than white children.

A small proportion of children are lead poisoned by eating paint chips from the walls of deteriorating inner-city dwellings. These children become ill and usually must be hospitalized. In most instances, however, childhood lead poisoning occurs from an accumulation of low levels of lead from household dust, and there are no immediate symptoms.

W. Reed (✉)
Department of Sociology, Virginia Tech, Blacksburg, VA, USA
e-mail: wornie@vt.edu

A.J. Lemelle et al. (eds.), *Handbook of African American Health: Social and Behavioral Interventions*,
DOI 10.1007/978-1-4419-9616-9_6, © Springer Science+Business Media, LLC 2011

A blood lead test is the only way to determine if a child is lead poisoned. The U.S. Centers for Disease Control and Prevention (CDC) defines a blood lead level of 10 micrograms (μg) per deciliter (dl) of blood as a level of concern, indicating that steps should be taken to reduce ongoing lead exposure. Recent research has found adverse health effects, including learning disabilities, at even lower levels of exposure.

Trends in Blood Lead Levels

In the 1999–2002 period, the National Health and Nutrition Examination Survey (NHANES) found that 1.4% of all children between 1 and 5 years of age had elevated blood lead levels (BLLs) – readings above 10 μg/dl. This was a decrease from 4.4% of children in the 1991–1994 period, and 8.6% in the 1988–1991 period (see Table 6.1).

The decline in BLLs is believed to be the result of efforts to remove lead from gasoline and residential paint. Figure 6.1 shows a strong correlation between the decrease in lead use in gasoline and the decline in blood lead levels.

There has been a substantial decline in the lead poisoning rates for blacks, whites, and Hispanics; however, the rates for blacks have continued to be greater than that of whites and Mexican Americans. In fact, the lead poisoning rates for blacks have been consistently almost three times that of whites.

There are strong efforts to get all children tested; however, only a third of children below the age of six are tested. This situation obtains despite federal regulations that require that all children

Table 6.1 Prevalence of elevated blood lead levels, ≥10 μg/dl, among children aged 1–5 years by race/ethnicity by year of NHANES surveys

Race/ethnicity	Years of NHANES surveys		
	1988–1991	1991–1994	1999–2004
Total	8.6%	4.4%	1.4%
Non-Hispanic Black	18.6	11.2	3.4
Mexican American	7.2	4.0	1.2
Non-Hispanic White	5.5	2.3	1.2

Source: Jones, R. L., Homa, D. M., Meyer, P. A., Brody, D. J., Caldwell, K. L., Pirkle, J. L., & Brown, M. J. (2009). Trends in blood lead levels and blood lead testing Among U.S. children aged 1 to 5 years, 1988–2004

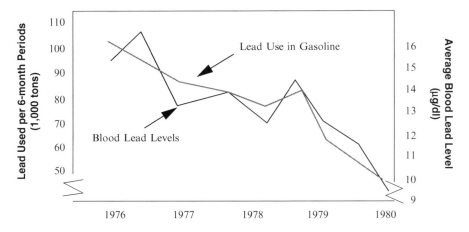

Fig. 6.1 Decline in leaded gasoline and blood lead levels. Source: Kovarik (2010)

enrolled in Medicaid must receive a blood lead screening test at ages 12 and 24 months, and all children ages 36–72 months who have not previously been screened must also receive a blood lead test.

Sources of Lead

Lead-Based Paint

Many health experts agree that exposure to lead-contaminated dust from deteriorated lead-based paint in older homes is the primary pathway for lead exposure in young children. Lead dust, which is invisible to the naked eye, is difficult to clean up. It settles on the floor where young children tend to play; thus, children are usually poisoned by normal hand-to-mouth activity.

All houses built before 1975 are likely to have lead, as up until that time lead was routinely included in paint. The United States government's Consumer Product Safety Commission finally banned lead paint in 1977. It was banned in France and many other countries prior to 1920.

Soil and Dust

Soil in the vicinity of the home can also be contaminated by flaking exterior lead-based paint or from previous exhausts from leaded gasoline. In yards where soil is contaminated with lead, children may ingest it through regular hand-to-mouth activity during normal play. Adults can track dust into homes, where regular child actions can result in exposure to lead.

Leaded Gasoline

Automobile emissions have been a significant source of lead exposure for urban residents, particularly in areas with congested traffic. Lead from gasoline has been labeled by some experts as the most important source of lead poisoning in the inner cities (Mielke, 1999). In 2010, an interdisciplinary team of scientists sought to determine the predominant recent historic source of lead exposure within a city. They concluded that leaded gasoline was responsible for about two-thirds of toxic lead that African American children in Cleveland ingested or inhaled during the latter two-thirds of the twentieth century (Robbins et al., 2010).

Tetra-ethyl lead (TEL) was blended with gasoline, primarily to boost octane levels, from the 1920s to the 1980s. In the 1920s, TEL won out over the safer ethyl alcohol (ethanol) for use as an antiknock ingredient for gasoline. In terms of engine performance there was little difference between the two additives. Three grams of TEL had about the same effect on antiknock as adding a pint and a half of ethanol to a gallon of gasoline (Thomas & Kwong, 2001). Ethanol is made from farm crops or cellulose, which can be blended with gasoline to boost octane (antiknock) ratings. TEL was an additive discovered by General Motors' researchers in 1921. Although several workers in plants producing TEL became violently ill and died, TEL was declared safe when diluted in gasoline. Pushed by General Motors, it won out over ethanol, which was already in use and known to be safe. Ethanol blends in gasoline have regained popularity in recent years, sometimes called "gasohol" and "ethanol enhanced" gasoline (Kovarik, 2003). Gasoline with TEL is considered one of the world's greatest environmental disasters (Kovarik).

The Environmental Protection Agency (EPA) began working to reduce lead emissions by issuing the first reduction standards in 1973. Effective in January 1, 1996, the Clean Air Act banned the sale of the small amount of leaded fuel that was still available in some parts of the country for use in on-road vehicles.

Following are some key dates in the history of the use of TEL in gasoline:

1922 – Public Health Service warns of dangers of lead production and leaded fuel.
1923 – Leaded gasoline goes on sale in selected markets.
1936 – 90% of gasoline sold in USA contains TEL.
1972 – EPA gives notice of proposed phase out of lead in gasoline.
1986 – Primary phase out of leaded gasoline in USA is completed.
1994 – Study shows that US blood-lead levels declined by 78% from 1978 to 1991.

Figure 6.1 shows the close relationship between the decrease in the sale and use of leaded gasoline and the decline in blood lead levels among children. A precipitous decline in blood lead levels followed the discontinuation of lead use in gasoline.

Old Housing

Approximately 40% of all US housing units (about 38 million homes) have some lead-based paint, and 25% of all US housing units (about 24 million homes) have significant lead-based paint hazards. Of units built before 1940, 68% have significant lead-based paint hazards, as do 43% of units built from 1940 to 1959. About 4 million units with some lead-based paint are occupied by families with children less than 6 years of age.

Effects of Lead in Children

As lead poisoning rates have declined nationally, the racial disparities of this disease have increased. African American children are at increased risk, when compared with both Hispanic and white children. In some communities, the rate of exposure is about five times the national average (Environmental Health Watch, 2008).

Some of the health effects of lead poisoning include

- Encephalopathy (a disease of the brain that alters brain function and structure)
- Colic (chronic digestive disorder, severe abdominal pain, obstinate constipation)
- Frank anemia (severe iron deficiency, decrease in levels of hemoglobin, which is responsible for transporting oxygen in the body)
- Decreased hemoglobin synthesis
- Erythrocyte protoporphyrin (condition of red blood cells, e.g., lack of iron)
- Developmental toxicity (lead passed from mother to fetus)
- Reduced nerve conduction velocity
- IQ, memory, learning
- Growth

Longtime problems from childhood lead exposure can include

- Low grades
- Absenteeism
- Reading disabilities

- Increased risk of not graduating from high school
- Increased evidence of depression
- Higher rate of hard drug use
- Increased risk for attention deficit disorder
- Increased risk for antisocial behavior

Blood lead concentrations, even those below 10 g/dl, are inversely associated with children's IQ scores at 3 and 5 years of age, and associated declines in IQ are greater at these concentrations than at higher concentrations. These findings suggest that more US children may be adversely affected by environmental lead than previously estimated.

Delinquency and Violence

Some researchers have suggested that lead continues to contribute significantly to socio-behavioral problems such as juvenile delinquency and violent crime (Needleman, 2002; Nevin, 2000). What had long been hypothesized was demonstrated to be the case in a study by Needleman, Riess, Tobin, Biesecker, and Greenhouse (1996). This study showed that youth with relatively high levels of lead in their bones were more likely to engage in aggressive acts and delinquent behavior than boys with less lead in their bones.

Needleman's earlier longitudinal studies had shown a relationship between lead and school behavioral problems such as hyperactivity, attention deficit disorders, impaired impulse control, and other learning disorders. Many observers had hypothesized that these behaviors – which predict delinquency and criminal behavior – were just intervening variables between lead exposure and delinquent or criminal careers. Needleman's findings show these links and suggest that some of the violence in our society could be the result of preventable environmental pollution by lead.

However, this information is not new. Just as we have known about the harmful effects of lead paint for 100 years – Germany banned lead from paint in the 1890s – we have known about the relationship between lead and delinquency a long time. In fact, more than 60 years ago, Randy Byers, a child neurologist at Boston Children's Hospital, linked acute lead poisoning in children to later "violent, aggressive behavioral difficulties, such as attacking teachers with knives or scissors" (Byers & Lord, 1943).

Treatment for Lead Poisoning

Treatment for lead poisoning involves removing the sources of lead and providing balanced nutrition. The first step is to reduce or eliminate exposure to lead. The second step is to reduce lead levels in the body. Lead-based paint and the dust and dirt that come from its decomposition should be removed by professionals. Balanced nutrition includes adequate amounts of vitamins and minerals such as iron, calcium, and vitamin C. A child who eats a balanced, nutritious diet absorbs less lead than one whose diet is inadequate.

If removing the source of lead and balancing nutrition do not reduce lead levels, or if the blood lead level is very high, chelation therapy may be used. Chelation therapy is a process that lowers the amount of lead stored in the body. Drugs called chelating agents cause metals like lead to bind to them, and then they are eliminated from the body through urine. Chelating agents increase the absorption of lead and other metals. Therefore, it is essential that sources of lead exposure be removed before a child is treated. Neurological damage from lead poisoning, however, is often incurable and may not improve with treatment.

Prevention

Except for severely poisoned children, there is no medical treatment for lead poisoning. Drug therapy can reduce high levels of lead in the body, such as might occur when a child eats paint chips; however, this therapy cannot undo the harm caused to developing organs and systems. Consequently, the focus is on preventing lead exposure.

More than 38 million US homes and apartments are burdened by lead-based paint, and more than 24 million of them contain substantial lead hazards. Interim controls like lead-safe painting and rehabilitation should become the minimum national norm to avoid creating lead hazards in properties now in good condition. The Environmental Protection Agency needs to develop and enforce rules to ensure that this occurs (Alliance for Healthy Homes, 2010).

Recommendations of the President's Task Force on Environmental Health Risks

In 2000, the President's Task Force on Environmental Health Risks and Safety Risks to Children concluded the following:

Lead poisoning is a completely preventable disease.
Residential lead paint hazards in homes of children can be virtually eliminated in 10 years.
Every child deserves to grow up in a home free of lead paint hazards.

Of course, 10 years later, lead poisoning has not been virtually eliminated. This task force also laid out some guiding steps that should be taken to accomplish the goal of having every child grow up in a home free of lead paint hazards: act before children are poisoned, identify and care for lead-poisoned children, conduct research, and measure progress and refine lead poisoning prevention strategies.

Act before children are poisoned. The Task Force suggested that federal grants should be provided for low-income housing owners to control lead paint hazards. This should be accompanied by promoting education for universal lead-safe panting, renovation, and maintenance work practices; and insuring compliance and enforcement of lead paint laws.

Identify and care for lead-poisoned children. There was a recommendation to expand blood lead level screening and follow-up services for at-risk children.

Conduct research. Relatively little research funding goes into improving prevention strategies and developing ways to drive down lead hazard control costs; however, without such funding lead hazard control will not be made more cost-efficient.

Measure progress and refine lead poisoning prevention strategies. The Task Force recognized the need to develop monitoring and surveillance programs for lead hazard control. Increased attention and reporting may set the stage for accomplishing the goals of lead-safe childhoods.

Primary, Secondary, and Tertiary Prevention

One way to look at lead poisoning prevention is with the public health framework of primary, secondary, and tertiary prevention. Primary prevention protects individuals in order to avoid disease prior to signs or symptoms of the disease. It includes activities, programs, and practices that operate on a fundamentally nonpersonal basis and alter the set of opportunities, risks, and expectations surrounding

Table 6.2 Proposed CDC intervention policy

Blood lead level (µg/dl)	Actions	Time frame for beginning intervention
<2	No action	
2–5	Provide caregiver lead education. Provide follow-up testing. Refer the child for social services to investigate possible sources of lead exposure	Within 30 days
5–10	Above actions, plus: If blood lead levels (BLLs) persist (i.e., 2 venous BLLs in this range at least 3 months apart) or increase, proceed according to actions for BLLs 10–20	Within 2 weeks
10–20	Above actions, plus: Provide coordination of care (case management). Provide clinical evaluation and care. Provide environmental investigation and control current lead hazards	Within 1 week
20–70	Above actions	Within 24 h
70 or higher	Above actions, plus hospitalize child for chelation therapy immediately	Within 24 h

Source: Landrigan et al. (2002)

individuals. Secondary intervention is essentially the early detection of disease, followed by appropriate intervention, such as health promotion or treatment. Tertiary prevention aims to reduce the impact of the disease and promote rehabilitation of persons with the disease. This is often referred to as treatment.

Tertiary Prevention (Intervention)

Tertiary prevention is involved when a child is already lead poisoned. It is oriented toward preventing cases from getting worse. By the time a child is identified as lead poisoned, the damage may already have been done, with possible irreversible consequences (Dietrich et al., 2004). Table 6.2 shows the list of actions proposed by the Centers for Disease Control when children are discovered through blood testing to have specific blood lead levels.

Secondary Prevention

The most prevalent activity in secondary prevention is testing of children for blood lead. However, secondary prevention does not prevent childhood lead poisoning, as it depends on blood screening. By that point it is too late. An elevated blood lead level signifies that exposure has already occurred. Prevention at that point is only concerned with preventing the disease from becoming any worse (i.e., the child ingesting more lead). Thus, more attention to primary prevention is needed.

Primary Prevention

Primary prevention of lead poisoning would require attention before children are exposed to lead in their environment, especially their home environment. Primary prevention is step one of the recommendations of the President's Task Force: act before children are poisoned. This would mean removing the lead from inside and around homes where young children live.

At least one state, Massachusetts, addresses a part of the issue of lead in homes. The Massachusetts "Lead Law" requires an owner to remove or appropriately cover lead paint hazards in homes built before 1978 if a child under six lives there. If there is lead in the home, the owner must remove or cover it. When a buyer is about to purchase a home built before 1978, the owner must provide a copy of any lead inspection report and a letter of compliance. This law also covers all owners of residential rental property, as well as owners of their own single or multifamily home (MassLegalHelp, 2008).

The abatement of lead from within houses addresses the problems of lead paint, while the abatement of lead outside of houses addresses lead in the soil which can be caused by paint as well as automobile exhausts and other emissions. Lead-contaminated soil is removed by digging and removing the topsoil to the depth of approximately one foot. While both approaches are needed (Reed, 1992), I will focus here on lead abatement within the home.

Lead Paint Abatement

Banned since 1978, lead-based paint has been a major source of lead poisoning for children. Lead-based paint removal costs an estimated $8–15 a square foot, which means removing all lead from a house of 1,200–2,000 ft^2 could cost as much as $9,600–$30,000, while the average removal project runs around $10,000 for a typical pre-1978 home. Obviously, lead abatement is expensive. One option is encapsulation (applying a liquid coating that forms a watertight jacket over lead paint) which on average costs less than 50 cents a square foot, or $600–$1,000 for 1,200–2,000 ft^2 (Costhelper, 2008).

In 2002 there were an estimated four million lead-contaminated houses in the USA. Using $7,000 as the average cost of lead abatement per house, the Committee on Environmental Health (2005) estimated that it would cost $28 billion to delead all of these homes.

Although lead abatement is expensive, some analysts suggest that it would be cost effective. Studies show that for every 1 µg/dl of blood lead children experience a .25 IQ point reduction; and other studies show that the loss of one IQ point is associated with an overall reduction in lifetime earnings of 2.39%. Based on this data, Landrigan, Schechter, Lipton, Fahs, and Schwartz (2002) argue that the present value of economic losses attributable to lead exposure in the birth cohort of 5-year-olds amounted to $43.4 billion per year. The Committee on Environmental Health suggested that lead abatement is cost-effective if it prevents even two-thirds of lead exposure for any single year's cohort of young children.

Conclusion

Blood lead levels have been steadily decreasing in the past two to three decades. This decline is generally attributed to the discontinuance of the use of leaded gasoline. However, this decreasing rate is expected to slow down, and lead poisoning is expected to continue as an issue, as the bans on lead-based paint and leaded gasoline might have already had the bulk of their effects. The rates are still much higher for African American children in urban areas. For example, in Cleveland, Ohio, a city with a majority black population the proportion of children with blood lead levels greater than 10 µg/dl was 14% in 2003 (Environmental Health Watch, 2008).

Despite increasing attention to lead abatement, the most prominent prevention activity for lead poisoning is testing. Blood lead level testing is obviously not a primary prevention technique. With testing of children it appears as if they are being used the way miners previously used canary birds.

Miners would send a canary down a mine to test for poisonous gases. If the bird came back that was a signal that there were no poisonous gases and it was safe for the men to enter the mine. If the bird did not come back that was a signal that there were poisonous gases and the bird had succumbed. Similarly with children, if we test them to determine whether their environments have lead we may find out too late, after they have been poisoned already.

Instead of testing the children, we need to practice more primary prevention and test and treat the environment – the home and the soil. Then we can get closer to assuring that we can act before children are poisoned.

References

Alliance for Healthy Homes. (2010). *Understanding new national data on lead poisoning.* Retrieved from http://www.afhh.org/chil_ar/chil_ar_lead_poisoning_BLL_data_factsheet.htm

Byers, R. K., & Lord, E. E. (1943). Late effects of lead poisoning on mental development. *American Journal of Diseases of Children, 66,* 471–494.

Committee on Environmental Health. (2005). Lead exposure in children: prevention, detection, and management. *Pediatrics, 116*(4), 1036–11046. Retrieved from http://pediatrics.aappublications.org/cgi/content/full/116/4/1036

CostHelper. (2008). *Lead paint abatement cost.* Retrieved from http://www.costhelper.com/cost/home-garden/lead-paint-abatement.html

Dietrich, K. N., Ware, J. H., Salganik, M., Radcliffe, J. K., Roban, W. J., Rhoads, G. G., et al. (2004). Effect of chelation therapy on the neuropsychological and behavioral development of lead-exposed children after school entry. *Pediatrics, 114*(1), 19–26.

Environmental Health Watch. (2008). *Childhood lead poisoning.* Retrieved from http://www.ehw.org/Lead/LEAD_home3.htm#ClevelandRates

Kovarik, W. (2003). *Ethyl: The 1920s environmental conflict over leaded gasoline and alternative fuels.* Paper presented at the annual conference of the American Society for Environmental History, Providence, RI. Retrieved from http://www.runet.edu/~wkovarik/ethylwar

Kovarik, W. (2010). *Ethyl: Henry Ford, Charles Kettering and the fight over leaded gasoline and the fuel of the future.* Retrieved from http://www.runet.edu/~wkovarik/ethylwar/

Landrigan, P. J., Schechter, C. B., Lipton, J. M., Fahs, M. C., & Schwartz, J. (2002). Environmental pollutants and disease in American children: estimates of morbidity, and costs for lead poisoning, asthma, cancer, and developmental disabilities. *Environmental Health Perspectives, 110*(7), 721–728.

MassLegalHelp. (2008). *Tenants' rights in Massachusetts: Private housing.* Retrieved from http://www.masslegal-help.org/housing/legal-tactics1

Mielke, H. W. (1999). Lead in the inner cities: Policies to reduce children's exposure to lead may be overlooking a major source of lead in the environment. *American Scientist, 87*(1), 62–73.

Needleman, H. L., Riess, J. K., Tobin, M., Biesecker, G., & Greenhouse, J. (1996). Bone lead levels and delinquent behavior. *Journal of the American Medical Association, 275*(5), 363–369.

Needleman, H. L. (2002). Bone lead levels in adjudicated delinquents: A case control study. *Neurotoxicology and Teratology, 24,* 711–717.

Nevin, R. (2000). How lead exposure relates to temporal changes in IQ, violent crime, and unwed pregnancy. *Environmental Research, 8*(1), 1–22.

Reed, W. L. (1992). Lead poisoning: A modern plague among African American children. In L. Braithwaite & S. E. Taylor (Eds.), *Health issues in the black community.* San Francisco: Jossey-Bass.

President's Task Force on Environmental Health Risks and Safety Risks to Children. (2000). *Eliminating childhood lead poisoning: a federal strategy targeting lead paint hazards.* Retrieved from http://www.epa.gov/lead/pubs/fedstrategy2000.pdf

Robbins, N., Zhang, Z., Sun, J., Ketterer, M. E., Lalumandier, J. A., & Shulze, R. A. (2010). Childhood lead exposure and uptake in teeth in the Cleveland area during the era of leaded gasoline. *The Science of the Total Environment, 408*(19), 4118–4127.

Thomas, V. M., & Kwong, A. (2001). Ethanol as a lead replacement: Phasing out lead in Africa. *Energy Policy, 29,* 1133–1143.

Chapter 7
Contemporary Interventions to Prevent and Reduce Community Violence Among African American Youth

Duane E. Thomas, Elizabeth M. Woodburn, Celine I. Thompson, and Stephen S. Leff

Introduction

While community violence in the United States has diminished since the early 1990s, when its levels peaked to epidemic proportions, it continues to be a major public health problem. Indeed, over the course of the last decade, American teens and young adults have continued to experience rates of violent crime that are much higher than those for any other age group (Bureau of Justice Statistics, 2007). According to the Centers for Disease Control and Prevention (CDC, 2009a, 2009b), in 2006, 5,958 young people between the ages of 10 and 24 were murdered, making homicide the second leading cause of death for youth in that age group. Additionally, in 2007, more than 668,000 young people aged 10–24 years were treated in emergency departments for injuries sustained from violence.

For African American youth specifically, recent violence statistics paint a particularly grim picture. Violence is the leading cause of mortality for African Americans between the ages of 10 and 24 years of age, while it is the second leading cause for Hispanics, and the third leading cause for Asian/Pacific Islanders and Alaska Natives (CDC, 2009a, 2009b). African American youth have been found to be victims of violence at rates higher than all other races, with reported rates of violent victimization against African Americans at 26 per 1,000 persons age 12 or older compared to 18 per 1,000 Caucasian persons, and 15 per 1,000 persons of other races (Bureau of Justice Statistics, 2007). Unfortunately, young Black males bear the brunt of violent victimization with the highest homicide victimization rates. Homicide rates among non-Hispanic, African American males 10–24 years of age (62.2 per 100,000) have been found to exceed those of Hispanic males (21.5 per 100,000) and non-Hispanic, White males in the same age group (3.4 per 100,000) (CDC, 2009a, 2009b).

Moreover, while community violence affects youth of all races, ethnicities, and socioeconomic groups in the USA, African American youth living in economically challenged, urban communities encounter community violence most frequently (Cooley-Strickland et al., 2009; Mathews, Dempsey, & Overstreet, 2009). According to Cooley-Strickland and colleagues (2009), over 80% of children living in urban areas have witnessed community violence, and as many as 70% of them report being victims of this violence (2009). The investigators also reported that, within a sample of adolescents

D.E. Thomas (✉)
Graduate School of Education, University of Pennsylvania, Philadelphia, PA, USA
e-mail: duanet@gse.upenn.edu

A.J. Lemelle et al. (eds.), *Handbook of African American Health: Social and Behavioral Interventions*, DOI 10.1007/978-1-4419-9616-9_7, © Springer Science+Business Media, LLC 2011

representative of the United States, 57% of the African American children in their sample had witnessed violence compared to 50% of the Latinos and 34% of the Caucasians. The community violence to which African American youth are frequently exposed is often chronic and severe, as opposed to single, nonrecurring violent episodes (Cooley-Strickland et al.), suggesting that it may have a continuous impact on youth's abilities to cope. Given the enormity of this problem for African American youth, the development of effective interventions to reduce and prevent community violence is a foremost and desirable goal of multiple disciplines (U.S. Department of Health and Human Services [USDHHS], 2001).

Considerable progress has been made toward the development of promising approaches to youth violence prevention. This chapter first establishes the critical role that developmental research has played in developing programs to reduce and prevent violence among African American youth. We then describe several contemporary violence prevention programs that have demonstrated effectiveness or promise for this population. This includes school-based aggression prevention programs that have demonstrated efficacy with varied student populations including African American children and youth. Additionally, we discuss school-based aggression prevention programs that were developed for and/or implemented specifically with this population. Finally, we discuss new directions in comprehensive prevention efforts that have emerged over the past few years aimed at reducing the incidence of community violence.

Developmental Risks and Youth Violence Prevention

Longitudinal research has shown that, across different racial/ethnic backgrounds, individuals who are aggressive during early childhood are at increased risk for long-term antisocial outcomes and for a range of personal and social difficulties in adolescence and adulthood, including juvenile offending and adult violence (Broidy et al., 2003; Loeber, Farrington, & Waschbusch, 1998; Loeber et al., 2001; Nagin & Tremblay, 1999). Some children who exhibit significant patterns of aggression in early childhood gradually escalate to more severe forms of aggression before and during adolescence; with roughly a quarter to a half of boys and over half of girls who fall into this category continuing their violent behavior into adulthood (Loeber, Farrington, & Waschbusch, 1998).

Exposure to community violence is another strong predictor of aggression and violent behavior among children and adolescents in studies that utilize both cross sectional and longitudinal data (Guerra, Huesmann, & Spindler, 2003; Spano, Vazsonyi, & Bolland, 2009). Such exposure not only affects youth who are direct victims, but also affects those who are indirect victims, such as bystanders, witnesses, or those who are familiar with the victims. These indirect victims of community violence are not only equally affected, but are also much more numerous (Cooley-Strickland et al., 2009).

One of the longest running prospective longitudinal studies examining predictors of violent behavior began 23 years ago with first, fourth, and seventh-grade boys (>50% African American) in inner-city Pittsburgh (Pittsburgh Youth Study; Loeber, Farrington, Stouthamer-Loeber, Moffitt, & Caspi, 1998). With yearly assessments, one of the primary goals of the project was to chart the progression of aggression and delinquency across time. Perhaps most notable was the role that risk played in the prediction of escalating aggression. An examination of the developmental impact of risk across the boys' lifespan suggested that a greater number of contexts in which boys experienced risks (e.g., school, community, home) was suggestive of poorer behavioral outcomes (Loeber, Farrington, Stouthamer-Loeber, Moffitt, & Caspi, 1998). Individual risk factors for escalating aggression and later antisocial behavior included temperamental factors, behavioral inhibition, as well as poor school performance (Loeber, Farrington, Stouthamer-Loeber, Moffitt, & Caspi, 1998; Loeber et al., 2001). Family variables associated with increased risk included poor parent–child communication (one of the strongest predictors), corporal punishment, poor supervision, and high parental stress (Loeber et al., 2001). Most importantly, risk factors at the youngest ages were predictive of later problems, highlighting the importance of prevention-based work to occur as early as possible in an individual's development.

The cumulative nature of both risk and aggressive behavior across a child's lifespan suggests the need for violence preventive programming that is developmentally focused and comprehensive. Developmental-ecological models that apply developmental principles first introduced by Bronfenbrenner's ecological systems model (1977), suggest that an individual's interaction with aspects of his or her environment (and their cross-interactions) drive developmental change. This developmental change may include increases or decreases in behaviors and circumstances forecasting violence. Models incorporating interactions between an individual and his or her environment have guided much of the contemporary work on youth violence prevention.

Specific to African American youth, the Phenomenological Variant of Ecological Systems Theory (PVEST; Spencer, 2006) offers a particularly useful framework for examining developmental processes that may lead to violence. PVEST is a cyclic recursive model of human development for racially and ethnically diverse individuals that provides a heuristic device for examining youths' cultural experiences in various interrelated contexts. It incorporates the development of stable identities through evolving stress engagement and management responses to context. For example, in a risky context, such as a violent neighborhood, a Black male youth may find it helpful to apply a hypermasculine persona (potentially maladaptive coping response and identity) that may be displayed through fighting and other forms of aggression in order to provide self-protection and/or survive in their surroundings (Spencer, 1999). This process has been used to describe precursors to conduct problems at school for African American male youth (Thomas, Coard, Stevenson, Bentley, & Zamel, 2009; Thomas & Stevenson, 2009) and contributors of risk for and protection against serious antisocial behaviors (Spencer & Jones-Walker, 2004).

Hence, these developmental models may be particularly appropriate for inner-city racial minority youth who face unique adversity at several levels of their socioenvironment (e.g., family stress, poverty, institutional racism) and, therefore, require interventions aimed at both the individual and the context (see Spencer, Dupree, Cunningham, Harpalani, & Muñoz-Miller, 2003; Swick & Williams, 2006). Taken together, developmental theory and research suggests that efforts to prevent or reduce violence among African American youth should begin as early as possible and target both individual-level and multiple contextual influences in its research design.

School-Based Violence Prevention Programming

Existing violence prevention programming is frequently implemented in school settings. Due to the amount of time youth spend in school, as well as the opportunity schools can provide to observe behavior in structured settings, the school setting has been one of the primary places in which behaviors that sow the seeds for violence have been addressed and violence prevention efforts have been designed and carried out. School-based violence prevention may be targeted at individual children and youth already exhibiting, or determined to be at heightened risk for, precursors to violent behavior, including, but not limited to, early and prolonged aggressive behavior problems (Broidy et al., 2003), social cognitive deficits (Guerra et al., 2003), comorbid affective disorders and academic failure (Cooley-Strickland et al., 2009), substance use (Botvin, Griffin, & Nichols, 2006; Cooley-Strickland et al., 2009), exposure to aggressive peer norms in classrooms (Henry, Guerra, Huesmann, Tolan, VanAcker, et al., 2000; Thomas, Bierman, & the Conduct Problems Prevention Research Group [CPPRG], 2006; Thomas, Bierman, Powers, & CPPRG, 2011), and heightened community violence exposure (Guerra et al.). Programming may also be universal, focusing on all students and classroom- and school-level rules and systems, or targeted to specific groups of students at particular risk of violence exposure. Regardless of the universal or targeted nature of the intervention, multicomponent violence prevention programs have been the most effective – aiming treatment at the child, school and parent level.

School-level violence prevention programming has had mixed success. Recent systematic reviews of the effectiveness of school-based youth violence interventions showed that universal prevention approaches were effective in reducing violence and associated behavioral issues (Hahn et al., 2007; Lochman & Wells, 2003). Other research has suggested greater benefits for violence prevention programming that is more selective in its scope and corresponding procedures, especially for students with extant elevated levels of aggressive behavior (Multisite Violence Prevention Project, 2009). However, the majority of recent research has suggested that a combination of universal and targeted programming may be most effective, changing both individual child factors and the environment (e.g., Leff, Power, Manz, Constigan, & Nabors, 2001). Such programs, delivered to preadolescent children and youth, have demonstrated effective reductions in aggression, disruption, and violent behavior as well as increases in social competence and prosocial decision-making skills. The stability of aggressive behavior and the propensity for its increase over time among a subset of youth suggests the need for programming aimed at prevention, through universal and targeted interventions to reduce behaviors considered to be precursors to later violence.

Following a review of universal school-wide violence prevention programs, the Taskforce on Community Preventive Services (CDC, 2007) determined that most programs were effective across a variety of neighborhood contexts (i.e., SES level, level of violence) and school type. For children living in low SES neighborhoods and schools with greater than 50% African American students, an average reduction of 17–29% in violent behavior was reported. The Taskforce recommended a closer study of the components of violence prevention programming that engender positive results, better study across ethnic, racial and socioeconomic groups, and programming that is carried out and evaluated more systematically.

Among programs with some demonstrated success, a focus on individuals' sociocognitive development is the most prevalent. The Social Information Processing (SIP; Crick & Dodge, 1994) model of childhood aggression suggests that deficiencies in cognitive processes (e.g., encoding problems and attribution biases, misrepresentation of social information, cue-utilization difficulties, response search and decision difficulties, and cognitive processes requiring the evaluation and mental enactment of an interpersonal experience) shape the responses of aggressive children. Interventions that have addressed individual risk factors through a SIP model have demonstrated success in reducing aggressive behavior problems (Boxer & Dubow, 2001). Furthermore, nesting these individually targeted programs within contexts such as classrooms, schools, and families have proven the most successful (e.g., Ozer, 2006). Discussed below are several notable school-based violence prevention programs that involve individual and contextual foci (in varying degrees) and target different predictors of youth violence (See Table 7.1).

Fast Track Project

One of the most comprehensive and evaluated programs of this type is FAST Track, a long-term prevention program targeting children at risk for serious delinquency and antisocial behavior in four diverse American communities (Durham, NC, Nashville, TN, Seattle, WA, and several rural counties in Pennsylvania) (CPPRG, 1992). Beginning in first grade and continuing into the secondary school years, selected high-risk children and their parents participate in a combination of social skills and anger-control training, academic tutoring, and parent training, respectively. At earlier ages, children also receive a teacher-led classroom curriculum called PATHS (Promoting Alternative

Table 7.1 Overview of school-based violence prevention programs

Program	Target participants	Target skills	Unique program aspects	Research findings	Future research needs
Fast track	First grade through high school	• Social skills • Anger control • Academic skills	• Parent component • Longitudinal and developmental focus • Diversity of participants	• Increases in sociocognitive skills • Improved peer likeability • Decreases in aggression and conduct problems • Decreases in harsh parenting among involved families	Evaluation of mechanisms of effects and separate program components Focus on ethnic and racial subgroups
Bullying prevention program	Elementary school through junior high	• Improvement in school climate • Reductions in victimization	• Focus on school climate and context • Effort to change overall acceptability of bullying	• Reductions in bullying behavior • Suppression of growth in students' aggressive behavior	A focus on individual as well as context. Fidelity evaluations as component of program
Coping power	Preadolescent girls and boys	• Increasing prosocial behavior • Decreasing aggression • Decreasing substance use	• Parent component • Contextual focus	• Higher teacher rated school functioning • Lower self-reported aggression • Lower parent-rated drug and alcohol use • Greater self-regulation and social competence	Studies of mechanisms of program effects Studies with more diverse samples, subgroup analyses
Second step (and steps to respect)	Kindergarten-middle school	• Decreasing aggression and risky behavior • Increasing positive social skills • Decreasing bullying	• Focus on protective factors • Work with both high and low-income students	• Decreased physical aggression (maintained at 6 months) • Increased knowledge and peer relations • Efficacy in low-income groups	Studies with control and comparison groups. Program effects with subgroups (racial, ethnic, and SES groups)

Thinking Strategies), which focus on emotional development, social problem-solving, and peer-related social skills. Moreover, home visits are included as part of the intervention to assist with the generalization of children's acquisition of skills beyond the school and improvement in parent–child communication and behavior management practices in the home.

The FAST Track project has demonstrated effectiveness in several main areas of violence prevention including increases in sociocognitive skills, improved peer likeability, decreases in aggression and hyperactive behavior, decreases in conduct problems and special needs referrals, improved classroom climate, and decreases in harsh parenting among involved families (CPPRG, 2002; Kaplow et al., 2002; McMahon, Greenberg, & CPPRG, 1995).

Bullying Prevention Program

Broader programs addressing overall school context have also demonstrated success at reducing early violence among youth. The Olweus Bullying Prevention Program (OBPP; Olweus, 1991) is a school-based intervention program targeting the school context, classroom-wide practices, and the individual child. Aimed at children in elementary school through junior high school, the program works to change the environment in which the bullying occurs, producing improvements in school climate and reductions in victimization (Olweus, Limber, & Mihalic, 1999). School administrations are provided with structured guidelines for setting strict rules related to bullying within their schools and teachers are trained to talk with their classrooms about the negative effects and serious nature of bullying and to develop rules and consequences to combat the behavior. At the individual level, children are referred for individual therapy if they are bullying or are the victim of bullying and families are consulted to share school rules. Significant reductions in bullying behavior have been found across a wide-range of cultures and countries within which the program has been implemented (Olweus, 2004). In the United States, studies have suggested that the program may have a suppression effect, slowing increases in students' aggressive, and bullying behaviors (Limber, Nation, Tracy, Melton, & Flerx, 2004; Olweus, 2005).

Coping Power Program

Evidence-based programs that have also demonstrated success with preadolescents and adolescents include the Coping Power program (Lochman & Wells, 1996). Developed as a program to prevent aggressive behavior in preadolescent children at the transition to middle school, Coping Power is sociocognitively oriented, with intervention aimed at multiple social-information processing steps to develop more prosocial cognitive processing among aggressive children. The program consists of 34 group sessions (complemented by intermittent individual sessions) delivered in school over approximately one and a half years. More recently, a parenting program was created to complement the youth program, which involves parents of the affected youth participating in a 16-session group format that includes periodic home visits from interventionists. Coping Power is targeted at reducing delinquency and substance abuse among aggressive youth through increased social competence and self-regulation skills.

Initial efficacy of Coping Power was established through demonstrated reductions in teacher-rated school functioning, self-reported aggression and parent-reported drug and alcohol use, as well as effects on boys' temperament and social information processing (Lochman & Wells, 2002a). Furthermore, measures of self-regulation (assessed through aggression, temperament, and regulation measures) and social competence (assessed through social behavior and cognitions) improved for children receiving the combined (universal and indicated) intervention (Lochman & Wells, 2002b). Coping Power has also demonstrated retention of some key program effects at 1-year follow-up (Lochman & Wells, 2003) including lower rates of substance abuse among moderate-risk children, lower self-reported delinquency, lower levels of covert behavior, and teacher-rated aggression.

Second Step

Second Step (Committee for Children, 2002) is a widely used, violence prevention program geared toward children from kindergarten through middle school. The program aims to decrease and prevent aggressive and risky behaviors while increasing and promoting positive skills. In the middle school years, the Second Step program works in conjunction with the Steps to Respect program, a subprogram that specifically addresses bullying prevention. Second Step has five main themes: empathy and communication, bullying prevention, emotion management and coping, problem solving/decision making, and substance abuse prevention (for full reviews of Second Step, see Fitzgerald & Edstrom, 2006; Frey, Hirschstein & Guzzo, 2000). While decreasing problem behaviors is the main focus of the program, increasing protective factors, including positive social skills and academic competence, is a major goal. Based upon social learning theory (Bandura, 1986) and SIP (Crick & Dodge, 1994), lessons are taught twice a week by teachers or school staff and focus on empathy, social problem solving, and impulse control (Frey et al., 2000).

Evaluations of the Second Step program among urban and suburban students in elementary school indicated a decrease in physical, some aggression (especially on the playground), improved peer relations, and suppression of aggression after completing the program (Cooke et al., 2007; Grossman et al., 1997). Relevant to the goals of this chapter, implementation of Second Step with low-income elementary school age children demonstrated an improvement in children's knowledge of social skills, and decreases in verbal aggression, disruptive behavior, and physical aggression over time (McMahon & Washburn, 2003). Unfortunately, although these results are positive, the lack of a control group in the study design makes interpretation of the results difficult.

Violence Prevention Programming for African American Youth

As demonstrated in the programs reviewed above, clear strides in youth violence prevention have been made. However, reviews of the extant programs aimed at violence prevention among youth find great variability in the systematic implementation, fidelity, and effectiveness of programs aimed at preventing the development of violent and antisocial behavior among adolescents in general and African American youth in particular (e.g., Limbos et al., 2007; Mytton et al., 2002; Thornton et al., 2000). Few of these programs address issues of race, ethnicity, social-economic status, and other sociocultural factors directly within their interventions – with few published programs explicitly targeting African American youth. Following are descriptions of several programs intended specifically for reducing risks and promoting protective factors to stem behavioral health-related problems facing African American youth (see Table 7.2).

Strengthening Families Program

Focusing particularly on African American youth, the Strengthening Families Program (SF) is a universal intervention that applies a biopsychosocial model – with children learning skills individually

Table 7.2 Overview of school-based violence prevention programs specifically targeting African American youth

Program	Target population	Focus	Components	Outcomes	Future directions
Strengthening families	10–14-year-old African American girls and boys	• Preventing drug and alcohol use and early antisocial behavior	• Includes families in intervention • Racial socialization a key component	• Lower risk cognitions • Increased parent–child communication	More efficacy studies needed
Sisters of Nia	5th–9th grade African American girls	• Planning future goals and increasing self-esteem • Peer relationships • Leadership • African American identity	• Ethnic identity component • Future goals planning • Leadership focus	• Increased ethnic identity and values • Increased self-concept • Lower relational aggression	More efficacy and effectiveness studies needed, more focus on peer relations
LEAD	10–12 year olds	• Self-esteem • Self-exploration • Expressive arts	• Arts curriculum • Focus on children at risk for juvenile justice system	• Increased behavioral control • Increased self-esteem • Increased resiliency	Need studies with greater number of participants, longitudinal research
Friend to friend	3rd and 4th grade African American relationally aggressive girls	• Understanding feelings • Increasing social skills • Peer relations • Leadership skills	• Developed through CBPR • Focus on African American girls • Small group intervention with added classroom component	• Increased peer likeability • Decreases in hostile attribution biases • Decreases in teacher rated aggression • High rates of program acceptability	Longitudinal, randomized comparisons
BRAVE	Middle and junior high school	• Preventing alcohol and drug use • Preventing violence	• Mentorship • Vocational training	• Lower alcohol and marijuana use • Trend toward lower violence (both victimization and perpetration)	Studies with broader participant groups (e.g., ages, urban/rural)

and in groups, and then joined by their families to practice family communication (Spoth, Reyes, Redmond & Shin, 1999). The Strengthening African American Families Program (SAAF; Brody et al., 2005) was recently developed out of the Strengthening Families program and was developed for African American children ages 10–14. Targeting rural African American children, the program is designed to prevent alcohol and drug abuse as well as early antisocial behavior. SF and SAAF focus on children and families with weekly parallel sessions for caregivers and children. SAAF focuses particularly on family tradition and practices, based upon research suggesting stronger familial influence over attitudes among African American families as compared with Caucasian families (Spoth et al., 1999). Group meetings focus on communication building across families. For caregivers, the focus is primarily on rule setting, expectations and boundaries, as well as racial socialization. For youth, the focus is on building skills to ward off peer pressure, developing future-oriented goals, and discussing negative effects of alcohol and drug abuse. The program has demonstrated decreases in youths' "risk cognitions" (e.g., their intentions, willingness, and images around alcohol use) through both caregiver and child participation (Gerrard et al., 2006). Relevant to the development of interventions aimed at increasing youth protective factors, improved parent–child communication was found to produce changes in both attitudes and behavior among the youth (Brody et al., 2006).

Sisters of Nia

Sisters of Nia is a cultural enrichment program for African American females in grades 5–9 (for a review see Belgrave, 2009). In order to accomplish their mission of helping girls plan their future and goals, program sessions include skill building in peer and romantic relationships, education about African American female role models, and discussions about health, school achievement, and leadership. The program aims to improve participants' self-esteem, expectations for the future, and relationships with peers through small group format. Groups meet once a week for approximately 4 months, while progression through several topics including relationships, African history and culture, self-concept, creativity, leadership, education, and faith.

In a study investigating the program's impact on girls age 10–12 in an urban school district, Sisters of Nia participants demonstrated higher levels of ethnic identity, stronger Africentric values, and had better self-concept as compared with girls who did not participate in the program (Belgrave, Chase-Vaughn, Gray, Addison, & Cherry, 2000). Girls participating in Sisters of Nia have also demonstrated some changes in their gender role beliefs, a quality that has been tied to beneficial outcomes (e.g., higher school achievement, less risky behavior) for adolescent females (Belgrave et al., 2004). Furthermore, the program has also demonstrated preliminary evidence for lowered relational aggression among African American girls (Belgrave et al.).

Leadership, Education, Achievement, and Development Program

Leadership, Education, Achievement, and Development (LEAD; Shelton, 2009) is a community-based prevention program for children at risk of entering the juvenile justice system. LEAD is conducted within an after-school program in rural middle schools. The 14-week program was developed in partnership with community-academic and school-based input and centers on self-esteem and self-exploration in a small group format within an expressive arts curriculum. In a 2-year study on its' effectiveness among 10–12-year-old African American children, the program demonstrated group effects on behavioral control for the treatment group as compared to a comparison group

(Shelton, 2008). Youth found the program enjoyable and outcomes favoring the treatment group were also present for youths' self-esteem and reports of resiliency (Shelton, 2009). Current research is underway to determine if the behavioral control extends to an avoidance of the juvenile justice system by participating youth, however, initial results suggest that, with expansion over a longer time period, the program may offer important benefit to at-risk African American youth in rural communities (Shelton, 2009).

Friend to Friend Program

Although many violence prevention programs have been developed for preadolescent children, almost all of these programs focus either specifically on boys, or on physical aggression exclusively (Leff et al., 2001). The Friend to Friend program is a preventative intervention for relationally aggressive 3rd and 4th grade girls in urban environments. Relational aggression (i.e., aggression targeting friendships or hurting social status, Crick & Grotpeter, 1995) is prevalent among inner-city female youth and is often predictive of negative outcomes for both aggressors and victims (Leff et al., 2009). Primarily targeted toward African American children and developed with considerable input from school stakeholders, the goal of the program is to increase social skills and peer relationships among girls identified as relationally aggressive by teachers and peers. Friend to Friend is delivered in a small group format, with groups of 8–10 girls meeting during the school day for 20 sessions that cover friendship-making skills, physiological arousal and calming strategies, aspects of SIP (including evaluations intentions), leadership skills, and building social problem solving/ strategies. The program also has a classroom component, allowing the participants from the small groups to develop leadership skills as they assist in leading classroom-wide delivery of the program components (for a review of the program, see Leff et al., 2007).

Initial effectiveness studies of Friend to Friend demonstrated that the program was highly acceptable to both the participating children and teachers. Additionally, an examination of effect size differences in change scores for participating girls versus attention control group participants indicated that the Friend to Friend girls demonstrated lower rates of teacher-rated relational and physical aggression (effect sizes were large and moderate to small for relational and physical aggression, respectively), increased peer likeability, greater decreases in hostile attribution biases, and an improvement in participants feelings of loneliness (Leff et al., 2009). Current research is examining the effects of Friend to Friend through a large-scale randomized design.

The Building Resiliency and Vocational Excellence Program

A similar program has recently been developed targeting African American children in middle school. The Building Resiliency and Vocational Excellence (BRAVE; Griffin et al., 2009) program is aimed at preventing alcohol, drug use, and violence among middle and junior-high school students. Through a mentorship model, youth meet for 90-min, two to three times a week across 9-weeks of the school year. Curriculum revolves around a life-skills building program, violence prevention, character building (e.g., behavioral maturity, gender expectations), career planning, and vocational training. Participants were also provided with mentors that they were able to meet with on a one-on-one basis in order to encourage generalizability outside the school system to the broader community. In a study of African American children ($N = 199$) in sixth through eight grade (Griffin et al., 2009), intervention effects were found for some substance use variables – including alcohol and marijuana use – and a small, trending (nonsignificant) effect on violence victimization and perpetration. The authors suggest that an expansion of the ages involved, as well as the length of time of the program may help to increase program effects (Griffin et al., 2009).

New Directions in Youth Violence Prevention Programming

New directions in violence prevention have moved further from focusing primarily on individuals and proximal factors to considering community-level factors in the design (Griffith et al., 2008). As part of this movement, community-based participatory research (CBPR) has received growing attention as an approach to address manifold public health concerns, especially in ethnic minority and other disadvantaged communities (Brownson, Riley, & Bruce, 1998; Israel et al., 2001; Viswanathan et al., 2004). CBPR is a research paradigm designed to ensure and establish structures for collaboration and participation in all aspects of the research process by engaging community members, representatives of community organizations, policy makers, and academic researchers. The goal of CBPR is to improve the health and well-being of communities by integrating feedback from key members of the community with empirically supported strategies and techniques (Nastasi et al., 2000; USDHHS, 2003). CBPR has particular relevance to ethnic minority and economically disadvantaged communities because it helps to ensure that the voice of the community is respected and also reflected in how the chosen violence prevention interventions are adapted, implemented, and evaluated.

This research paradigm differs from conventional research in several fundamental ways, most notably in its reliance on a nonhierarchical partnership between community members and academic researchers (see Leff, Costigan, & Power, 2004). All partners are engaged in implementing the intervention and helping to translate results into action. Within this framework, community members are active participants in the research process, as opposed to subjects on whom the research is conducted. Further, academic researchers and community partners both are viewed as experts and new learners and bi-directional teaching is an integral part of the CBPR process. CBPR utilizes valuable key stakeholder feedback within the context of best practice proven intervention strategies to help ensure that the resulting programs are culturally sensitive, meaningful, and help to promote sustainability (Leff et al., 2004; Nastasi et al., 2000).

A CBPR project to develop a multicomponent violence prevention program for urban African American adolescents within a number of after-school settings (e.g., recreation centers, church-based programs, school-based programs), the PARTNERS Program, is instructive for thinking through additional future next steps in violence prevention efforts (Leff et al., in press). Sponsored by a cooperative agreement with the Centers for Disease Control and Prevention, the PARTNERS Program has entailed academic researchers and community leaders forming research teams to systematically review best practice interventions on violence prevention programming among youth and to provide suggestions for designing and/or adapting a violence prevention curriculum to best meet the needs of urban African American teenagers. Although the content of many traditional programs was viewed as being relevant and important to the local community from the perspective of the participating community leaders, they also identified that leadership promotion strategies were largely absent from many best practice programs. More specifically, community stakeholders indicated that teaching youth social cognitive strategies (to include social information processing) to prevent violence within after-school contexts would not be sufficient without also preparing these individuals for applying these strategies to become future leaders within their community.

The PARTNERS Program is now being evaluated as part of community-based clinical trial to determine program acceptability and impact. As has been demonstrated in other recent violence prevention efforts (see Griffith et al., 2008), the use of a CBPR model as part of the PARTNERS Program helps to ensure that resulting violence prevention programming for African Americans will be empirically based and meaningful for participants. Further, preliminary findings from the program suggest that future interventions designed to address violence prevention among African American youngsters should focus upon ways to increase resiliency and leadership among youth while also trying to reduce levels of aggression and associated problematic behaviors that foreshadow violence.

Conclusion

Community violence continues to be a major public health issue. While violence impacts all communities, it has disproportionately dire consequences for inner-city African American communities and, above all, its youth. Although significant gains in violence prevention programming have been made, few of these efforts attend directly to the contextual and cultural realties of African American youth and address factors that render this population more vulnerable to community violence. However, the programs mentioned in this chapter demonstrate the promise of early intervention to reduce violence among youth. Indeed, all of them demonstrate that any attempts for solutions will require comprehensive multilevel approaches that consider multiple contexts (family–school–community) in their designs and involve reductions in aggressive behaviors and the promotion of protective factors that range from sociocognitive skills to academic and social skills. Moreover, expansion of additional programs to include more diverse populations and partnership-based methodology, and future research on the specific factors relevant to intervention success among African American inner-city youth within a developmental-ecological framework, would add crucial elements to the growing evidence favoring early and comprehensive interventions to reduce and prevent youth violence.

References

A. Bandura, *Social foundations of thought and action: A social cognitive theory.* Englewood Cliffs, NJ: Prentice-Hall, Inc. (1986)

F.Z. Belgrave, *African American Girls: Reframing Perceptions and Changing Experiences. Advancing Responsible Adolescent Development* (Springer Science, New York, 2009)

F.Z. Belgrave, G. Chase-Vaughn, F. Gray, J. Dixon-Addison, V.R. Cherry, The effectiveness of a culture and gender specific intervention for increasing resiliency among African American pre-adolescent females. Journal of Black Psychology **26**(2), 123–147 (2000)

F.Z. Belgrave, M.C. Reed, L.E. Plybon, D.S. Butler, K.W. Allison, T. Davis, An evaluation of Sisters of Nia: A cultural program for African American girls. The journal of Black Psychology **30**(3), 329–343 (2004)

G. Botvin, K.W. Griffin, T.D. Nichols, Preventing youth violence and delinquency through a universal school-based prevention approach. Prevention Science **7**(4), 403–408 (2006)

P. Boxer, E.F. Dubow, A social-cognitive information-processing model for school-based aggression reduction and prevention programs: Issues for research and practice. Applied & Preventive Psychology **10**(3), 177–192 (2001)

G.H. Brody, V.M. Murry, Y. Chen, S.M. Kogan, A.C. Brown, Effects of family risk factors on dosage and efficacy of a family-centered preventive intervention for rural African Americans. Prevention Science **7**(3), 281–291 (2006)

G.H. Brody, V.M. Murry, L. McNair, Y. Chen, F.X. Gibbons, M. Gerrard et al., Linking changes in parenting to parent-child relationship quality and youth self-control: The strong African American families program. Journal of Research on Adolescence **15**(1), 47–69 (2005)

L.M. Broidy, D.S. Nagin, R.E. Tremblay, J.E. Bates, B. Brame, K.A. Dodge et al., Developmental trajectories of childhood disruptive behaviors and adolescent delinquency: A six-site, cross-national study. Developmental Psychology. Special Issue: Violent children **39**(2), 222–245 (2003)

U. Bronfenbrenner, Toward an experimental ecology of human development. American Psychologist **32**(7), 513–531 (1977)

R.C. Brownson, P. Riley, T.A. Bruce, Demonstration projects in community based prevention. Journal of Public Health Management Practice **4**, 66–77 (1998)

Bureau of Justice Statistics. (2007). [Data file]. *Homicide trends in the U.S.: Age, gender, and race trends.* Retrieved November 14, 2009, from http://www.ojp.usdoj.gov/bjs/homicide/ageracesex.html

Centers for Disease Control and Prevention, National Center for Injury Prevention and Control, *Youth violence: facts at a glance* (Centers for Disease Control and Prevention, Division of Violence Prevention, Atlanta, GA, 2009)

Centers for Disease Control and Prevention. The effectiveness of universal school-based programs for the prevention of violent and aggressive behavior: A report on recommendations of the Task Force on Community Preventive Services. Morbidity and Mortality Weekly Report, 56, (pp. 1–12). Centers for Disease Control and Prevention, Division of Violence Prevention, Atlanta, GA (2007)

Centers for Disease Control and Prevention, National Center for Injury Prevention and Control (2009a). [Online]. *Web-based Injury Statistics Query and Reporting System.* Retrieved November 14, 2009, from http://www.cdc.gov/injury/wisqars/index.html

Committee for Children. Secondstep: A violence prevention curriculum grades 4–5 teacher 5 guide (3d Ed.). Seattle, WA: author (2002)

Conduct Problems Prevention Research Group, Evaluation of the first 3 years of the Fast Track prevention trial with children at high risk for adolescent conduct problems. Journal of Abnormal Child Psychology **30**, 19–36 (2002)

Conduct Problems Prevention Research Group, A developmental and clinical model for the prevention of conduct disorders: The FAST Track Program. Development and Psychopathology **4**, 509–527 (1992)

M.B. Cooke, J. Ford, J. Levine, C. Bourke, L. Newell, G. Lapidus, The effects of city-wide implementation of "*Second Step*" on elementary school students' prosocial and aggressive behaviors. Journal of Primary Prevention **28**, 93–115 (2007)

M. Cooley-Strickland, T.J. Quille, R.S. Griffin, E.A. Stuart, C.P. Bradshaw, D. Furr-Holden, Community violence and youth: Affect, behavior, substance use, and academics. Clinical Child and Family Psychology Review **12**(2), 127–156 (2009)

N.R. Crick, K.A. Dodge, A review and reformulation of social information-processing mechanisms in children's social adjustment. Psychological Bulletin **115**(1), 74–101 (1994)

N.R. Crick, J.K. Grotpeter, Relational aggression, gender and social-psychological adjustment. Child Development **66**, 710–722 (1995)

P. Fitzgerald, L.V.S. Edstrom, Second Step: A violence prevention curriculum. In S. R. Jimerson, & M. J. Furlong (Eds.), *The handbook of school violence and school safety: From research to practice* (pp. 383–394). Mahwah, NJ: Erlbaum (2006)

K.S. Frey, M.K. Hirschstein, B.A. Guzzo, Second Step: Preventing aggression by promoting social competence. Journal of Emotional & Behavioral Disorders **8**, 102–112 (2000)

M. Gerrard, F.X. Gibbons, G.H. Brody, V.M. Murry, M.J. Cleveland, T.A. Wills, A theory-based dual-focus alcohol intervention for preadolescents: The strong African American families program. Psychology of Addictive Behaviors **20**(2), 185–195 (2006)

D.M. Griffith, J.O. Allen, M.A. Zimmerman, S. Morrel-Samuels, T.M. Reischl, S.E. Cohen et al., Organizational empowerment in community mobilization to address youth violence. American Journal of Preventive Medicine **34**, 89–99 (2008)

J.P. Griffin, R.C. Holliday, E. Frazier, R.L. Braithwaite, The BRAVE (building resiliency and vocational excellence) program: Evaluation findings for a career-oriented substance abuse and violence preventive intervention. Journal of Health Care for the Poor and Underserved **20**(3), 798–816 (2009)

D.C. Grossman, H.J. Neckerman, T.D. Koepsell, P.Y. Liu, K.N. Asher, K. Beland, K. Frey, F.P Rivara, Effectiveness of a violence prevention curriculum among children in elementary school: A randomized control trial. Journal of the American Medical Association **227**(20), 1605–1611 (1997)

N.G. Guerra, L.R. Huesmann, A. Spindler, Community violence exposure, social cognition, and aggression among urban elementary school children. Child Development **74**(5), 1561–1576 (2003)

R. Hahn, D. Fuqua-Whitley, H. Wethington, J. Lowy, A. Crosby et al., Effectiveness of universal school-based programs to prevent violent and aggressive behavior: A systematic review. American Journal of Preventive Medicine **33**, 114–129 (2007)

D. Henry, N. Guerra, R. Huesmann, P. Tolan, R. VanAcker, L. Eron, Normative influences on aggression in urban elementary school classrooms. American Journal of Community Psychology **28**(1), 59–81 (2000)

B.A. Israel, R. Lichtenstein, P. Lantz, R. McGranaghan, A. Allen, J.R. Guzman et al., The Detroit Community-Academic Urban Research Center: development, implementation, and evaluation. J Public Health Manag Pract. **7**, 1–19 (2001)

J.B. Kaplow, P.J. Curran, K.A. Dodge, The Conduct Problems Prevention Research Group, Child, parent, and peer predictors of early-onset substance use: A multisite longitudinal study. Journal of Abnormal Child Psychology **30**, 199–216 (2002)

S.S. Leff, J. Angelucci, A.B. Goldstein, L. Cardaciotto, M.S. Paskewich, M.B. Grossman, Using a participatory action research model to create a school-based intervention program for relationally aggressive girls: The Friend to Friend Program, in *Handbook of Prevention and Intervention in Peer Harassment, Victimization, and Bullying (pp. 199–218)*, ed. by J. Zins, M. Elias, C. Maher (Haworth, New York, 2007)

S.S. Leff, T.E. Costigan, T.J. Power, Using participatory-action research to develop a playground-based prevention program. Journal of School Psychology **42**, 3–21 (2004)

S.S. Leff, R.L. Gullan, B.S. Paskewich, S. Abdul-Kabir, A.F. Jawad, M. Grossman et al., An initial evaluation of a culturally-adapted social problem solving and relational aggression prevention program for urban African American relationally aggressive girls. Journal of Prevention and Intervention in the Community **37**, 1–15 (2009)

S.S. Leff, T.J. Power, P.H. Manz, T.E. Costigan, L.A. Nabors, School-based aggression prevention programs for young children: Current status and implications for violence prevention. School Psychology Review **30**(3), 344–362 (2001)

S.S. Leff, D.E. Thomas, N. Vaughn, N. Thomas, J.P. MacEvoy, et al., Using community-based participatory research to develop the PARTNERS violence prevention program. *Progress in Community Health Partnerships: Research, Education, and Action* **4**(3), 207–216 (2010)

S.P. Limber, M. Nation, A.J. Tracy, G.B. Melton, V. Flerx, Implementation of the Olweus bullying prevention program in the southeastern united states, in *Bullying in schools: How successful can interventions be?* ed. by P.K. Smith, D. Pepler, K. Rigby (Cambridge University Press, New York, 2004), pp. 55–79

M.A. Limbos, L.S. Chan, C. Warf, A. Schneir, E. Iverson, P. Shekelle et al., Effectiveness of interventions to prevent youth violence: A systematic review. American Journal of Preventive Medicine **33**(1), 65–74 (2007)

J.E. Lochman, K.C. Wells, A social-cognitive intervention with aggressive children: Prevention effects and contextual implementation issues, in *Preventing childhood disorders, substance abuse, and delinquency*, ed. by R.D. Peters, R.J. McMahon (Sage, Thousand Oaks, CA, 1996), pp. 111–143

J.E. Lochman, K.C. Wells, Contextual social-cognitive mediators and child outcome: A test of the theoretical model in the coping power program. Development and Psychopathology **14**(4), 945–967 (2002a)

J.E. Lochman, K.C. Wells, The coping power program at the middle-school transition: Universal and indicated prevention effects. Psychology of Addictive Behaviors **16**(4), S40–S54 (2002b)

J.E. Lochman, K.C. Wells, Effectiveness of the coping power program and of classroom intervention with aggressive children: Outcomes at a 1-year follow-up. Behavior Therapy. Special Issue: Behaviorally Oriented Interventions for Children with Aggressive Behavior and/or Conduct Problems **34**(4), 493–515 (2003)

R. Loeber, D.P. Farrington, M. Stouthamer-Loeber, T.E. Moffitt, A. Caspi, The development of male offending: Key findings from the first decade of the Pittsburgh youth study. Studies on Crime & Crime Prevention **7**(2), 141–171 (1998a)

R. Loeber, D.P. Farrington, M. Stouthamer-Loeber, T.E. Moffitt, A. Caspi, D. Lynam, Male mental health problems, psychopathy, and personality traits: Key findings from the first 14 years of the Pittsburgh youth study. Clinical Child and Family Psychology Review **4**(4), 273–297 (2001)

R. Loeber, D.P. Farrington, D.A. Waschbusch, Serious and violent juvenile offenders, in *Serious and Violent Juvenile Offenders: Risk Factors and Successful Interventions*, ed. by R. Loeber, D.P. Farrington (Sage, Thousand Oaks, CA, 1998b), pp. 13–29

T. Mathews, M. Dempsey, S. Overstreet, Effects of exposure to community violence on school functioning: The mediating role of posttraumatic stress symptoms. Behaviour Research and Therapy **47**, 586–591 (2009)

R.J. McMahon, M.T. Greenberg, Conduct Problems Prevention Research Group, The Fast Track Program: A developmentally focused intervention for children with conduct problems. Clinician's Research Digest, Supplemental Bulletin **13**, 1–2 (1995)

S.D. McMahon, J.J. Washbum, Violence prevention: An evaluation of program effects with urban African American students. Journal of Primary Prevention **24**, 43–62 (2003)

Multisite Violence Prevention Project, The ecological effects of universal and selective violence prevention programs for middle school students: A randomized trial. *Journal of Consulting and Clinical Psychology*, **77**(3), 526–542 (2009)

J.A. Mytton, C. DiGuiseppi, D.A. Gough, R.S. Taylor, S. Logan, School-based violence prevention programs: Systematic review of secondary prevention trials. Archives of Pediatrics & Adolescent Medicine **156**(8), 752–762 (2002)

D. Nagin, R.E. Tremblay, Trajectories of boys' physical aggression, opposition, and hyperactivity on the path to physically violent and nonviolent juvenile delinquency. Child Development **70**, 1181–1196 (1999)

B.K. Nastasi, K. Varjas, S.L. Schensul, K.T. Silva, J.J. Schensul, P. Ratnayake et al., The participatory intervention model: A framework for conceptualizing and promoting intervention acceptability. School Psychology Quarterly **15**, 207–232 (2000)

D. Olweus, Bully/victim problems among schoolchildren: Basic facts and effects of a school based intervention program, in *The development and treatment of aggression*, ed. by D.J. Pepler, K.H. Rubin (Erlbaum, Hillsdale, NJ, 1991), pp. 411–448

D. Olweus, The Olweus bullying prevention programme: Design and implementation issues and a new national initiative in Norway, in *Bullying in schools: How successful can interventions be?* ed. by P.K. Smith, D. Pepler, K. Rigby (Cambridge University Press, New York, 2004), pp. 13–36

D. Olweus, A useful evaluation design, and effects of the Olweus bullying prevention program. Psychology, Crime & Law. Special Issue: Working with Aggression and Violence. Assessment, Prevention and Treatment **11**(4), 389–402 (2005)

D. Olweus, S. Limber, S. Mihalic, *Blueprints for Violence Prevention: Book Nine – Bullying Prevention Program* (University of Colorado, Boulder, 1999)

E.J. Ozer, Contextual effects in school-based violence prevention programs: Conceptual framework and empirical review. Journal of Primary Prevention **27**, 315–340 (2006)

D. Shelton, Translating theory into practice: Results of a 2-year trial for the LEAD programme. Journal of Psychiatric and Mental Health Nursing **15**(4), 313–321 (2008)

D. Shelton, Leadership, education, achievement, and development: A nursing intervention for prevention of youthful offending behavior. Journal of the American Psychiatric Nurses Association **14**(6), 429–441 (2009)

R. Spano, A.T. Vazsonyi, J. Bolland, Does parenting mediate the effects of exposure to violent behavior? An ecological-transactional model of community violence. Journal of Adolescence **32**, 1321–1341 (2009)

M.B. Spencer, Social and cultural influences on school adjustment: The application of an identity-focused cultural ecological perspective. Educational Psychologist **34**(1), 43–57 (1999)

M.B. Spencer, Phenomenology and ecological systems theory: Development of Diverse Groups, in *Handbook of Child Psychology,* ed. by R.M. Lerner, W. Damon. Theoretical models of human development, vol. 1, 6th edn. (Wiley, Hoboken, NJ, 2006), pp. 829–893

M.B. Spencer, D. Dupree, M. Cunningham, V. Harpalani, M. Muñoz-Miller, Vulnerability to violence: A contextually-sensitive, developmental perspective on African American adolescents. Journal of Social Issues. Special Issue: Youth perspectives on violence and injustice **59**(1), 33–49 (2003)

M.B. Spencer, C. Jones-Walker, Interventions and services offered to former juvenile offenders reentering their communities: An analysis of program effectiveness. Youth Violence and Juvenile Justice **2**(1), 88–97 (2004)

R. Spoth, M.L. Reyes, C. Redmond, C. Shin, Assessing a public health approach to delay onset and progression of adolescent substance use: Latent transition and log-linear analyses of longitudinal family preventive intervention outcomes. Journal of Consulting and Clinical Psychology **67**(5), 619–630 (1999)

K.J. Swick, R.D. Williams, An analysis of Bronfenbrenner's bio-ecological perspective for early childhood educators: Implications for working with families experiencing stress. Early Childhood Education Journal **33**(5), 371–378 (2006)

D.E. Thomas, K.L. Bierman, The Conduct Problems Prevention Research Group, The impact of classroom aggression on the development of aggressive behavior problems in children. Development and Psychopathology **18**(2), 471–487 (2006)

D.E. Thomas, K.L. Bierman, C.J. Powers, The Conduct Problems Prevention Research Group, The impact of peer aggression and classroom climate on the development of aggressive behavior problems. Child Development **82**(3), 751–757 (2011)

D.E. Thomas, S. Coard, H. Stevenson, K. Bentley, P. Zamel, Race and emotional factors predicting teacher observations of classroom behavioral adjustment for African American male youth. Psychology in the Schools **46**(2), 184–196 (2009)

D.E. Thomas, H. Stevenson, Gender risks and education: The particular classroom challenges for urban, low-income African American boys. Review of Research in Education: Special Issue on Risk, Schooling, and Equity **33**, 160–180 (2009)

T.N. Thornton, C.A. Craft, L.L. Dahlberg, B.S. Lynch, K. Baer, *Best practices of youth violence prevention: A sourcebook for community action* (Centers for Disease Control, Atlanta, GA, 2000)

U. S. Department of Health and Human Services (2001). *Youth Violence: A Report of the Surgeon General. Final Report.* Washington, DC: USDHHS, Office of the Surgeon General.

U. S. Department of Health and Human Services, *The role of community-based participatory research: creating partnerships, improving health* (Agency for Healthcare Research and Quality, Rockville, MD, 2003)

M. Viswanathan, A. Ammerman, E. Eng, G. Gartlehner, K.N. Lohr, D. Griffith et al., *Community-based participatory research: assessing the evidence, Summary, evidence report/technology assessment* (Agency for Healthcare Research and Quality, Rockville, MD, 2004)

Chapter 8
Factor Structure and Expression of Depressive Symptoms in a Community Sample of African American Adolescents Living in Urban Public Housing

Von E. Nebbitt, Andridia Mapson, and Ajita Robinson

Introduction

The last two decades have seen an increased interest in minority youth mental health. Researchers have sought to understand and explicate the expression and structure of depression in minority youth. Researchers have questioned whether urban minority youth express depressive symptoms similar to nonminority urban youth (Davis & Stevenson, 2006; Roelofs, Meesters, Mijke ter Huurne, Lotte Bamelis, & Muris, 2006; Shaffer, Forehand, Kotchick, & The Family Health Project Research Group, 2002). Researchers have also questioned whether the structure of depression differs by race and ethnicity and how, or whether, the structure of depression changes across the span of adolescence (Gullone, Ollendick, & King, 2006; Schraedley, Gotlib, & Hayward, 1999; Wichstrom, 1999; Wight, Aneshensel, Botticello, & Sepulveda, 2005). Using a sample of 788 African American youth, this chapter contributes to knowledge on the expression and factor structure of depressive symptoms in urban African American youth, living in urban public housing developments by evaluating the structural equivalences of depression using the Center for Epidemiologic Depression Scale (CES-D). This chapter also assesses differences between females and males and across three age groups of adolescents (early, middle, and late).

Review of the Literature

Prevalence and Service Use

The mental health of youth is a major public health concern (HHS, 2000). According to *Healthy People 2010*, one in five youth between the ages 9 and 17 years currently has a diagnosable mental disorder (HHS, 2000). Approximately 9% of adolescents in the United States suffer from major depression disorder (MDD) at any given time (Birmaher, Ryan, & Wiliamson, 1996; Office of Applied Studies, 2005). Lifetime prevalence of MDD for adolescents has been estimated at 14% (Office of Applied Studies). Research shows that 50% of all lifetime mental illness began by age 14 (NIMH, 2009). Approximately 90% of the MDD episodes remit within 2 years, and the average length of a MDD episode being between 6 and 7 months (Birmaher et al.). More than half of

V.E. Nebbitt (✉)
School of Social Work, Howard University, Washington, DC, USA
e-mail: vnebbitt_@howard.edu

A.J. Lemelle et al. (eds.), *Handbook of African American Health: Social and Behavioral Interventions*,
DOI 10.1007/978-1-4419-9616-9_8, © Springer Science+Business Media, LLC 2011

all youth with MDD experience a relapse 1–2 years after treatment has ended: relapse is more the rule than the exception (Lagged & Dunn, 2003). Among adolescents aged 12–17 who reported experiencing a Major Depression Episode (MDE) within the previous year, less than half (40.3%) reported having received treatment for depression during that time (The NSDUH Report, 2005). Seventy percent of all adolescents with MDD experience a relapse within 5 years post treatment Franko et al., (2005).

Gender Differences

During adolescence, girls are twice as likely as boys to develop MDD (13.0% versus 5.0%) and the symptoms of depression increase from childhood to adolescence (Birmaher et al., 1996; Cicchetti & Toth, 1998; Hankins et al., 1998; Nolen-Hoeksema & Girgus, 1994; Office of Applied Studies, 2005; Wichstrom, 1999). Franko and colleagues looked at whether adolescent girls' age was associated with ethnicity and depressive symptoms and found that age was a moderating factor (Franko et al., 2005). White adolescent girls' depressive symptoms showed decreasing depression scores with increasing age; whereas, African American girls depression scores were similar across ages (Franko et al.). Depression among African American adolescent boys has been linked to having perceived fewer future opportunities (Hawkins, Hawkins, Sabatino, & Ley, 1998), low neighborhood social capital, and kinship social support (Stevenson, 1998). Additional research is needed to fully understand gender differences in expressive of depressive symptoms.

Ethnic Differences

Though the literature on childhood and adolescent depression has grown exponentially over the last decade, a glaring limitation in the literature is the persistent lack of studies on the expression and development of depression among minority youth (Shaffer et al., 2002; Tandon & Solomon, 2009). The limited research results that exists on depressive symptoms in African American youth are inconsistent. In a review of the outcomes facing African American youth, Taylor (1995) concluded that many studies found lower rates of depressive symptomatology in African American adolescents compared to White adolescents. Schraedley and colleagues (1999) found lower rates of depressive symptoms in African American adolescents compared to counterparts from other ethnic groups (Tandon & Solomon). In contrast, others (Franko et al., 2005; Roberts, Chen, & Solovitz, 1995; Roberts, Roberts, & Chen, 1997) have found higher rates of depressive symptoms in African American adolescents compared to their White counterparts, whereas Schraedley, Gotlab, and Hayward (1999) found no significant difference between African American adolescents and White adolescents. Wight and colleagues (as cited in Tandon & Solomon) conducted a more recent study that found higher depressive symptoms among African American 7th–12th graders.

Causes and Correlates

There is no mono-causal explanation for the onset of depression in most adolescents; rather, a combination of environmental, neurological, and genetic variables are responsible for depressive symptoms (Lagged & Dunn, 2003; NIMH, 2009). Several factors increase the risk of depression, including a family history of mood disorders and stressful life events (NAMI, 2010). Youth with depressed parents may be at risk for depression and suffer the negative psychological effects of having a depressed parent whose symptoms may decrease responsiveness and increase negative evaluations (Lagged & Dunn). Both family functioning and parent–child bonding are weakened by maternal depression, and impaired family functioning, in the form of parental rejection, is associated with depression in adolescents (Muris, Schmidt, Lambrichs, & Meesters, 2001). Parental psychopathology consistently has been found as the strongest risk factor for adolescent depression (Kessler, Avenevoli, & Merikangas, 2001). Depressive disorders co-occur at a high rates with other psychological problems in children and adolescents (Hammen & Compas, 1994). Between 40 and 70% of depressed children have at least one comorbid diagnosis (Birmaher et al., 1996). The most frequently cited comorbid diagnoses include anxiety and conduct disorders (Hammen & Compas). The co-occurrence of mental health disorders is also true for community-based nonclinical populations (i.e., youth for whom symptoms do not meet clinical criteria), suggesting that the co-occurrence of depression with other disorders probably exist on a continuum and is not exclusive to disorders at levels of clinical significance (cf., Compas et al., 1993).

Several risk factors for depression in adolescents have been identified in the empirical literature. These risk factors include community risk factors (social isolation, poverty, and affiliation with antisocial peers), family risk factors (low levels of parental warmth and family dysfunction), and individual level factors (gender, temperament, and antisocial behavior) (Garber, 2006; Levisohn et al., 1998). The most salient risk factor specific for depression in African American adolescents is low socioeconomic status (Tandon & Solomon, 2009). Additionally, studies that looked at depression and family functioning, and family structure found associations between these variables (Tandon & Solomon). Zimmerman and colleagues (2000) examined the role that familial factors play in moderating the effects of depressive symptoms in African American males; they found that parental support buffered the effect of stressful events on depressive symptoms. Nebbitt and Lombe (2010) found community cohesion provided similar buffering effects.

This review of the literature provides a sound empirical foundation and justification for a continuous investigation of depressive symptoms in African American youth. However, sound empirical evidence on depression within African American youth must be built on reliable measures. This chapter attempts to contribute this body of knowledge by examining the factor structure of depression using the CES-D in a sample of African American youth within the context of urban public housing.

Significance of Context: African American Youth in Public Housing

Much of human activity takes place in the social context of daily life (Bandura, 1997). The social context plays a critical role in adolescent's mental health and development. African American youth are disproportionately over-represented in neighborhoods marked by poverty, alternative market activities, and chronic levels of community violence (National Center for Child Poverty, 2001; Urban Institute, 1997). It is not unusual that they also experience poorer outcomes compared to other groups of youth. It is important to note, however, that even within challenging environments, like urban public housing, many African American youth manage to avoid life-compromising situations and become well-functioning adults (Furstenberg, Cook, Eceles, Elder, & Sameroff, 1999; Smith, Lizotte, Thornberry, & Krohn, 1995).

Methods

Research Settings

This study was conducted in location-based family public housing developments in four large cities. Adolescents living in elderly and disabled housing and Section 8 apartments were not included in this sample.

Site 1 is large housing development located in a large Northeast city. Site 1 is comprised of 96 six-story buildings with 3,142 apartments occupying six square city blocks. Approximately 3,000 families reside in Site 1. African American (60%) and Latino (33%) families comprise over 90% of the population. Seventy-five percent of the residents are under the age of 18 and 60% are between the ages 10 and 18. In 2006, the median household income was slightly over $20,000 (Department of Resident Service, 2007).

Site 2 comprised two smaller housing developments located in a large Mid-Atlantic city. The first housing development in site 2 consists of 58 two-story barrack style buildings with 234 units. The second housing development in site 2 consists of 108 two-story barrack style buildings comprising 432 apartments. Both developments are located within close proximity of each other. Two hundred and twenty-three families reside in development one and 426 families reside in development two. African American families comprise 98% of the population in these two developments. Fifty-eight percent of the residents are under the age of 18. In 2006, the median household income was approximately $10,200 (Office of Resident Services, 2006).

Site 3 included two housing developments (one two-story barrack style housing development and two 17 story highrise developments) in a large Northeast city. The first development in Site 3 consist of 43 building containing 535 units and the second development hosted 499 units in two 17 story highrise buildings. The two developments had approximately 2,230 residents, 63% under the age of 21. Ninety-eight percent of the residents were African American ($N=2,185$). The 2007 median household income in the two housing developments was approximately $7,500.

Site 4 included three housing developments: one mixed high-rise and low-rise development and two barrack style developments. The 2005 median household income in the three housing developments was $6,864. Over 75% of the residents had incomes below the official poverty line. Approximately 90% of the households were female-headed. The three developments housed approximately 3,500 residents, 47% are under the age of 18. Ninety-six percent of the residents were African American (St. Louis Housing Authority, 2006).

Procedures

Youth were eligible to participate if they were between the ages of 11 and 21, resided in one of the target housing developments, could demonstrate the capacity to give informed consent and were able to provide both youth assent and parental written informed consent. The local housing authorities in each city approved this exploration. Advertisement of the study was done using flyers and announcements at local social service agencies and community centers. Research assistants posted flyers in the housing developments, in community centers, and in agencies around the housing developments. The flyers included a brief overview of the study, the date and location for data collection, and contact information for the PI and research assistant. The department of recreation provided space in community centers located in each housing development where youth were screened, provided consent and the survey was administrated.

Once the initial group of youth came to the community center in response to our announcements, we used respondent driven sampling (RDS) (Heckathorn, 1997). RDS is an excellent method to use when conducting research in communities that are highly stigmatized, has mistrust for outsiders, and has strong privacy concerns, leading to low participation in research or giving unreliable answers to protect their privacy (Heckathorn). Examples include populations living in blighted urban areas and concentrated poverty, like public housing projects. RDS is a form of chain-referral sampling that correct sampling biases typically associated with snowball and chain-referral sampling by producing a sample that is independent of the initial participants from which sampling begins (Heckathorn). IRB approval was obtained from Howard University (IRB # 06-SW-05).

Data Collections

Once an adequate sample was recruited, youth who met the inclusion criteria were asked to meet at the designated data collection sites. During this meeting the PI provided an overview of the study, its risk and benefits, and explained the rights of human participants in research. The PI emphasized that participants could refuse to answer any questions on the survey and that they could dropout of the study at anytime without consequences. Youth were provided parental consent and youth assent forms. After providing youth assent and parental consent, youth were administered the Capacity-to-Consent Screen (CSS). The CCS is a screening tool that assesses youths' mental capacity to give informed assent. A score above 8 indicates a minimum capacity to give informed consent. Only youth who score above 8 on the CCS and who provided parental consent and youth assent (18 and younger) and informed consent (18 and older) were administrated the survey instrument for this study.

After consent was established and screening was completed, youth met in groups of 10–15 to complete the survey. The survey was composed of several standardized measures to assess youths' perception of their housing development and their parents' behavior. The instrument also assessed youths' health-risk behavior and mental health symptoms. Two African American graduate students administrated the survey: one student read the questions and the other student read the possible responses. Youth circled the desired response. The survey took approximately 40 min to complete. Youth received $15 and a snack for their participation.

Measure

Depressive symptoms were assessed using the Center for Epidemiologic Studies Depression Scale (CES-D). The CES-D was developed at the Center for Epidemiologic Studies, a division of the National Institutes of Mental Health (Radloff, 1977). The CES-D is a self-report scale developed from existing depressive inventories (see, for example, Beck et al., 1961; MMPI, 1960; Zung, 1965). CES-D includes 20 items that survey mood, somatic complaints, interactions with others, and motor functioning. Responses are rated on a four-point Likert scale, ranging from 0 to 3, with anchor points in terms of days per week (less than 1 day) to (5–7 days). The theoretical range is 0–60, with higher scores representing greater symptoms. Adults with a final score of 16 or higher are typically identified as a depressive "case." This generally represents someone that has reported at least six items to be frequently present over the course of the previous week, or most of the 20 items to be present for a shorter duration. The 16-cutoff point has been used in adult samples, but this cutoff point has yield estimated prevalence of 50% or more in adolescents (Nebbitt & Lombe, 2007; Rushton, Forcier, & Schectman, 2002). Roberts et al., (1991) suggest a cutoff of 24 for adolescents on the basis of improved ability to detect DSM-IV defined depression. Roberts et al., (1991) suggest categorizing youth according to level of depressive symptoms. They suggest reporting results as minimal depressive symptoms (0–15), mild depressive symptoms (16–23), and moderate/severe depressive symptoms (24+).

CES-D (Radloff, 1977) has been the workhorse of depression epidemiology (Comstock & Helsing, 1976; Radloff & Locke, 1986). It is understandable and accessible to underserved populations such as the economically disadvantaged groups. The scale is one of the most widely used instruments in the field of psychiatric epidemiology (Murphy, 2002; Naughton & Wiklund, 1993; Nezu et al., 2002; Snaith, 1993). A recent PubMed search yielded 890 articles indexed under the keywords "Center for Epidemiologic Studies Depression Scale."

Among community samples, internal consistency estimates range from 0.8 to 0.9; test–retest reliability ranging from 2 weeks to 1 year, reported between 0.4 and 0.7 (Devins et al., 1988; Nebbitt & Lombe, 2007; Radloff, 1977). Four factors – depressed affect, positive affect, somatic and retarded activity, and interpersonal – have consistently, but not always, been reported for the CES-D (Devins et al.; Golding & Aneshensel, 1989; Radloff, Sheehan et al., 1995). The factors appear to be generally robust across time (Sheehan et al.), populations varying in ethnicity (Golding et al., 1991; Golding & Aneshensel), and health (Devins et al.). Measuring the prevalence of depressive symptoms among specific subgroups of the community, such as the homeless (Wong, 2000), adolescents (Goodman & Whitaker, 2002), and the elderly population (Beekman, Geerlings, Deeg et al., 2002) has also been reported. Despite the CES-D's widespread use, there is little published research on the expression and development of depressive symptoms on African American youth living in public housing using the CES-D (see Nebbitt & Lombe for exception) and no research exist on the factor structure of depression using CES-D in this vulnerable subgroup of urban youth.

Analytic Procedures

Principal component factor analysis was the primary analytic procedure. To ensure that the assumptions of the test are not violated, data were evaluated using frequency distribution and casewise diagnostics. The preliminary diagnosis revealed that the variable was normally distributed, that 3% of the observations were missing and that four youth had standardized residuals that were three standard deviations above the mean. Transformations were not needed, outliers were removed, and listwise deletion was employed. In addition to principal component factor analysis, descriptive statistics, t-test, and one-way ANOVA procedures were performed. To examine factor loadings across adolescence, the sample was divided into early adolescence (11–14), middle adolescence (15–17), and late adolescence (18–21).

Results

Sample Characteristics

The sample included 788 adolescents from public housing in four large US cities: 30% from St. Louis, 19% from Philadelphia, 21% from Washington, D.C., and 30% from New York to Queens. The sample reported an average age of 15.46 with a standard deviation of 2.7 years. Ages ranged from 11 to 21 years. Thirty-eight percent reported being in early adolescence (11–14), 37% reported being in middle adolescence (15–17), and 25% reported being in late adolescence (18–21). Females composed 48% of the sample. Ninety percent of the sample reported being African American; 8% reported being mixed (parents from different racial groups), and the remaining 2% reported being Latino (see Table 8.1).

Table 8.1 Sample characteristics

Variables	Mean (SD)	Percentage
Age	15.46 (2.7)	
Age groups		
• Early		38
• Middle		37
• Late		25
Gender		
• Female		48
• Male		52
Race		
• African American		90
• Latino		02
• Mixed		08

Univariate Descriptors

Respondents reported a mean depressive symptom score of 17.53 with a standard deviation of 10 points. Depressive symptoms ranged from 0 to 51. The sample reported a 28% prevalence of depression based on the 24 cutoff point and a 47% prevalence of depression based on the 16 cutoff point. Fifty-three percent of the sample reported minimal depressive symptoms (0–15), 19% reported mild depressive symptoms (16–23), and 28% reported severe depressive symptoms (24 and above). The scale demonstrated acceptable internal consistency with this sample ($\alpha=0.91$). See Table 8.2 for results.

Mean Comparisons

Males reported significantly higher symptoms than females ($t=-2.72$, $p<0.05$). Symptoms of depression did not differ across age group. However, depressive symptoms differed significantly across research sites, $F(780,3)=13.17$, $p<0.001$. Youth in New York and D.C. reported significantly lower symptoms of depression than youth in St. Louis and Philadelphia. Symptoms did not differ between New York and D.C.; neither did symptom differ between St. Louis and Philadelphia (see Table 8.2).

Factor Loadings for Entire Sample

Principal components factor analysis using a varimax rotation was conducted to determine the underlying constructs of depression. Four criteria were used to determine the number of underlying domains that would be retained: e.g., eigenvalue, variance, scree plot, and residuals. To have epidemiological applications, CES-D must have similar factor structures within subgroups in a population. Therefore, the analysis was conducted to examine factor loadings by gender (e.g., male and female) and across adolescence (e.g., early, middle and late adolescents). Results from the analyses are presented in Tables 8.3–8.9. In addition to principal components factor analysis, Cronbach alphas were calculated for the sample at large and for each subgroup.

Results from the item analysis suggest that the internal consistency does not differ between the sample at large and the subsamples of youth. The Cronbach alpha for the sample at large was 0.89, while the alpha score for the subsamples ranged from 0.89 to 0.91.

Table 8.2 Ranges, means, standard deviations, and Cronbach's alpha by gender and age groups

	Sample (n=788)				Males (n=411)				Females (n=374)			
Variables	Range	M	SD	α	Range	M	SD	α	Range	M	SD	α
Depressive symptoms	0–51	17.53	10.00	0.90	0–51	18.21[**]	9.89	0.91	03–51	16.61	9.79	0.89

[**]$p<0.00$

Table 8.3 Ranges, means, standard deviations, and Cronbach's alpha by age groups

	Early adolescence (n=298)				Middle adolescence (n=296)				Late adolescence (n=194)			
Variables	Range	M	SD	α	Range	M	SD	α	Range	M	SD	α
Depressive symptoms	0–49	16.79	9.97	0.91	02–51	17.82	10.27	0.91	03–51	17.53	10.00	0.89

Table 8.4 Varimax rotated factor loadings of CES-D for entire sample (n=788)

CES-D items	(Factor 1) negative affects	(Factor 2) somatic complaints	(Factor 3) positive affects
Felt hopeful	0.498		
Life been failure	0.568		
Felt fearful	0.492		
Talked less	0.620		
Felt lonely	0.670		
People unfriendly	0.614		
Crying spells	0.671		
Felt sad	0.749		
People disliked me	0.676		
Could not get going	0.714		
Bothered by things		0.613	
Poor apatite		0.663	
Can't shake blues		0.733	
Trouble concentrating		0.626	
Felt depressed		0.570	
Restless sleep		0.469	
Felt as good as others			0.654
Everything was effort			0.656
Was happy			0.630
Enjoyed life			0.775
Eigenvalues	7.65	1.69	1.08
Variance explained	24.02%	17.45%	10.73%

Results from the principal components factor analysis using the sample at large identified a three factors model (see Table 8.4). This finding differs from the four factors model found by Radloff (1977) and others (Hertzog et al., 1990; Knight et al., 1997). There was no evidence of an Interpersonal Factor with the sample at large. Factor 1, which explained 24% of the variance in depressive symptoms, contained items found by Radloff (1977) to load as interpersonal, somatic, and negative affect. Factor 2, which explained 17% of the variance, also contained a mix of interpersonal, somatic and negative affect items. Only Factor 3, explaining 11% of the variance, contained items that loaded as positive affect. However, unlike the original positive affect factor found by Radloff, our third factor included the item *"Everything was an effort."* We found similar factor loadings for the female (see Table 8.5), male (see Table 8.6), early adolescent (see Table 8.7), middle adolescent (see Table 8.8) and late adolescent (see Table 8.9) subgroups. That is, a three-factor model with no

Table 8.5 Varimax rotated factor loadings of CES-D for female sample ($n=374$)

CES-D items	(Factor 1) negative affects	(Factor 2) somatic complaints	(Factor 3) positive affects
Felt hopeful	0.498		
Life been failure	0.568		
Felt fearful	0.492		
Talked less	0.648		
Felt lonely	0.703		
People unfriendly	0.593		
Crying spells	0.661		
Felt sad	0.709		
People disliked me	0.605		
Could not get going	0.722		
Restless sleep	0.469		
Bothered by things		0.676	
Poor apatite		0.613	
Can't shake blues		0.739	
Trouble concentrating		0.631	
Felt depressed		0.515	
Felt as good as others			0.731
Everything was effort			0.749
Was happy			0.572
Enjoyed life			0.735
Eigenvalues	7.23	1.84	1.13
Variance explained	24.75%	14.98%	11.27%

Table 8.6 Varimax rotated factor loadings of CES-D for male sample ($n=411$)

CES-D items	(Factor 1) negative affects	(Factor 2) somatic complaints	(Factor 3) positive affects
Felt hopeful	0.484		
Talked less	0.589		
Felt lonely	0.648		
People unfriendly	0.620		
Crying spells	0.679		
Felt sad	0.776		
People disliked me	0.708		
Could not get going	0.689		
Bothered by things		0.603	
Poor apatite		0.684	
Can't shake blues		0.715	
Trouble concentrating		0.634	
Felt depressed		0.622	
Life been failure		0.570	
Felt fearful		0.428	
Restless sleep		0.592	
Felt as good as others			0.554
Everything was effort			0.500
Was happy			0.676
Enjoyed life			0.797
Eigenvalues	8.09	1.54	1.12
Variance explained	22.92%	21.14%	9.77%

Table 8.7 Varimax rotated factor loadings of CES-D for early adolescent sample ($n=298$)

CES-D Items	(Factor 1) negative affects	(Factor 2) somatic complaints	(Factor 3) positive affects
Felt hopeful	0.484		
Talked less	0.589		
Felt lonely	0.648		
People unfriendly	0.620		
Crying spells	0.679		
Felt sad	0.776		
People disliked me	0.708		
Could not get going	0.689		
Bothered by things		0.603	
Poor apatite		0.684	
Can't shake blues		0.715	
Trouble concentrating		0.634	
Felt depressed		0.622	
Life been failure		0.570	
Felt fearful		0.428	
Restless sleep		0.592	
Felt as good as others			0.554
Everything was effort			0.500
Was happy			0.676
Enjoyed life			0.797
Eigenvalues	7.83	1.63	1.11
Variance explained	26.86%	15.05%	11.06%

Table 8.8 Varimax rotated factor loadings of CES-D for middle adolescent sample ($n=201$)

CES-D Items	(Factor 1) negative affects	(Factor 2) somatic complaints	(Factor 3) positive affects	(Factor 4) interpersonal
Felt hopeful	0.633			
Talked less		0.716		
Felt lonely		0.679		
People unfriendly	0.595			
Crying spells	0.635			
Felt sad	0.736			
People disliked me	0.602			
Could not get going	0.785			
Bothered by things				0.830
Poor apatite				0.560
Can't shake blues	0.572			
Trouble concentrating	0.637			
Felt depressed	0.687			
Life been failure	0.705			
Felt fearful	0.724			
Restless sleep	0.621			
Felt as good as others		0.822		
Everything was effort		0.740		
Was happy			0.647	
Enjoyed life		0.742		
Eigenvalues	7.64	2.01	1.15	1.09
Variance explained	28.74%	11.72%	9.06%	9.43%

Table 8.9 Varimax rotated factor loadings of CES-D for late adolescent sample ($n = 137$)

CES-D Items	(Factor 1) negative affects	(Factor 2) somatic complaints	(Factor 3) positive affects	(Factor 4) interpersonal
Felt hopeful		0.684		
Talked less	0.576			
Felt lonely	0.708			
People unfriendly	0.568			
Crying spells	0.763			
Felt sad	0.772			
People disliked me	0.682			
Could not get going	0.698			
Bothered by things			0.813	
Poor apatite			0.543	
Can't shake blues			0.518	
Trouble concentrating		0.499		
Felt depressed		0.676		
Life been failure		0.647		
Felt fearful		0.377		
Restless sleep			0.439	
Felt as good as others				0.456
Everything was effort				0.633
Was happy				0.688
Enjoyed life				0.787
Eigenvalues	6.29	1.94	1.49	1.12
Variance explained	18.71%	13.84%	10.94%	10.77%

clear cut distinction among Negative Affect, Positive Affect, Somatic, and Interpersonal. Furthermore, *"Everything was an effort"* continued to load with the positive affect items with the female, male, and early adolescent subgroups.

Results from the principal components factor analysis using the middle and late adolescence samples identified a four factors model (not shown). Although a four-factor model was identified, the loadings differ from the four factors model reported by Radloff (1977) and others (Knight et al., 1997). As with the previous models, there was no evidence of an Interpersonal Factor within these subsamples. Also, *"Everything was an effort"* continued to load with the positive affect items with the middle and late adolescent subgroups. A salient finding within the Middle Adolescence subgroup is that 12 items loaded on a single domain, which explained 39% of the total variance. Another unique loading within this subgroup is that "was happy" loaded with "talked less" and "felt lonely." Factor loadings for the late adolescence subgroup were closer to the loadings reported for national samples (Radloff). However, items loaded in domains that may be specific to African American youth living in urban public housing communities.

Discussion

Contrary to existing evidence, African American males in urban public housing experience heightened depressive symptoms relative to their female counterpart (Birmaher et al., 1996; Cicchetti & Toth, 1998; Hankins et al., 1998; Nolen-Hoeksema & Girgus, 1994; Office of Applied Studies, 2005; Wichstrom, 1999). This finding highlights the need for further investigations on the development and expression of depression by gender among urban adolescents living in public housing.

In addition to gender differences, depressive symptoms differed across research sites. Youth in New York and D.C. had lower symptoms of depression than youth in St. Louis and Philadelphia.

However, symptoms did not differ between New York and D.C.; neither did symptoms differ between St. Louis and Philadelphia. These differences in research sites may be explained by variations in the housing structures and characteristics of the neighborhood, the family, the peer, and the individual domains. Further investigations are needed to identify factors contributing to disparities in depressive symptoms among youth living in urban public housing. It should be noted that depressive symptoms did not differ across adolescence.

Data also suggest that the factor structure of depression in urban African American youth differs from their nonminority youth counterpart. When using the sample at large, a three-factor model was identified unlike the four-factor model reported by Radloff (1977). The Middle Adolescence subgroup had 12 items load on a single domain, which included "was happy," "talked less," and "felt lonely." The three-factor model had no clear distinction among Negative Affect, Positive Affect, Somatic, and Interpersonal as reported by others (Radloff). Also, there was no evidence of an interpersonal factor in this sample of youth.

The structure of depression changed across the span of adolescence. The middle and late adolescence samples identified a four factors model. Notwithstanding this finding, the four-factor model differed from that of Radloff (1977) and others (Knight et al., 1997). Not only did the loadings differ there was still no evidence of an Interpersonal Factor within these subsamples. The late adolescence subgroup loadings were closer to the loadings reported for national samples.

Though beyond the scope of these data, the following speculations may help to understand our findings. The differences across the span of adolescence could be attributed to the early adolescence subgroup not grasping the effects their neighborhoods may have on their future and the daily stressors there family has to deal with economically. They are sheltered and their focus is on attending school and interacting with peers. Also, depression may not be a very complex phenomenon that they can grasp and understand during early adolescence. However, once youth reach middle adolescence, they are able to see and comprehend what is going on around them and see a compromised opportunity structure, low neighborhood socioeconomic status, and minimal support from nonfamily members. This would be the likely period where depression would begin to manifest. The late adolescence subgroup is no longer shielded by the community and neighborhood supports and has to deal with going out in the real world and surviving in any way they can. They still may have some form of guidance but they are now responsible for working so they can assist in providing for their siblings and parental household. Even when this subgroup is experiencing symptoms of depression, it is a feeling that they have to internalize and repress since their focus has to be on surviving. Unfortunately, it goes undetected until the depressive symptoms affect their daily level of functioning and adolescents in this subgroup act out as a result of not being able to manage their feelings.

Limitations. It is important to note that certain limitations exist. First, the chapter is based upon self-reported data; therefore, the veracity of the data is only as accurate as youth honestly report and recall their symptoms. Second, results are not based on a nationally representative sample. Generalizing the results to youth living in suburban public housing and urban African American youth not living in public housing should be done with caution. Third, the statistical procedures used were preliminary and exploratory rather than confirmatory, which only identifies factors but do not confirm a model. Fourth, the chapter does not identify causes and correlates of depressive symptoms.

Implications in Research

The exploration has several implications to our understanding of the expression and structure of depressive symptoms among African American adolescents living in urban public housing. One important implication of this study is that it provides public health workers and mental health practitioners with basic prevalence data and information of gender differences in depressive symptoms in an underserved population of minority youth. Mental and public health services within public housing communities should target males and interventions should be developed to address the increased depressive symptoms within the male population. Interventions should also take into account racial and environmental differences that may impact increased depressive symptoms among males.

Another key implication is that depression does not become a complex phenomenon within this population until later in adolescence. This is important information considering that certain domains of depression may go undetected until a youth enters late adolescence. The late detection of depression may have far reaching and deleterious consequences in the lives of this already vulnerable population of youth. For example, African American youth living in public housing may be in the chronic stages of depression before they actually manifest domain-specific symptoms typically associated with chronic depression. Mental and public health practitioners within public housing settings may consider adjusting diagnostic tools to detect depression while these youth are in early adolescence. For example, MAYSI-2 (Massachusetts Youth Screening Instrument) may be an effective tool to be used in school systems in these neighborhoods to detect depression. Although this tool has been used mainly in the juvenile correctional system to screen youth for special mental health needs, the instrument has been effective in detecting mental health issues among youth.

The last implication of this exploration is to the measurement of depression using CES-D with African American youth living in public housing settings. A consistent internal structure across populations and cultural groups is critical to the validity of any measure (Bollen & Lennox, 1991). Furthermore, psychometric properties, in particular internal consistency, should be similar across populations (Perreira, Deeb-sossa, Harris & Bollen, 2005). If a measure is not invariant across populations and setting the measure's ability to validly detect the construct in question should be questioned. In this exploratory investigation, we did not find evidence that CES-D demonstrated a similar internal structure with African American youth in public housing as others have reported elsewhere (Knight et al., 1997; Radloff, 1977). This finding, though preliminary, has implications to measures used to assess depressive symptoms with African American youth in public housing settings. This chapter suggests both a need to develop a more precise understanding of why the internal structure of depression differs for urban youth in public housing and the need to develop measures that validly and reliably assesses depression in this vulnerable population of youth.

Conclusion

The Department of Health and Human Services has identified the mental health of young people as a major public health concern (Healthy People, 2010). This concern is particularly salient in vulnerable populations of youth, such as youth living in our nation's only public neighborhoods (e.g., public housing). Research has found that minority youth in public housing with elevated depressive symptoms are significantly more vulnerable to other risk factors and that these youth do not express depressive symptoms similar to national samples (Nebbitt & Lombe, 2007, 2008).

Research is needed to determine the degree to which differences in interpersonal factors emerge in late adolescence and/or the degree to which cultural and background may account for gender differences. The results also highlight the heightened risk for depressive symptoms among males relative to their female peers. Further research is needed to uncover the extent of depression among African American males in urban public housing so that effective preventive interventions may be developed to prevent the onset or decrease depressive symptoms. Lastly, there is a need to understand the structure and expression of depression in African American youth living in public housing and to develop measures to accurately detect depression in this vulnerable population of youth.

References

Bandura, A. (1997). *Self efficacy: The exercise of control*. New York: Freeman.

Beck, A.T., Ward, C., & Mendelson, M. (1961). Beck Depression Inventory (BDI). *Archive of General Psychiatry, 4*, 561–571.

Beekman, A. T., Geerlings, S. W., Deeg, D. J., Smit, J. H., Schoevers, R. S., de Beurs, E., et al. (2002). The natural history of late-life depression: A 6-year prospective study in the community. *Archive of General Psychiatry, 59*, 605–611.

Birmaher, B., Ryan, N. D., & Williamson, D. E. (1996). Depression in children and adolescents: Clinical features and pathogenesis. In K. Schulman, M. Tohen, & S. P. Kutcher (Eds.), *Mood disorders across the life spans* (pp. 51–82). New York: Wiley.

Bollen, K., & Lennox, R. (1991). Conventional wisdom on measurement: A structural equation on perspective. *Psychological Bulletin, 110*(2), 305–314.

Cicchetti, D., & Toth, S. L. (1998). The development of depression in children and adolescents. *American Psychologist, 53*, 221–241.

Compas, B. E., Ey, S., & Grant, K. E. (1993). Taxonomy, assessment, and diagnosis of depression during adolescence. *Psychological Bulletin, 114*, 323–344.

Comstock, G. W., & Helsing, K. J. (1976). Symptoms of depression in two communities. *Psychological Medicine, 6*(4), 551–63.

Davis, G. Y., & Stevenson, H. C. (2006). Racial socialization experiences and symptoms of depression among Black youth. *Journal of Child and Family Studies, 15*(3), 293–307.

Department of Resident Service. (2007). Annual Report. North Eastern Housing Authority. Prepared by the Department of Resident Services, New York Housing Authority.

Devins, G. M., Orme, C. M., Costello, C. G., Binik, Y. M., Frizzell, B., Stam, H. J., et al. (1988). Measuring depressive symptoms in illness populations: Psychometric properties of the Center for Epidemiologic Studies Depression (CES-D). *Psychology and Health, 2*, 139–156.

Franko, D. L., Striegel-Moore, R. H., Bean, J., Barton, B. A., Biro, F., Kraemer, H. C., et al. (2005). Self-reported symptoms of depression in late adolescence in early adulthood: A comparison of African American and Caucasian females. *Journal of Adolescent Health, 37*, 526–529.

Furstenberg, F. F., Cook, T. D., Excels, J., Elder, G. H., & Sameroff, A. (1999). *Managing to make it: Urban families and adolescent success*. Chicago: University of Chicago Press.

Garber, J. (2006). Depression in children and adolescents: Linking risk research and prevention., *31*. *American Journal of Preventive Medicine, 31*(Suppl. 1), S104–125.

Golding, J. M., & Aneshensel, C. S. (1989). Factor structure of the Center for Epidemiologic Studies Depression Scale among Mexican Americans and non-Hispanic Whites. *Psychological Assessments, 1*, 163–168.

Golding, J. M., Aneshensel, C. S., & Hough, R. L. (1991). Responses to depression scale items among Mexican Americans and non-Hispanic Whites. *Journal of Clinical Psychology, 47*, 61–75.

Goodman, E., & Whitaker, R. C. (2002). A prospective study of the role of depression in the development and persistence of adolescent obesity. *Pediatrics, 109*, 497–504.

Gullone, E., Ollendick, T. H., & King, N. J. (2006). The role of attachment representation in the relationship between depressive symptomatology and social withdrawal in middle childhood. *Journal of Child and Family Studies, 35*(3), 293–307.

Hammen, C., & Compas, B. (1994). Unmasking unmasked depression in children and adolescents: The problem of co-morbidity. *Clinical Psychology Review, 14*, 585–603.

Hankins, B., Abramson, L., Moffit, T., Silva, P., McGee, R., & Angell, K. (1998). Development of depression from preadolescence to young adulthood: Emerging gender differences in a 10-year longitudinal study. *Journal of Abnormal Psychology, 107*, 128–140.

Hawkins, W., Hawkins, M., Sabatino, C., & Ley, S. (1998). Relationship of perceived future opportunity to depressive symptomatology of inner-city African American adolescents. *Children and Youth Service Review, 20*(9), 757–764.

Heckathorn, D. D. (1997). Respondent-driven sampling: a new approach to the study of hidden populations. *Social Problems, 44*, 174–199.

Hertzog, C., Van Alsline, J., Usala, P. D., Hultsch, D. P., & Dixon, R. (1990). Measurement properties of the Center for Epidemiological Studies Depression Scale (CES-D) in older populations. *Psychological Assessment, 2*, 64–72.

HHS, (2000). U.S. Department of Health and Human Service, The State of the American Child: The Impact of Federal Policies on Children, Retrieved from http://www.hhs.gov/asl/testify/2010/07/t20100729a.html, on March 15, 2010.

U.S. Department of Health & Human Services. (2001). *Healthy People 2010: Healthy people in healthy communities.* Washington, D.C.: U.S. Government Printing Office.

Kessler, R. C., Avenevoli, S., & Merikangas, K. R. (2001). Mood disorders in children and adolescents: An epidemiologic perspective. *Biological Psychiatry, 49*, 1002–1014.

Knight, R. G., Williams, S., McGee, R., & Olaman, S. (1997). Psychometric properties of the Centre for Epidemiologic Studies Depression Scale (CES-D) in a sample of women in middle life. *Behaviour Research and Therapy, 35*(4), 373–380.

Lagged, A. M., & Dunn, D. W. (2003). Depression in children and adolescents. *Neurological Clinics, 21*, 953–960.

Levisohn, P. M., Rhode, P., & Seeley, J. R. (1998). Major depressive disorder in older adolescents: Prevalence, risk factors, and clinical implications. *Clinical Psychology Review, 18*, 765–794.

MMPI. (1960). *Minnesota Multiphase Personality Inventory.* Minneapolis, MN: University of Minnesota Press.

Muris, P., Schmidt, H., Lambrichs, R., & Meesters, C. (2001). Protective and vulnerability factors of depression in normal adolescents. *Behaviour Research and Therapy, 39*(5), 555–565.

Murphy, J. M. (2002). Symptom scales and diagnostic schedules in adult psychiatry. In M. T. Tsuang & M. Tohen (Eds.), *Textbook in Psychiatric Epidemiology* (pp. 273–332). New York: Wiley-Liss.

National Alliance on Mental Illness (NAMI). (2010). Depression in children and adolescents. Retrieved April 12, 2004, from http://www.nami.org/Template.cfm?Section=Depression&Template=/ContentManagement/ContentDisplay.cfm&ContentID=89198

National Center for Child Poverty (2001). Retrieved April 12, 2004, from http://www.nccp.org/main1.html

Naughton, M. J., & Wiklund, I. (1993). A critical review of dimension-specific measures of health related quality of life in cross-cultural research. *Quality of Life Research, 2*(6), 397–432.

Nebbitt, V. E., & Lombe, M. (2010). Urban African American adolescents and adultification. *Families in Society: The Journal of Contemporary Social Services., 91*(4), 234–240.

Nebbitt, V. E., & Lombe, M. (2008). Assessing the moderating effects of depressive symptoms among urban youth in public housing. *Child and Adolescent Social Work Journal, 2*(5), 409–424.

Nebbitt, V. E., & Lombe, M. (2007). Environmental correlates of depressive symptoms among African American adolescents living in public housing. *Journal of Human Behavior in the Social Environment, Special Issue of African American Perspective, 15*(2/3), 435–454.

Nezu, A. M., Nezu, C. M., McClure, K. S., & Zwick, M. L. (2002). Assessment of depression. In I. H. Gotlib & C. L. Hammen (Eds.), *Handbook of Depression* (pp. 61–85). New York: The Guilford Press.

NIMH (2009). *Treatment of children with mental disorders.* NIH publication No. 09–4702. http://www.nimh.nih.gov

Nolen-Hoeksema, S., & Girgus, J. S. (1994). The emergence of gender differences in depression during adolescence. *Psychological Bulletin, 115*, 424–443.

Office of Applied Studies (2005). *Substance abuse and mental health administration. National survey on drug use and health.* The NSDUH report: Depression among adolescents. Retrieved from http://www.oas.samhsa.gov/2k5/youthdepression/youthdepression.htm, on March 12, 2010.

Office of Resident Services. (2006). *Asset management plan: Analysis of city and public housing characteristics in the District: Toward an enhanced resident service model.* Washington, D.C.: Housing Authority.

Perreira, K. M., Deeb-Sossa, N., Harris, K., & Bollen, K. (2005). What are we measuring? *An evaluation of the CES-D across race/ethnicity and immigrant generation. Social Forces., 83*, 1567–1602.

Radloff, L. S. (1977). The CES-D scale: A self-report depression scale for research in the general population. *Applied Psychological Measurement, 1*, 385–401.

Radloff, L. S., & Locke, B. (1986). The community mental health assessment survey and the CES-D scale. In M. Weissman, J. Myers, & C. Ross (Eds.), *Community surveys of psychiatric disorders* (pp. 177–189). New Jersey: Rutgers University Press.

Roberts, R. E., Lewinsohn, P. M., & Seely, J. R. (1991). Screening for adolescent depression: a comparison of depression scales. *Journal of the American Academy of Child and Adolescent Psychiatry, 30*, 58–66.

Roberts, R., Chen, Y., & Solovitz, B. (1995). Symptoms of DSM-III-R major depression among Anglo, African and Mexican American adolescents. *Journal of Affective Disorders, 36*, 1–9.

Roberts, R., Roberts, C., & Chen, Y. (1997). Ethnocultural differences in the prevalence of adolescent depression. *American Journal of Community Psychology, 25*, 95–110.

Roelofs, J., Meesters, C., Mijke ter Huurne, M., Lotte Bamelis, M., & Muris, P. (2006). On the links between attachment style, parental rearing behaviors, and internalizing and externalizing problems in non-clinical children. *Journal of Child and Family Studies, 15*(3), 331–344.

Rushton, J. L., Forcier, M., & Schectman, R. M. (2002). Epidemiology of depressive symptoms in the National Longitudinal Study of Adolescent Health. *Journal of American Child Adolescent Psychiatry, 41*(2), 199–205.

Saint Louis Housing Authority. (2006). *St. Louis Housing Authority, Annual report*. St. Louis: Office of Information Technology.

Schraedley, P. K., Gotlib, I. H., & Hayward, C. (1999). Gender differences in correlates of depressive symptoms in adolescents. *Journal of Adolescent Health, 25*, 98–108.

Shaffer, A., Forehand, R., Kotchick, B. A., & The Family Health Project Research Group. (2002). A longitudinal examination of correlates of depressive symptoms among inner-city African American children and adolescents. *Journal of Child and Family Studies, 11*(2), 151–164.

Sheehan, T. J., Fifield, J., Reisine, S., & Tennen, H. (1995). The measurement structure of the Center for Epidemiologic Studies Depression Scale. *Journal of Personality Assessment, 64*(3), 507–521.

Smith, C., Lizotte, A., Thornberry, T., & Krohn, M. (1995). Resilient youth: Identifying factors that prevent high-risk youth from engaging in delinquency and drug use. *Current Perspectives. Aging Life Cycle, 4*, 217–247.

Snaith, P. (1993). What do depression rating scales measure? *British Journal of Psychiatry, 163*, 293–298.

Stevenson, H. C. (1998). Raising safe villages: Cultural-ecological factors that influence the emotional adjustment of adolescents. *Journal of Black Psychology, 24*(1), 44–59.

Tandon, D. S., & Solomon, B. S. (2009). Risk and protective factors for depressive symptoms in urban African American adolescents. *Youth Society, 41*, 80–99.

Taylor, R. L. (1995). Black youth in United States: An overview. In R. L. Taylor (Ed.), *African American youth: Their social and economic status in the United States* (pp. 3–36). Westprot, CT: Praeger.

Urban Institute. (1997). Segregation by design [Online]. Retrived April 12, 2008, from http://urban.org

Wichstrom, L. (1999). The emergence of gender difference in depressed mood during adolescence: The role of intensified gender socialization. *Developmental Psychology, 35*, 232–245.

Wight, R. G., Aneshensel, C. S., Botticello, A. L., & Sepulveda, J. E. (2005). A multilevel analysis of ethnic variation in depressive symptoms among adolescents in the United States. *Social Science & Medicine, 60*, 2073–2084.

Wong, Y. I. (2000). Measurement properties of the Center for Epidemiological Studies – Depression scale in a homeless population. *Psychological Assessment, 12*(1), 69–76.

Zimmerman, M., Ramirez-Valles, J., Zapert, K., & Maton, K. (2000). A longitudinal study of stress-buffering effects for urban African American male adolescent problem behaviors and mental health. *Journal of Community Psychology, 28*(1), 17–33.

Zung, W. (1965). A self-rating depression scale. *Archive General Psychiatry, 12*, 63–70.

Chapter 9
Rites of Passage: Cultural Paths for HIV/AIDS Prevention in African American Girls

Donna Shambley-Ebron

New medical technologies, diagnostic methods, medications, and treatments have ushered in the twenty-first century as scientists continue the quest to improve health and quality of life for all. Although health science and technology continue to advance at astounding rates, health disparities are still occurring between various populations in the USA. This problem has been well recognized and its elimination has been identified as a goal for our nation in Healthy People (2020). Particularly, troubling is the trend that HIV/AIDS has taken with African American people who are contracting the disease and dying at a much higher rate than White Americans (Centers for Disease Control and Prevention, 2006). Specifically, African American women contract HIV at about 23 times that of White American women (Centers for Disease Control and Prevention, 2008). The incidence and prevalence of HIV among African American women strongly suggest the need to develop culturally specific prevention interventions targeted toward young African American girls who are at risk for becoming newly infected.

In various cultures, past and present, formal initiation into adulthood or rites of passage has served to help adolescents make developmental transitions with the support of their families and communities. These rites of passage have the potential to create benefits for African American girls and boys that can be health promoting and lead to responsible decision making during the critical adolescent years leading to adulthood. Choices that adolescents make during this time can influence their risks for HIV/AIDS, other sexually transmissible infections, unplanned pregnancies, and unmet life goals. Although there have been a number of HIV/AIDS prevention interventions developed for African American adolescents, contemporary rites of passage have not been explored (Dancy, Crittenden, & Talashek, 2006; DiClemente et al., 2004; Dilorio et al., 2006; Jemmott, Jemmott, & Fong, 1998). The purpose of this chapter is to discuss how traditions of African culture, especially rites of passage in adolescence, have the potential to promote health and reduce HIV/AIDS risk in African American girls. An example of such a program will be presented. The role that African American community-based organizations, particularly churches, can play in developing, implementing, and sustaining such programs will also be discussed.

D. Shambley-Ebron (✉)
College of Nursing, University of Cincinnati,
Cincinnati, OH, USA
e-mail: donna.shambley-ebron@uc.edu

A.J. Lemelle et al. (eds.), *Handbook of African American Health: Social and Behavioral Interventions*,
DOI 10.1007/978-1-4419-9616-9_9, © Springer Science+Business Media, LLC 2011

Background and Significance

HIV/AIDS in Heterosexual African American Women

HIV/AIDS appeared in the USA in the 1980s, primarily affecting homosexual males. Leaving thousands dead in its wake, the intravenous drug using population became the next group of those who were greatly impacted. The HIV/AIDS epidemic in America has now settled heavily into African American communities. Now in the twenty-first century, heterosexual African American women, those who bear children and transmit culture, are bearing an excess burden of disease that is about 20 times greater than that of White American women (Centers for Disease Control and Prevention, 2008).

How this deadly virus has proliferated so rapidly within one population should concern all Americans. Reasons why nondrug using, heterosexual African American women have been so disproportionately impacted by HIV/AIDS have been speculated upon by those who study disease transmission and trends. Some explanations relate to the fact that talking openly about HIV/AIDS and particularly homosexuality have been taboo topics in African American communities (Belgrave & Allison, 2006). Generally, both homosexuality and HIV/AIDS are stigmatized among African Americans. Because of this, men who covertly have sex with other men may lead dual lives, and have socially acceptable heterosexual relationships with women who are unaware of their homosexual activities (Gilbert & Wright, 2003).

African American men also are disproportionately represented in the US penal system. According to (Hattery & Smith, 2007), African American prisoners compose almost 2/3 of the male prison population, even though they represent only 13% of the entire U.S. population. High risk prison behaviors such as "survival sex" tattooing, and drug use by inmates, place women at risk when men who have been incarcerated are released back into the community where they may again resume heterosexual relationships (Gilbert & Wright, 2003). Finally, women who have sex with men who have used needles to inject drugs are at high risk for HIV infection (Centers for Disease Control and Prevention, 2008).

Young girls living in impoverished conditions are especially at risk for exposure to HIV/AIDS due to a combination of factors that can be present in poor neighborhoods. The U.S. Census Bureau reported that in 2006, 24% of African Americans were living at the poverty level as compared to 8% of non-Hispanic White Americans (2008). In addition to the stressors associated with racism and discrimination, low socioeconomic status in African Americans is often accompanied by hopelessness, depression, substance abuse, lack of access to quality health care, and present-time orientation (Gilbert & Wright, 2003). These factors, individually and collectively translate into increased risk for poor health. As young girls who live in poverty move from childhood to adolescence, many have had first-hand exposures to, and experiences with violence, sex, and other ravages of poor communities.

In spite of recognizable barriers to sexual health promotion in African American girls in poor communities, there are cultural strengths, some of which remain untapped, that have potential to reverse the trends of early sexual activity and its associated negative health consequences. Medical science and technology cannot fully address certain issues of health and illness that are buried in the depth of African American communities, are rooted and grounded in experiences of racism, oppression, and discrimination, and are often influenced by poverty. African American communities, together with community nurses and other professionals can identify cultural traditions, values, and strengths, and purposefully and formally introduce them to pre-adolescent and adolescent girls in community settings through rites of passage programs.

Rites of Passage

Rites of passage represent formal or informal processes, rituals or ceremonies that mark the movement of humans through various stages of life (Van Gennep, 2004). These rites may mark biological processes such as birth, menstruation, pregnancy, menopause, or even death. Other rites mark symbolic transitions, such as baptisms, circumcisions, and marriage. Although a plethora of types of rites of passage ceremonies have existed in different cultures and societies, the transition to adulthood is often recognized and celebrated. Warfield-Coppock (1992) defines the adolescent rites of passage as "a supervised developmental and educational process whose goal is to assist young people in attaining the knowledge and accepting the responsibilities, privileges, and duties of an adult member of a society" (p. 472). These rituals are usually grounded in cultural tradition and are influenced by spiritual and or religious belief systems.

In contemporary American society, the transition to adulthood can be conferred upon adolescent girls in various ways. There are formal cultural recognitions of "coming of age" such as the Bat Mitzvah in Jewish tradition, or the Quincenera for Latina girls. Cotillions and debutante balls for those girls from more affluent families are sponsored by sororities or women's clubs, and serve to socialize adolescent girls into expected roles. Although these events have their origins in Europe, they have a long history among the African American upper class (Lynch, 1999). Other events that may serve as initiations into adulthood are, recognition of the onset of puberty or menstruation, graduation from middle or high school or participation in adult behaviors such as the first sexual intercourse, or pregnancy and parenthood. A culturally appropriate planned formal process that serves to initiate young African American girls into appropriate adult roles has the potential to reduce unhealthy and self-destructive entrées into adulthood.

Van Gennep (2004), the European anthropologist who studied these life transitions in depth, identified three dimensions of rites of passage; separation, transition, and incorporation. Separation refers to removal of the individuals to be initiated away from society. Transition is the process by which the initiates are transformed into their new societal roles. This transition usually involves teaching and indoctrination by the elders of the society that will prepare them for their new roles. Incorporation is the stage by which the initiates are re-introduced to the society as full-fledged members in their new roles, prepared to be responsible, contributing members of their communities.

Historical Perspectives

Warfield-Coppock (1992), detailed the origin of African rites of passage in ancient Egypt. The process was imbedded within the formal system of education and stressed not only liberal arts and science education, but also the development of ten specific virtues. They were (1) control of thought, (2) control of action, (3) devotion to purpose, (4) faith in the Master's ability to teach the truth, (5) faith in one's ability to assimilate the truth, (6) faith in one's self to wield the truth, (7) freedom from resentment under persecution, (8) freedom from resentment under wrong, (9) the ability to distinguish right from wrong, and (10) the ability to distinguish the real from the unreal (Warfield-Coppock, 1992). The spiritual and moral component of developing and preparing individuals for life were recognized as essential within this cultural process of initiation. These ten virtues can be translated into contemporary ideals that are applicable to developing African American adolescents (Table 9.1).

Delaney (1995) described various rites emanating from African countries that traditionally served to initiate adolescents into adulthood. Tribal rites of certain tribes such as the Okieks and Orika initiated adolescent girls and boys between the ages of 14 and 16 years of age. These rituals

Table 9.1 Ten virtues taught in ancient Egyptian rites of passage translation to contemporary ideals

Goal	Learning
Control of thought	Teaches the learner discipline in thinking that is informed, critical, and positive in nature
Control of action	Teaches the learner self-control and acting after careful thought and with intention
Devotion to purpose	Teaches goal setting and consistent and intentional progress to reach goals
Faith in the Master's ability to teach the truth	Teaches the learner respect for elders and those who hold knowledge from which one can learn
Faith in one's ability to assimilate the truth	Teaches self-confidence and belief in oneself to learn from one's teachers
Faith in one's self to wield the truth	Teaches belief in one's ability to pass on knowledge to others
Freedom from resentment under persecution	Development of moral strength to withstand discrimination, oppression, and bigotry
Freedom from resentment under wrong	Development of moral strength to withstand wrong treatment without retaliation or excessive anger
The ability to distinguish right from wrong	Development of moral and ethical discernment and behaviors
The ability to distinguish the real from the unreal	Development of discernment of truth and reality from those ideas and material goods that only appear to represent the truth

involved separation of males and females, where knowledge was transmitted by same-sex elders. Spiritual aspects as well as elaborate ceremonies that served to usher adolescents safely into adulthood were included. Likewise, Watson & Montgomery (1999) described rites of passage in traditional African peoples, specifically seven tribal groups from Kenya. They described the "coming of age" and initiation period as the most significant event in the lives of individuals. Similar to the ceremonies previously described, the initiates were between the ages of 12 and 18; the process occurred over 1–2 months; and it served to teach tribal customs and adult roles. All of these rites were consistent with Van Genneps's stages of separation, transition, and incorporation.

Groce, Mawar, & McNamara (2006) discussed the importance of including AIDS messages in rites of passage ceremonies in tribal societies. They cited traditional ceremonies in African cultures in Togo and in Xhosa and Zulu communities. Although some of these ceremonies included circumcision and scarification rites, young women and men were introduced into their roles apart from their families and underwent instruction related to adulthood. These rites of passage were often lengthy, and played a significant role in situating both young males and females in their family and community roles. Rites of passage programs for contemporary African American adolescents would necessarily look different from African tribal traditions, while still emphasizing African cultural roots. Lengthy processes of initiation that may take years to complete may not be practical in today's society, however, principles similar to these ancient models can be adapted for contemporary use.

Contemporary Perspectives

Warfield-Coppock (1992) explored contemporary rites programs for African American adolescents and described six models. They were (1) community-based programs, (2) agency or organizationally based programs, (3) school-based programs, (4) church-based programs, (5) therapeutic programs, and (6) family-based programs. These models primarily differed by the origin of their sponsorships and their inclusion criteria. For example, therapeutic programs generally focused on youth who were in treatment for mental health issues or drug use and abuse problems. Family-based programs included models whereby several families collaborated to provide a structured program for their same-sex adolescent children. Scott cites specific developmental elements that are included in contemporary rites of passage programs. They are sexuality, societal relationships, personal status and esteem, identity, skill development, religious duty, spiritual values, and consideration of mortality (Scott, 1998).

Warfield-Coppock reviewed 20 contemporary programs and found that these programs were designed primarily to assist African American youth in addressing the social issues that they faced and most used some form of an African-centered framework (1992). Although these programs involved the initiation of both males and females, recent literature revealed more programs that have been directed toward the transition of African American males than females (Alford, 2000; Cooper, Groce, & Thomas, 2003; Harvey & Hill, 2004; Harvey & Rauch, 1997).

Adolescent Girls in Need of Cultural Guidance

During the developmental stage of adolescence, girls most often begin to explore their sexuality, and when sexually active are at the greatest risk for contracting sexually transmissible diseases and HIV/AIDS (Burstein & Murray, 2003). How young girls experience and adapt to the physiologic and emotional changes associated with puberty can be shaped by appropriate cultural messages from elders and even from older girls who have successfully navigated this stage of living. In rites of passage programs, girls can receive cultural socialization and sound information about bodily changes, sexual health, and avoiding sexually transmissible diseases including HIV/AIDS. When girls are allowed to express themselves freely, ask questions, and discuss the important issues of growing up in a culturally safe and trusting environment away from their parents, they may be more likely to draw on a solid foundation of knowledge when faced with making future choices related to sexuality. The blend of cultural immersion with the guidance and wisdom of female elders and the infusion of cultural values and strengths have the potential to grow healthier African American girls and healthier African American communities.

For some African American girls, initiation into young womanhood occurs through the first sexual intercourse or an unwanted pregnancy instead of a planned, positive process through the intervention of wise elders in the community. These girls move quickly into adulthood without knowledge of cultural strengths, sexual health, and the skills needed to navigate the complexity of their worlds. Lewis-Cooper (2001) stated that these experiences (early sexual activity and unwanted pregnancies), "are not conducive to the creation of confident and whole individuals with the ability to manage their own lives and contribute to the well-being of the community" (p. 64). Schools are not adequately equipped to address critical social and cultural needs of young African American girls. Young parents who may be overwhelmed with life stressors, including working and child rearing may lack the time, community support, and knowledge to address the needs of their young daughters. Thus, more female centered rites programs are clearly needed to address the unique needs of African American girls and help them successfully navigate the transitions from girlhood to womanhood and to promote their sexual health. These programs would most likely be successful within a community and cultural context such as the African American church.

The Role of the African American Church

African American churches are in a unique position to develop, sponsor, and maintain rites of passage programs for youth in their own communities. Historically, the African American church has played a vital and respected role in shaping the lives of African American people. In past and present times, the church, a collective community in itself, has served as a venue for corporate worship, political activism, leadership development, and socialization of its members. Concern for guiding and directing youth has been a consistent purpose for the church (Lincoln & Mamiya, 1990).

Throughout the USA, African American churches of various denominations are prominent and visible in predominantly African American communities. From small urban "store front" churches to large elaborate edifices, these houses of worship are known to serve all members of the community regardless of church membership (Giger, Appel, Davidhizar, & Davis, 2008; Pinkett, 1993). In recent years, larger African American churches have once again taken on the role of educating its youth through church-based schools. Values that represent the African worldview are transmitted, such as, spirituality, respect for elders, harmony with nature, collective responsibility, and community pride (Belgrave & Allison, 2006). These same values have served to maintain the survival of people of African descent throughout history who live in a culturally different and sometimes oppositional environment characterized by discrimination and oppression (Warfield-Coppock, 1992). Engaging community members in rites of passage programs for girls through the African American church may serve to strengthen communities by reinforcing these same cultural values. Also, churches are consistently present in most communities where African American people dwell, and are a trusted and safe environment for parents to leave their children for a few hours to a few days.

Public health nurses and other professionals, such as social workers, are in a strategic position to develop relationships with church pastors, women's groups, and other church leaders to plan, develop, implement, and evaluate rites of passage programs for African American girls. Moreover, public health nurses can serve as resources and partners to churches for the delivery of age-appropriate sexual health messages as a part of these programs.

My Sister, Myself: A Model from Nursing

The three stages of rites of passage according to Van Gennep (2004) were enacted in a nursing and community collaborative project, "My Sister, Myself: Culture and Health for Africana Girls", in an urban community in the Midwest (Shambley-Ebron, 2009). A group of eight African American girls between the ages of 8 and 13 met weekly for 3 h each week for 8 weeks for an African American and woman-centered rites of passage project. A group which included parents, grandparents, community members, and African American nurses in the community collaborated to plan and implement this project in one particular church which had the physical resources to support the project.

As consistent with the first stage of rites of passage, "separation"; the sessions were held in a community church classroom that was converted to an African and woman-inspired sacred space. This space was adorned with African wall hangings, women's affirmations, and pictures of historically famous African American women. African and feminist inspired music helped to create an atmosphere of shared cultural identification. Although the girls were not removed from their homes for an extended period, the time spent at the Africana girls' room created time away from their everyday lives to become immersed in an environment to facilitate transformation. Parents were purposely not involved in the sessions so the girls felt free to participate fully and to bond with the other girls.

The second stage, "transition" was accomplished by the planned weekly activities. The themes for each week focused on Africentric principles of developing individual and collective identity and responsibility. The overall goal included developing body knowledge, understanding healthy and unhealthy relationships, developing life skills, developing positive mental and emotional health, and planning for successful adult womanhood.

Girls participated in reflective journaling, life mapping, and goal setting, as well as musical activities, spiritual dance, games, food, and fellowship. The girls also participated in lessons about African American women's history, and were encouraged to select an African American female role model with whom they might identify. Lessons about sexual health and behaviors were infused in the 8-week program with messages and stories about HIV/AIDS, sexually transmissible diseases, and unplanned pregnancy. All sessions were conducted by African American "women elders," that is, informed, knowledgeable, and experienced women who were respected in the community. Some of the "women elders" were school nurses, public health nurses, and other professional women. These women were interviewed and selected by the community members and project director to insure that they were knowledgeable, nonjudgmental, and supportive of adolescent girls and their healthy development.

The final session, "incorporation" was a program of formal presentation of the girls back to their community. The girls planned this program to which they invited their parents, families, and important community members. Each girl was given the opportunity to speak about what she had gained from her experience participating in the 8-week project in the African and African American tradition of "testimony." As a symbol of their new knowledge, transformation, and cultural identities, the girls were presented colorful African scarves and certificates of completion. They each wore personally designed African bead necklaces which were a representation of the values of knowledge, collective responsibility, harmony, and self-respect. The girls received encouragement and a charge to move forward positively in their lives from a young woman community speaker. Families and the communities shared a celebratory feast culminating the event.

Conclusion

Preventing HIV/AIDS in the African American community must involve knowledge development and behavior change in both males and females. Most rites of passage programs however separate males and females, as their needs, issues, and concerns are different. Because of the rapidly growing rates of HIV/AIDS in African American heterosexual women, this project was developed to place its focus on girls specifically. Consistent with historical rites of passage programs; knowledge about sexuality, responsible and irresponsible behaviors, and dangers of making unwise choices were discussed frankly by knowledgeable community women. Similar community programs focused on boys should also be developed.

A large scale clinical trial and longitudinal studies are needed to determine if consistent community participation in these types of rites programs for girls will indeed lead to a reduction in the incidence and prevalence of HIV/AIDS in African American women. Booster sessions might also be helpful to reinforce learnings from the initial project.

A rites of passage model such as "My Sister, Myself," can easily be enhanced and replicated in other African American communities, with churches as centers for these projects. Ideally, all adolescent girls in African American communities would have access to a rites of passage programs in their communities, and would eagerly anticipate their participation in this celebration of entry into young womanhood.

African American communities can actively participate in socializing their girls and transforming their communities at their hearts, the girls who will grow up to give life to future generations. African American girls who have formal instruction and preparation for womanhood can help to educate, indoctrinate, and model healthy behaviors for their peers.

Public health nurses are in a unique position to impact African American communities with positive health messages for growing girls. With the combination of indigenous community and evidence-based knowledge, negative health trends have the potential to be reversed. HIV/AIDS is one of the many perils that African American girls are facing in the twenty-first century. Reconnecting African American girls with strong cultural traditions and values through traditional rites of passage programs, have the potential to strengthen families, restore communities, and improve health outcomes.

References

Alford, K. (2000). Cultural themes in rites of passage: Voices of young African American males. *Journal of African American Studies, 7*(1), 3–26.

Belgrave, F. Z., & Allison, K. W. (2006). *African American psychology: From Africa to America.* Thousand Oaks, CA: Sage.

Burstein, G. R., & Murray, P. J. (2003). Diagnosis and management of sexually transmitted diseases among adolescents. *Pediatrics in Review, 24,* 119–127.

Centers for Disease Control and Prevention. (2008). HIV/AIDS among African Americans. *CDC Fact Sheet.* Retrieved October 24, 2008, from http://www.cdc.gov/hiv/topics/aa/resources/factsheets/aa.htm

Centers for Disease Control and Prevention. (2006). Racial/ethnic disparities in diagnoses of HIV/AIDS – 33 States, 2001–2004. *Morbidity and Mortality Weekly Report, 55*(5), 121–125.

Cooper, R., Groce, J., & Thomas, N. D. (2003). Changing direction: Rites of passage programs for African American older men. *Journal of African American Studies, 7*(3), 3–14.

Dancy, B. L., Crittenden, K. S., & Talashek, M. (2006). Mothers' effectiveness as HIV risk reduction educators for adolescent daughters. *Journal of Health Care for the Poor and Underserved, 17,* 218–219.

Delaney, C. H. (1995). Rites of passage in adolescence. *Adolescence, 30*(120), 891–897.

DiClemente, R. J., Wingood, G. M., Harrington, K. F., Lang, D. L., Davies, S. L., Hook, E. W., et al. (2004). Efficacy of an HIV prevention intervention for African American adolescent girls: A randomized control trial. *Journal of the American Medical Association, 292,* 171–179.

Dilorio, C., Resnicow, K., McCarty, F., De, A. K., Dudley, W. N., Wang, D. T., et al. (2006). Keepin' it R.E.A.L! Results of a mother-adolescent HIV prevention program. *Nursing Research, 55*(1), 43–51.

Giger, J. N., Appel, S. J., Davidhizar, R., & Davis, C. (2008). Church and spirituality in the lives of the African American community. *Journal of Transcultural Nursing, 19*(4), 375–383.

Gilbert, D. J., & Wright, E. M. (Eds.). (2003). *African American women and HIV/AIDS: Critical Responses.* Westport, CT: Praeger.

Groce, N., Mawar, N., & McNamara, M. (2006). Inclusion of AIDS educational messages in rites of passage ceremonies: Reaching young people in tribal communities. *Culture, Health & Sexuality, 8*(4), 303–315.

Harvey, A. R., & Hill, R. B. (2004). Africentric youth and family rites of passage program: Promoting resilience among at-risk African American Youths. *Social Work, 49*(1), 65–74.

Harvey, A. R., & Rauch, J. B. (1997). A comprehensive Afrocentric rites of passage program for Black male adolescents. *Health & Social Work, 22*(1), 30–37.

Hattery, A., & Smith, E. (2007). *African American Families.* Thousand Oaks: Sage.

Healthy People. (2020). Retrieved August 4, 2008, from http://www.healthypeople.gov

Jemmott, J. B., III, Jemmott, L. S., & Fong, G. T. (1998). Abstinence and safer sex HIV risk-reduction intervention for African American adolescents: A randomized controlled trial. *Journal of the American Medical Association, 279,* 1529–1536.

Lincoln, C. E., & Mamiya, L. H. (1990). *The Black church in the African American experience.* Durham, NC: Duke University Press.

Lewis-Cooper, R. M. (2001). Some Jamaican rites of passage: Reflections for the twenty-first century. *Black Theology in Britain, 6,* 53–71.

Lynch, A. (1999). *Dress, gender, and cultural change.* Oxford, UK: Berg.

Pinkett, J. (1993). Spirituality in the African American community. In L. Goddard (Ed.), *An African-centered model of prevention for African-American youth at high risk* (pp. 79–86). Rockville, MD: US Department of Health and Human Services.

Scott, D. G. (1998). Rites of passage in adolescent development: A reappreciation. *Child & Youth Care Forum, 27*(5), 317–335.

Shambley-Ebron, D. Z. (2009). My sister, myself: A culture and gender-based approach to HIV/AIDS prevention. *Journal of Transcultural Nursing, 20,* 28–36.

U.S. Census Bureau. (2008). Retrieved September 24, 2008, from http://www.census.gov/

Van Gennep, A. (2004). *The rites of passage.* London: Routledge, Taylor & Francis Group.

Warfield-Coppock, N. (1992). The rites of passage movement: A resurgence of African-centered practices for socializing African American youth. *Journal of Negro Education, 61*(4), 471–482.

Watson, M. A., & Montgomery, S. (1999). *Instructor's manual to accompany rites of passage: Videocases of traditional African peoples.* Englewood Cliffs, NJ: Prentice Hall.

Part V
Urgent Interventions for Women

Chapter 10
Black–White Disparities in Birth Outcomes: Is Racism-Related Stress a Missing Piece of the Puzzle?

Paula Braveman

Black–White Disparities in Preterm Birth and Low Birth Weight: What Could Explain them?

For decades, large disparities in birth outcomes have been observed between babies born to African-American (black) women and those born to European-American (white) women. Adverse birth outcomes – being born "too early" (premature or preterm birth, before 37 completed weeks of pregnancy) or "too small" (low birth weight, less than 5½ pounds) – are powerful predictors not only of infant survival, but also of child health, development, and serious disability (Institute of Medicine, 2007). Recent research reveals that low birth weight and premature birth also are strong predictors of chronic disease in adulthood, including cardiovascular disease and diabetes, which are major causes of premature mortality (Barker, 2006; Phillips, Jones, & Goulden, 2006; Whincup et al., 2008). As shown in Figs. 10.1 and 10.2, the disparities generally have been persistent, until recently when relative disparities began to narrow somewhat, for undesirable reasons: the rates of both preterm birth (PTB) and low birth weight (LBW) worsened among white women, with little (PTB) or no (LBW) improvement among black women. (For simplicity, throughout this chapter "black" and "white" are used to refer only to non-Hispanic women.)

The known causes of adverse birth outcomes do not explain the disparities. LBW can be due to PTB or intrauterine growth retardation (IUGR, inadequate growth at a given gestational age), which are thought to have distinct etiologies (Goldenberg, Culhane, Iams, & Romero, 2008; Kramer, 1987). Research has linked both PTB and LBW to use of tobacco, excessive alcohol (particularly in the first trimester), or cocaine, and to low pre-pregnancy weight, inadequate weight gain during pregnancy, very short maternal stature, and chronic disease (Institute of Medicine, 2007; Kramer & Hogue, 2009); of these, only tobacco has been definitively identified as causal. Studies taking these factors into account, however, have still observed black-white disparities (Lu & Halfon, 2003). Overall and among both black and white women, rates of PTB and LBW vary according to income and education (Blumenshine, Egerter, Barclay, Cubbin & Braveman, 2010); racial disparities persist, however, even after taking income or education into account (Institute of Medicine, 2007; Lu & Halfon, 2003; P. Braveman et al., unpublished data from the California Maternal and Infant Health Assessment, 2007).

P. Braveman (✉)
Department of Family and Community Medicine, Center on Social Disparities in Health, San Francisco, CA, USA
e-mail: braveman@fcm.ucsf.edu

A.J. Lemelle et al. (eds.), *Handbook of African American Health: Social and Behavioral Interventions*, DOI 10.1007/978-1-4419-9616-9_10, © Springer Science+Business Media, LLC 2011

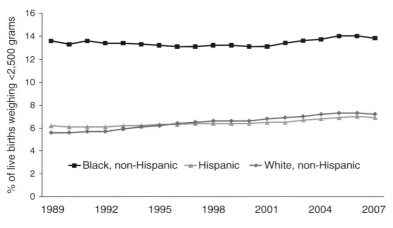

Source: National Vital Statistics Report, National Center for Health Statistics, 2009

Fig. 10.1 Racial/ethnic disparities in low birth weight: trends over time

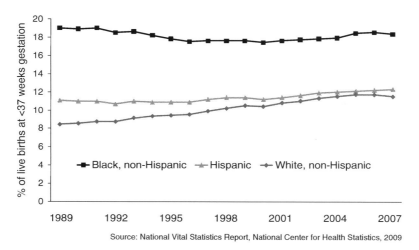

Source: National Vital Statistics Report, National Center for Health Statistics, 2009

Fig. 10.2 Racial/ethnic disparities in preterm birth: trends over time

A number of other causes have been suspected, but to date, no definitive evidence has established any of them. Many researchers have hypothesized that reproductive tract or periodontal infections were the cause (Institute of Medicine, 2007); these infections are more common among black women (Albandar, 2005; Hitti et al., 2007; Horton et al., 2008; Klatt, Cole, Eastwood, & Barnabei, 2010; Newton, Piper, Shain, Perdue, & Peairs, 2001). This seems unlikely, however, because experiments in which these infections have been successfully treated have not demonstrated consistently improved birth outcomes (Institute of Medicine, 2007; Lopez, 2007; McDonald, Brocklehurst, & Gordon, 2007; Michalowicz et al., 2006), suggesting that unmeasured factors associated with the infections may be the actual causal agents (Wadhwa et al., 2001). Some scientists have thought that exposure to certain environmental toxins might be the answer, and others have implicated work that is physically demanding – e.g., requiring one to be on one's feet for extended periods of time during pregnancy – but neither hypothesis has consistent evidence to support it (Institute of Medicine, 2007; Savitz & Murnane, 2010) .

Another widely held theory is that the differences are genetic in nature. No one, however, has identified a "PTB" or "LBW" gene or set of genes. The processes involved in PTB in particular are likely to be complex, involving cascades of factors that may interact with multiple other factors (Institute of Medicine, 2007). It is reasonable to question whether such complex cascades of factors would be likely to sort out through the process of natural selection along racial/ethnic lines, particularly given the extensive mixing of gene pools that has occurred for all but a very few small, isolated population groups (David & Collins, 2007).

Another issue that casts doubt on the genetic etiology hypothesis is that black immigrants to the US from Africa and the Caribbean have had much more favorable PTB and/or LBW rates than those of US-born black women (Acevedo-Garcia, Soobader, & Berkman, 2005; David & Collins, 1997; Howard, Marshall, Kaufman & Savitz, 2006; Singh & Yu, 1996); a study following multiple generations found evidence that the birth outcomes of the US-born daughters and granddaughters of those immigrants, however, become less favorable with successive generations (Collins, Wu, & David, 2002). These patterns suggest an "environmental" cause, in the broadest sense of environment – some factor(s) in the social or physical environment to which black women are exposed when they are born and raised in the US – rather than a genetic cause. The worsening of birth outcomes with successive generations in the US is consistent with the notion of some health-damaging exposure in the US context. While a purely or primarily genetic cause is apparently not supported by the observed social patterns, gene–environment interactions cannot be ruled out.

A number of researchers (Dominguez, Dunkel-Schetter, Glynn, Hobel & Sandman, 2008; Hogan, Njoroge, Durant & Ferre, 2001; Hogue & Bremner, 2005) strongly suspect that a key reason for the racial disparities in birth outcomes may be chronic stress and other disadvantages (e.g., poorer nutrition, health-damaging psychosocial and physical exposures in housing and neighborhoods, experiences related to racial discrimination) in childhood that are not frequently measured in health studies. We believe this explanation better fits the observed social patterns than other explanations. The evidence supporting this view is discussed further below.

Examining the Evidence Supporting a role for Racism-Related Stress

Good birth outcomes among Black immigrants

In several studies, Black African and Afro-Caribbean immigrants have demonstrated relatively good birth outcomes; in one study, the birth outcomes of their US-born descendants worsened with successive generations. This suggests an important role for social factors. As noted previously, black immigrants to the US from Africa and the Caribbean have birth outcomes far more favorable than those of US-born black women (Acevedo-Garcia et al., 2005; David & Collins, 1997; Howard et al., 2006; Pallotto, Collins, & David, 2000; Singh & Yu, 1996). Similarly, a 1990 study found that birth outcomes of North African immigrants to France or Belgium (who were not citizens) were at least as favorable as those of French or Belgian women who were native-born or who acquired citizenship (Guendelman et al., 1999). If the primary cause were genetic, one would expect the birth outcomes of black immigrants to be at least as unfavorable as those of native-born black women because the gene pool – at least of African immigrants – would be less diluted with genetic material from people of primarily European descent. Furthermore, as noted earlier, in the only relevant study we are aware of, the birth outcomes of the US-born daughters and granddaughters of black immigrants start to look increasingly like those of African-American (i.e., other US-born) women (Collins et al., 2002). It is very difficult to explain those patterns primarily with genetic causes.

A similar pattern has been observed for some time among Latinas (women of Latin American background), particularly those of Mexican-American or Central American background. These Latina immigrants have good birth outcomes (low rates of PTB and LBW), better than would be expected based on their relatively low incomes and educational levels (Acevedo-Garcia, Soobader,

Table 10.1 Ratio of low birth weight rates among Blacks vs. Whites at different income levels

Family income in relation to the federal poverty level[a]	Black to White ratio
Poor: at or below the poverty line	1.3 times
Near-poor:1–2 times the poverty line	1.6 times
Not low-income: more than 2 times the poverty line	Around 2.5 times

Source: P. Braveman et al., unpublished data from the California Maternal and Infant Health Assessment (MIHA), 1999–2005
[a] During 1999–2005, federal poverty level for a family of four was around $17,000–20,000

& Berkman, 2007; Collins & Shay, 1994); however, the daughters and granddaughters of Latina immigrants, are less likely than immigrant mothers to have favorable birth outcomes (Collins & David, 2004; Guendelman, Gould, Hudes, & Eskenazi, 1990). The favorable birth outcomes for both black and Latina immigrants may partly reflect "healthy immigrant" selection, meaning that immigrants are generally an unusually healthy group; emigration is challenging. It could also reflect the fact that immigrants tend to have healthier behaviors – regarding smoking, diet, alcohol, drugs – than the US-born (Lucas, Barr-Anderson, & Kington, 2005; Ojeda, Patterson, & Strathdee, 2008; Park, Neckerman, Quinn, Weiss, & Rundle, 2008; Singh & Hiatt, 2006). Studies considering smoking and alcohol use have still found favorable birth outcomes among black and Latina immigrants (Acevedo-Garcia et al., 2005; Acevedo-Garcia et al., 2007; Guendelman et al., 1990; Guendelman et al., 1999; Howard et al., 2006), however, and in any case the good outcomes among immigrants indicate that inherent genetic makeup is not the "rate-limiting step."

Is there something "toxic" in the exposure to growing up and coming of age as a woman of color in the US? The observed patterns certainly raise that question. Gene–environment interactions cannot be ruled out. If gene–environment interactions were involved, however, the practical implications would be the same as if the cause were entirely environmental. This is so not only because no one has identified the suspect genes, but also because, despite massive investment in genetic research, even where apparently causal genes for particular illnesses have been identified, there has been little yield to date in practical medical therapies (Pollack, 2010). The rational approach would be to identify and address the modifiable harmful social or physical exposures in the environment for US-born women of color.

Generally when the term "environment" is used in this chapter, it refers to characteristics of either the social or physical environment. The physical environment includes housing quality, sidewalks, parks, traffic, bike paths, other features of urban/suburban design, and pollution, for example. Features of the social environment could include, for example, presence of crime or gangs, concentrated poverty, family instability, or housing insecurity, hopelessness, and feelings of social exclusion or marginalization, including a widespread perception of belonging to a social group that is valued less by society in general.

Birth outcomes of affluent and highly educated African-American women

The relative disparity in birth outcomes between black and white women is largest among the most educated, affluent women; it is relatively small among the poor. This also suggests social factors are at play. Among both black and white women, PTB and LBW rates decline (improve) with increasing income or education. However, the *relative difference* (the ratio of the rates) between black and white birth outcomes actually *increases* (worsens) with higher income or education. For example, as shown in Table 10.1, recent statewide data from California (where one in seven US births occur) demonstrates that among poor women, blacks had 1.3 times the rate of LBW as whites; however, among women with incomes over two times the poverty level, black women were more than twice

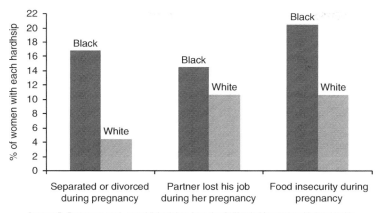

Source: P. Braveman et al., unpublished data from the California Maternal and Infant Health Assessment (MIHA) 2002-2004(*n* = 10,750)

Fig. 10.3 Selected hardships during pregnancy: disparities by race

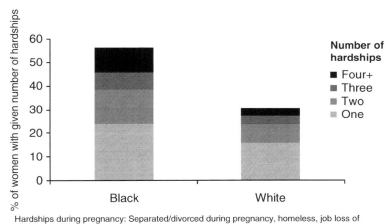

Hardships during pregnancy: Separated/divorced during pregnancy, homeless, job loss of spouse/partner, involuntary job loss of respondent, food insecurity, incarceration of respondent or her spouse/partner, domestic violence, hard to live on her family income, unpaid bills, no practical support, no emotional support. Source: P. Braveman et al., unpublished data from the California Maternal and Infant Health Assessment (MIHA) 2003-2004 (*n* =7,272)

Fig. 10.4 Total number of hardships during pregnancy: disparities by race

(2.5) times as likely as white women to have a LBW birth (P. Braveman et al., unpublished data from the California Maternal and Infant Health Assessment, 2007). A similar pattern has been seen in national data (Starfield et al., 1991), and patterns are similar for PTB. As with the favorable birth outcomes of immigrants and the unfavorable outcomes of their US-born daughters, it is also difficult to explain this pattern as primarily genetically based.

Why would higher income/education black women fare worse relative to their white counterparts with similar levels of income and education? How could this perhaps counter-intuitive pattern be explained? Two explanations seem reasonable, both having to do with stress: stress related to unmeasured financial hardship or insecurity, and stress related to awareness of racial discrimination.

Being poor or near-poor – i.e., having income below 200% of the federal poverty level – is stressful (Braveman et al., 2010). Black women are more likely to be poor or near-poor during pregnancy than their white counterparts (Braveman et al., 2010). They are more likely to experience stressful circumstances related to financial hardship, as illustrated in Figs. 10.3 and 10.4. Experiences of chronic stress, particularly during childhood, may have the most potential for damaging physiologic systems with potential implications for PTB (Hogue & Bremner, 2005; Lu & Halfon, 2003). Health studies rarely measure socioeconomic experiences in childhood, and black women of a given *current* income or education level are more likely than their white counterparts with similar levels of current income/education to have experienced worse socioeconomic conditions as children (Braveman et al., 2005). Black and white women of a given current education/income level also are likely to differ in socioeconomic characteristics of the neighborhoods where they have lived, and this, too, could affect birth outcomes. There may be more relative disparity in childhood and neighborhood conditions among black and white women of currently high education/income levels, than among those who are poor. Worse socioeconomic conditions could be stressful in themselves, and contribute to family strife and disruption, which then adds to the stress. Relatively affluent black women may face more stress than similarly affluent white women due to greater responsibilities to financially support family, friends, or partners. College-educated black women face the added stress, compared with their white counterparts, of having fewer similarly educated black men with whom they might partner, given the low rates of college graduation among black men in the US.

There is another dimension to consider as well. In addition to the stress of financial hardship and associated social stressors, chronically experiencing or anticipating discriminatory treatment could be stressful. Being aware of racial discrimination, and being vigilant to be prepared to respond to it if it occurs, also could be quite stressful. In focus groups with African-American women in California, my colleagues and I were struck by the extent to which black women – both low-income and not low-income – reported carried around with them a constant, gnawing awareness and anxiety about when the next incident, overt or subtle, might occur, not only to them but also to their children. Ironically, more educated and affluent African-American women may be more exposed to experiences of racial discrimination, because they are more likely to be working, shopping and residing with whites than are their less educated/affluent black counterparts. Regardless of whether these more educated and affluent African-American women experience more incidents of interpersonal discrimination, they may be more pervasively vigilant because they are more frequently in contact with whites. This theory must be tested empirically, but it is biologically plausible given what we know about the physiology of stress, which is discussed below.

How could stress lead to adverse birth outcomes?

There has been a marked growth in knowledge regarding the physiology of stress over the past 15 or so years. "Stress" refers to experiences in response to challenges ("stressors") taxing one's ability to cope. We now know that stress (of many varieties) can trigger neuroendocrine, sympathetic nervous system, inflammatory, immune, and/or vascular responses in the body. Physiologic pathways have been traced from the hypothalamus (one part of the brain) to the anterior pituitary (another) and from there to the adrenal glands, which secrete cortisol, potentially affecting multiple organs and systems. Acute stress may not necessarily result in bodily harm; however, over time, chronic, sustained stress, even if not dramtic, can result in harmful physiologic changes, including processes thought to be involved in PTB and potentially in LBW as well. It is therefore plausible that if a woman was exposed to chronic stress in childhood or generally before her pregnancy, she may be at higher risk of PTB, even if her pregnancy itself is relatively stress-free, because the physiologic systems involved in controlling when labor begins could have been dysregulated by her experience of chronic stress as a child (Lu & Halfon, 2003). Thus, if chronic economic hardship and/or experiences related to discrimination cause chronic stress, this could lead to premature aging or "weathering" (Geronimus, 1996), which may contribute to black women's risk of PTB. Dominguez discusses how racism-related stress may contribute to the racial disparities in birth outcomes (Dominguez et al., 2008). Biomedical research is shedding increasing light on the phenomena and structures involved in the health effects of chronic stress (McEwen & Gianaros, 2010).

African-Americans generally experience more stressful circumstances, which are not often measured

A number of ways have been mentioned above in which African-American women are likely to experience more chronically stressful circumstances chronically than their white counterparts, even those of apparently similar income and educational levels. At a given income level, blacks have a fraction of the accumulated wealth that whites have; wealth can buffer one from the effects of temporary losses of income. At a given educational level, blacks have lower incomes. As noted above, at a given current educational level, among women who have recently given birth in California, a black woman is more likely to have grown up in a socioeconomically worse-off household than her white counterpart of similar education (Braveman et al., 2005). At a given current income level, blacks are more likely to live in disadvantaged neighborhoods (Braveman et al., 2005); disadvantaged neighborhoods have more crime, social disarray, and fewer services than more advantaged communities. All of these socioeconomic circumstances are likely to be associated with more stress. In addition to socioeconomic hardship, it is important also to consider experiences of racial discrimination, which can be present at any socioeconomic level, as discussed briefly earlier. The effects of multiple sources of stress may accumulate over time, with particularly adverse physical effects.

Living in a society in which blacks have less wealth, influence, prestige, and social acceptance also can be chronically stressful

As noted above, my own research has suggested that African-American women of diverse socioeconomic levels may experience a constant concern and anxiety in anticipation of incidents – or attitudes – in which they will be judged and potentially treated in a biased manner because of their race (Nuru-Jeter et al., 2009). This constant vigilance over time could activate physiologic systems involved in the stress response, potentially resulting in significant damage to vital organs and systems, as mentioned in the discussion of stress (above). This could occur even in the absence of overt incidents of clearly unfair treatment.

What Are the Solutions?

No one has definitive knowledge of the causes of racial disparities in birth outcomes, but we do know enough to know that there are no simple solutions. The patterns are social, and the solutions therefore must be social, whether or not new biomedical therapies can make any additional contributions. The patterns strongly suggest a role for chronic social disadvantage, both related to economic hardship and its social consequences, and related to living in a society where racial discrimination still exists, perpetuated by societal structures such as racial residential segregation, even when there may no longer be conscious intent to discriminate. The solutions to racial disparities in PTB may, in fact, address most racial disparities in health – initiatives that will bring economic and social opportunities to communities that are marginalized.

Because conditions in neighborhoods can be such an important – and modifiable – determinant of a person's ability to escape poverty and its adverse health effects, efforts like the Department of Education's "Promise Neighborhoods" initiative (http://www.promiseneighborhoodsinstitute.org/) – combining early childhood development programs, improving schools, supporting families, and engaging communities – will be crucial for breaking the intergenerational cycle of poverty and despair that is one of the most important underlying factors of racial disparities in health in this country. Public dialogue about race and racism will also be important, but cannot take the place of concrete measures to change the material and social conditions of African Americans. Achieving more equality in social and economic opportunities will ultimately contribute more to racial equality – in health overall, and in PTB in particular – than discussions of racism.

References

Acevedo-Garcia, D., Soobader, M. J., & Berkman, L. F. (2007). Low birthweight among US Hispanic/Latino subgroups: The effect of maternal foreign-born status and education. *Social Science & Medicine, 65*(12), 2503–2516.

Acevedo-Garcia, D., Soobader, M. J., & Berkman, L. F. (2005). The differential effect of foreign-born status on low birth weight by race/ethnicity and education. *Pediatrics, 115*(1), e20–e30.

Albandar, J. M. (2005). Epidemiology and risk factors of periodontal diseases. *Dental Clinics of North America, 49*(3), 517–532, v–vi.

Barker, D. J. (2006). Adult consequences of fetal growth restriction. *Clinical Obstetrics and Gynecology, 49*(2), 270–283.

Blumenshine, P., Egerter, S., Barclay, C. J., Cubbin, C., & Braveman, P. (2010). Socioeconomic disparities in adverse birth outcomes: A systematic review. *American Journal of Preventive Medicine, 39*(3), 263–272.

Braveman, P., Marchi, K., Egerter, S., Kim, S., Metzler, M., Stancil, T., et al. (2010). Poverty, near-poverty, and hardship around the time of pregnancy. *Maternal and Child Health Journal, 14*(1), 20–35.

Braveman, P. A., Cubbin, C., Egerter, S., Chideya, S., Marchi, K. S., Metzler, M., et al. (2005). Socioeconomic status in health research: One size does not fit all. *Journal of the American Medical Association, 294*(22), 2879–2888.

Collins, J. W., Jr., & David, R. J. (2004). Pregnancy outcome of Mexican-American women: The effect of generational residence in the United States. *Ethnicity & Disease, 14*(3), 317–321.

Collins, J. W., Jr., & Shay, D. K. (1994). Prevalence of low birth weight among Hispanic infants with United States-born and foreign-born mothers: The effect of urban poverty. *American Journal of Epidemiology, 139*(2), 184–192.

Collins, J. W., Wu, S. Y., & David, R. J. (2002). Differing intergenerational birth weights among the descendants of US-born and foreign-born Whites and African Americans in Illinois. *American Journal of Epidemiology, 155*(3), 210–216.

David, R. J., & Collins, J. W., Jr. (2007). Disparities in infant mortality: What's genetics got to do with it? *American Journal of Public Health, 97*(7), 1191–1197.

David, R. J., & Collins, J. W., Jr. (1997). Differing birth weight among infants of U.S.-born blacks, African-born blacks, and U.S.-born whites. *The New England Journal of Medicine, 337*(17), 1209–1214.

Dominguez, T. P., Dunkel-Schetter, C., Glynn, L. M., Hobel, C., & Sandman, C. A. (2008). Racial differences in birth outcomes: The role of general, pregnancy, and racism stress. *Health Psychology, 27*(2), 194–203.

Geronimus, A. T. (1996). Black/white differences in the relationship of maternal age to birthweight: A population-based test of the weathering hypothesis. *Social Science & Medicine, 42*(4), 589–597.

Goldenberg, R. L., Culhane, J. F., Iams, J. D., & Romero, R. (2008). Epidemiology and causes of preterm birth. *Lancet, 371*(9606), 75–84.

Guendelman, S., Buekens, P., Blondel, B., Kaminski, M., Notzon, F. C., & Masuy-Stroobant, G. (1999). Birth outcomes of immigrant women in the United States, France, and Belgium. *Maternal and Child Health Journal, 3*(4), 177–187.

Guendelman, S., Gould, J. B., Hudes, M., & Eskenazi, B. (1990). Generational differences in perinatal health among the Mexican American population: Findings from HHANES 1982–84. *American Journal of Public Health, 80*(S), 61–65.

Hitti, J., Nugent, R., Boutain, D., Gardella, C., Hillier, S. L., & Eschenbach, D. A. (2007). Racial disparity in risk of preterm birth associated with lower genital tract infection. *Paediatric and Perinatal Epidemiology, 21*(4), 330–337.

Hogan, V. K., Njoroge, T., Durant, T. M., & Ferre, C. D. (2001). Eliminating disparities in perinatal outcomes–lessons learned. *Maternal and Child Health Journal, 5*(2), 135–140.

Hogue, C. J., & Bremner, J. D. (2005). Stress model for research into preterm delivery among black women. *American Journal of Obstetrics & Gynecology, 192*(5), S47–S55.

Horton, A. L., Boggess, K. A., Moss, K. L., Jared, H. L., Beck, J., & Offenbacher, S. (2008). Periodontal disease early in pregnancy is associated with maternal systemic inflammation among African American women. *The Journal of Periodontology, 79*(7), 1127–1132.

Howard, D. L., Marshall, S. S., Kaufman, J. S., & Savitz, D. A. (2006). Variations in low birth weight and preterm delivery among blacks in relation to ancestry and nativity: New York City, 1998–2002. *Pediatrics, 118*(5), e1399–e1405.

Institute of Medicine, Committee on Understanding Premature Birth and Assuring Healthy Outcomes, Board on Health Sciences Policy. (2007). *Preterm birth: causes, consequences, and prevention.* Washington, DC: The National Academies Press.

Klatt, T. E., Cole, D. C., Eastwood, D. C., & Barnabei, V. M. (2010). Factors associated with recurrent bacterial vaginosis. *The Journal of Reproductive Medicine, 55*(1–2), 55–61.

Kramer, M. R., & Hogue, C. R. (2009). What causes racial disparities in very preterm birth? A biosocial perspective. *Epidemiological Reviews, 31*, 84–98.

Kramer, M. S. (1987). Determinants of low birth weight: Methodological assessment and meta-analysis. *Bulletin of the World Health Organization, 65*(5), 663–737.

Lopez, R. (2007). Periodontal treatment in pregnant women improves periodontal disease but does not alter rates of preterm birth. *The Journal of Evidence-Based Dental Practice, 8*(2), 38.

Lu, M. C., & Halfon, N. (2003). Racial and ethnic disparities in birth outcomes: A life-course perspective. *Maternal and Child Health Journal, 7*(1), 13–30.

Lucas, J. W., Barr-Anderson, D. J., & Kington, R. S. (2005). Health status of non-Hispanic U.S.-born and foreign-born black and white persons: United States, 1992–95. *Vital and Health Statistics, 10*(226), 1–20.

McDonald, H. M., Brocklehurst, P., & Gordon, A. (2007). Antibiotics for treating bacterial vaginosis in pregnancy. *Cochrane Database of Systematic Reviews*, 1, CD000262.

McEwen, B. S., & Gianaros, P. J. (2010). Central role of the brain in stress and adaptation: Links to socioeconomic status, health, and disease. *Annals of the New York Academy of Sciences, 1186*, 190–222.

Michalowicz, B. S., Hodges, J. S., DiAngelis, A. J., Lupo, V. R., Novak, M. J., Ferguson, J. E., et al. (2006). Treatment of periodontal disease and the risk of preterm birth. *The New England Journal of Medicine, 355*(18), 1885–1894.

Newton, E. R., Piper, J. M., Shain, R. N., Perdue, S. T., & Peairs, W. (2001). Predictors of the vaginal microflora. *American Journal of Obstetrics &Gynecology, 184*(5), 845–853, discussion 853–855.

Nuru-Jeter, A., Dominguez, T. P., Hammond, W. P., Leu, J., Skaff, M., Egerter, S., et al. (2009). "It's the skin you're in": African American women talk about their experiences of racism. An exploratory study to develop measures of racism for birth outcome studies. *Maternal and Child Health Journal, 13*(1), 29–39.

Ojeda, V. D., Patterson, T. L., & Strathdee, S. A. (2008). The influence of perceived risk to health and immigration-related characteristics on substance use among Latino and other immigrants. *American Journal of Public Health, 98*(5), 862–868.

Pallotto, E. K., Collins, J. W., Jr., & David, R. J. (2000). Enigma of maternal race and infant birth weight: A population-based study of US-born Black and Caribbean-born Black women. *American Journal of Epidemiology, 151*(11), 1080–1085.

Park, Y., Neckerman, K. M., Quinn, J., Weiss, C., & Rundle, A. (2008). Place of birth, duration of residence, neighborhood immigrant composition and body mass index in New York City. *International Journal of Behavioral Nutrition and Physical Activity, 5*, 19.

Phillips, D. I., Jones, A., & Goulden, P. A. (2006). Birth weight, stress, and the metabolic syndrome in adult life. *Annals of the New York Academy of Sciences, 1083*, 28–36.

Pollack, A. (2010, June 14). Awaiting the genome payoff: The genome at 10. *New York Times*.

Savitz, D. A., & Murnane, P. (2010). Behavioral influences on preterm birth: A review. *Epidemiology, 21*(3), 291–299.

Singh, G. K., & Hiatt, R. A. (2006). Trends and disparities in socioeconomic and behavioural characteristics, life expectancy, and cause-specific mortality of native-born and foreign-born populations in the United States, 1979–2003. *International Journal of Epidemiology, 35*(4), 903–919.

Singh, G. K., & Yu, S. M. (1996). Adverse pregnancy outcomes: Differences between US- and foreign-born women in major US racial and ethnic groups. *American Journal of Public Health, 86*(6), 837–843.

Starfield, B., Shapiro, S., Weiss, J., Liang, K. Y., Ra, K., Paige, D., et al. (1991). Race, family income, and low birth weight. *American Journal of Epidemiology, 134*(10), 1167–1174.

Wadhwa, P. D., Culhane, J. F., Rauh, V., Barve, S. S., Hogan, V., Sandman, C. A., et al. (2001). Stress, infection and preterm birth: A biobehavioural perspective. *Paediatric and Perinatal Epidemiology, 15*(S2), 17–29.

Whincup, P. H., Kaye, S. J., Owen, C. G., Huxley, R., Cook, D. G., Anazawa, S., et al. (2008). Birth weight and risk of type 2 diabetes: A systematic review. *Journal of the American Medical Association, 300*(24), 2886–2897.

Chapter 11
African American Women and Breast Cancer: Interventions at Multiple Levels

Sarah Gehlert, Eusebius Small, and Sarah Bollinger

Introduction

Breast Cancer Incidence and Mortality Among African American Women

Cancer of the breast is the second leading cause of cancer death among women in the USA (McGregor & Antoni, 2009), with over 200,000 cases diagnosed annually (National Cancer Institute, 2009). Approximately 40,460 women died of the disease in 2007 alone (American Cancer Society, 2009). Whereas white women are more likely than African American women to develop breast cancer (130.6 per 100,000 white women vs. 117.5 per 100,000 African American women), African American women are 37% more likely to die from the disease (Ries et al., 2008). Although a notable annual decline in aggregate breast cancer mortality has been registered for all women since the 1990s, the disparity ratio gap between African American and white women continues to widen. The gap is particularly pronounced among women younger than 50 years of age, with African American women of this age group being 77% more likely to die from the disease than their white counterparts (Carey et al., 2006).

The unique situation of African American women who are at risk for or have been diagnosed with breast cancer warrants interventions that take into account disease biology and their social environment. In this chapter, after providing an overview of breast cancer among African American women and reviewing existing psychosocial interventions, we will frame African American and white mortality disparities within a larger biopsychosocial context, and then propose a new neighborhood- and community-level intervention for African American women. We will outline our own work with African American women newly diagnosed with breast cancer living on the South Side of Chicago, and present our novel approach to choosing the targets of intervention based on the community-based, multilevel investigations conducted at the Center for Interdisciplinary Health Disparities Research.

S. Gehlert (✉)
George Warren Brown School of Social Work,
Washington University, St. Louis, MO, USA
e-mail: sgehlert@wustl.edu

A.J. Lemelle et al. (eds.), *Handbook of African American Health: Social and Behavioral Interventions*,   165
DOI 10.1007/978-1-4419-9616-9_11, © Springer Science+Business Media, LLC 2011

Breast Cancer Differences in African American Women

Breast cancer affects all population groups. African American women, however, bear a disproportionate burden in terms of mortality and reduced survivorship compared to white women (Underwood, 2006). In addition, they are twice as likely to die from breast cancer developed before menopause than white women (Eley et al., 1994). Researchers attribute these disparities to factors such as late diagnosis of cancer, differences in access to screening, socioeconomic factors such as poverty and neighborhood degradation, and biological differences in the cancer tumors (Li, Malone, & Darling, 2003; Watlington, Byers, Mouchawar, Sauaia, & Ellis, 2007). However, a definitive explanation and understanding of the differences in African American and white disparity and survival rates remains unclear (Carey et al., 2006).

African American women do exhibit some unique breast cancer characteristics. As an example, they frequently are diagnosed at a much younger age (under 45 years) than their white counterparts (Newman, 2005). It is interesting to note that in West Africa, from where it is believed the majority of African Americans originate, breast cancer is seen as a lethal disease for young women. According to Huo et al. (2009), women in West Africa are more likely to develop the disease prior to menopause, whereas in the USA, it is considered a post-menopausal phenomenon.

Having breast cancer earlier in life may result in significantly poorer psychosocial outcomes for women. Younger women with breast cancer are thought to have significantly lower quality of life and higher levels of psychological morbidity, compared to older, post-menopausal women (Avis, Crawford, & Manuel, 2005; Ganz, Greendale, Peterson, Kahn, & Bower, 2003; Turner, Kelly, Swanson, Allison, & Wetzig, 2005). Unfortunately, although we know that this younger group of women typically faces greater challenges in coping with the disease, little work has been done to understand the specific psychosocial needs of women in this age group, especially for those who are of racial and ethnic minority status (Zebrack, Mills, & Weitzman, 2007).

A second way in which African American women may be unique biologically has to do with breast cancer subtype. Breast cancer is a heterogeneous disease whose subtypes vary significantly (Carey et al., 2006). Notably, they vary by race and age, with young African American women being more likely to experience aggressive forms of breast cancer more frequently than their white counterparts. An important example of this is the so-called triple-negative breast cancer, a particularly aggressive form of the disease that is overrepresented among pre-menopausal, African American women (National Cancer Institute, 2007). The term triple-negative refers to three biomarkers, namely estrogen receptors (ER), progesterone receptors (PR), and human epidermal growth factor receptor-2 (HER-2). When tumors lack these three hormone receptors, and thus are said to be triple-negative, typical targeted therapeutic treatment is rendered less effective (Schneider et al., 2008).

Triple-negative breast cancer has much overlap with an aggressive molecular breast cancer known as the basal-like subtype (Huo et al., 2009; Vona-Davis & Rose, 2009). The basal-like subtype is most often negative on all three hormone receptors, as is the case with triple-negative breast cancer, but also is defined by a specific gene array profile. The process of identifying the basal-like profile is more complex and often difficult to accomplish in clinical settings. The triple-negative subtype is often used as a proxy for basal-like breast tumors, even though the two classifications fail to overlap perfectly. Despite these difference, it is critical to note that the basal-like subtype also is concentrated among pre-menopausal African American women, compared to post-menopausal African American women and non-African American women (39 vs. 14 and 16%, respectively; $p < 0.001$) (Anders & Carey, 2008). The presence of this aggressive cancer subtype predicts early recurrence and poor survival prognosis (Li et al., 2003; Morris et al., 2007; Watlington et al., 2007).

A third way in which the breast cancer of African American women is unique is that they are likely to have larger primary tumors (Vona-Davis & Rose, 2009) and tumors of higher histological grade at the time of diagnosis than white women (Li et al., 2003; Martinez et al., 2007). Their tumors likewise are more likely to be node positive, meaning that at the time of diagnosis there is usually lymph node involvement (Newman, 2005). The tumors in African American women are of high mitotic activity, consistent with the more advanced disease at diagnosis, a consequence of rapid tumor growth rather than a delay in diagnosis (Porter et al., 2004). There is some debate about the relative contributions of determinants of the disparity in stage and grade of cancer between African American and white women. Some researchers attribute the difference primarily to access to care, while others consider biology to contribute.

Living in poverty and differential exposure to environmental toxins are two additional factors that disproportionately affect African American women. Bruce McEwen, in a seminal article published in 1998, observes that continual exposure to stressful physiological and environmental stimuli, such as social instability, job loss, and psychological stress, may increase the incidence of disease. He asserts that, "the core of the body's response to a challenge – whether it is a dangerous situation, an infection, living in a crowded and unpleasant neighborhood, is twofold, turning on an allostatic response that initiates a complex adaptive pathway, and then shutting off this response when the threat is past," (p. 172). In the ensuing two decades since the publication of this work, the knowledge base about how stress affects disease has increased. Nevertheless, the basic concept outlined by McEwen remains the same.

There is evidence that neighborhoods characterized by high rates of violence and crime, by fostering social isolation and depression, in time produce changes in biology and rates of disease (Chida & Hamer, 2009). The negative events that occur in certain neighborhoods may destabilize the body's homeostasis, causing allostatic overload (McEwen, 2008). Extreme stressors are associated with altered stress hormone response and may alter the chemistry of the body's DNA, causing epigenetic changes (Cacioppo et al., 2000).

Theories of the Origins of Breast Cancer Disparities Among African American Women

The Psychological Impacts of Cancer

Systematic stressors often are experienced by those at the bottom of economic and social strata. Stressors such as unpaid bills, jobs that do not pay enough to cover basic expenses, unsafe living conditions, exposure to environmental hazards, lack of control over work and schedule, worries over children, isolation, and few available resources, ultimately contribute to acute and chronic physiological stress that can lead to disease in a number of ways. Herbert and Cohen (1993) conducted a meta-analysis of the empirical literature linking stress and immunity, and found substantial evidence to link the two. Their study focused on the association between negative life events, operationalized as objective discrete events (e.g., bereavement, clinical examinations) and self-report of cumulative stressful events (e.g., life events, daily hassle). The authors concluded that negative events (i.e., stressors) lead to negative affective states (distress) that may ultimately relate to alterations in human immunity (Herbert & Cohen). Lowered immunity is associated with disease.

With these psychosocial stressors in mind, cancer diagnosis and cancer treatments are inherently negative events that cause tremendous emotional distress for those involved, regardless of race, age, ethnicity, and social economic status. According to Burgess et al. (2005), the prevalence of depression among women with breast cancer during the first year after diagnosis is twice as high as that of the general female population. Additionally, the prevalence of affective disorder and anxiety for women during the first year after a breast cancer diagnosis is said to be 25–33% higher than that of the general population (Härter et al., 2001). Treatment of psychological issues such as depression in women with breast cancer is of utmost importance in maintaining or increasing quality of life, and may possibly increase survivorship (Reich, Lesur, & Perdrizet-Chevallier, 2008). Women with breast cancer who have high levels of emotional support, and a strong social support system are less likely to experience depression than are those who lack these supports (Wong-Kim & Bloom, 2005); however, given the high prevalence of systematic stressors that affect vulnerable populations, these protective factors may not be as readily available for all women.

Social Determinants

The effect of the social environment on breast cancer incidence, mortality, and survival is well documented. Poverty, for example, is linked to all three indicators. A review of Surveillance Epidemiology and End Results (SEER) data from 1975 to 2000 reveals that the 5-year survival rate for breast cancer is lowest for women living in census tracks with 20% or greater population below the poverty level and highest for those living in census tracks with less than 10% population below poverty level (Datta et al., 2006). Freeman and Chu (2005) for example, conceptualized "barriers" to breast cancer screening, diagnosis, and treatment that might explain racial and ethnic disparities in healthcare. Gerend and Pai (2008) postulate that these "social barriers" interact with genetic, biological, and environmental factors to produce poorer outcomes among African American women with breast cancer.

Adverse upstream factors, such as social stressors at the neighborhood and community levels, may activate downstream biochemical pathways that increase the survival of malignant cancer cells, providing a fertile ground for the growth of cancer cells. A study done by Vona-Davis and Rose (2008) among lower socioeconomic status (SES) white women living in West Virginia found unusually high rates of triple-negative breast cancer. This group of women had increased prevalence rates of high-grade, estrogen receptor negative (ER-) tumors, similar to those of triple-negative breast cancers observed among African American women. Nineteen percent of the 620 breast cancer patients in their study were affected. Forty-five percent of women with this tumor type were under 50 years.

Biological Determinants

Stress contributes to multiple cancer relevant biological processes (McGregor & Antoni, 2009). The physiological stress produced by environmental stressors may produce epigenetic changes associated with breast cancer occurrence. Stressors associated with increased body mass index (BMI) may occur due to increased consumption of sweet foods and high fat foods (O'Connor, Jones, Conner, McMillan, & Ferguson, 2008), which ultimately may lead to decrements in physical activity. In turn, visceral fat is highly vascular and thus more susceptible to factors in the blood such as cortisol (McGregor & Antoni). Individuals who are depressed and anxious also are more likely to self-medicate with alcohol and other drugs (Andersen, Kiecolt-Glaser, & Glaser, 1994). Increased body weight, particularly central adiposity, has been linked to breast cancer (O'Connor et al.). Conzen et al. found that isolated SV40 Tag transgenic mice have different patterns of fat distribution than do their group housed peers (Williams et al., 2009).

Physiological stress is also believed to be associated with changes in gene function and to lead to DNA damage and poorer DNA repair crucial in the etiology of breast cancer. Stress interferes with the body's immune system; and chronic exposure to stress may contribute to poor sleep quality (O'Connor et al., 2008), which has been associated with unhealthy behaviors such as smoking or alcohol consumption. The cascading causal processes that begin with upstream forces affect downstream clinical and biological outcomes (Gehlert et al., 2008).

Access to Healthcare

A number of researchers have argued that access to healthcare is the primary cause of African American and white breast cancer disparities (Orsi, Margellos-Anast, & Whitman, 2010). African Americans on the whole have poorer access to quality health care, in part because they are less likely to have health insurance than whites (U.S. Department of Health and Human Services, 2010). Even in situations of equal access in healthcare, however, such as among women in the military who receive care through the United States Department of Defense, marked differences in survival from breast cancer are seen between African American and white women (Sarker, Jatoi, & Becher, 2007). Albain, Unger, Crowley, Coltman, and Hershman (2009) found that African Americans in clinical trials had higher mortality from breast, ovarian, and prostate cancer than white women, despite uniform treatment. Sarker et al. concluded that while differences in access to healthcare could play a factor, the "disparity in outcome after diagnosis of breast cancer should not be entirely ascribed to inequalities to access to health care" (p. 136).

Problem Conceptualization

The idea of studying social support to understand societal health arguably began with the work of Emile Durkheim 100 years ago (Cohen, Underwood, & Gottlieb, 2000). Durkheim hypothesized that the breakdown in family, community, and work that occurred during the Industrial Revolution, causing workers' migration to industrial areas, would be detrimental to their psychological well-being, because it produced a loss of family and community resources. Subsequent studies have found that people who participate and are actively engaged in their communities have better health outcomes than their more isolated counterparts (Bell, LeRoy, & Stephenson, 1982; Miller & Ingram, 1979).

Social relationships can influence health through a variety of processes. One such process involves the exchange of emotional, informational, and instrumental resources in response to the perception that others are available (Cohen et al., 2000). Another process involves social interaction. Here, others can influence cognitions, emotions, behaviors, and biological responses through the formation of human relationships. Social circumstances such as crime in neighborhoods instill fear among community residents that may cause them to isolate themselves, obviating the possibility of support and creating a sense of alienation and isolation.

Interventions for Women with Breast Cancer

The successful treatment of cancer requires several steps on the diagnostic/treatment continuum. Delays in the process (such as drop out incidents or inadequate therapy at a given point) can produce catastrophic consequences (Gorin, Heck, Cheng, & Smith, 2006; Gwyn et al., 2004). Differences by race can occur at each step of the process. A number of studies support the notion that African American women are less likely to receive treatment than white women, and to receive treatment that is of lesser quality. This alone can be very detrimental in breast cancer outcomes. A good example is chemotherapy. Therapeutic regimens should be tailored to specific patients and must be followed carefully (Goldhirsch et al., 2005). If these regimens are not prescribed accordingly or cannot be followed, as often is the case among poor, uninsured populations, prognosis will be affected adversely.

Gehlert et al. (2008) have noted that determinants at the social and environmental levels may significantly influence events at the molecular and genetic levels. The authors argue that adverse environmental factors may influence and change hormone and metabolic expression, which in turn may affect the body's ability to repair the spontaneous mutations that occur over the life course (Gehlert et al.). They assert, "The upstream environments that change the way DNA and cells throughout the body function include not only a person's physiology, but also his or her behavior and physical and social environments. Such high-level epigenetic triggers are central to the primary downward causal model of breast cancer in which multiple environments at different levels interact to regulate gene expression" (p. 342). Because so few cancers are due to hereditary mutations of breast cancer genes, understanding how social environmental factors might cause sporadic mutations has critical implications for the prevention and treatment of breast cancer, especially among African American and other minority women.

Successful interventions may occur at multiple levels of influence. On the individual level, they might target health behaviors. These might include health behaviors, such as cigarette smoking and diet. Yet, while individual risk factors are important to consider, they almost certainly are insufficient to reduce health disparities (Chin, Walters, & Cook, 2007). A comprehensive approach requires interventions at multiple levels. The model to be presented targets one level and, by virtue of empirical evidence of the links between determinants at various levels, outlines the effect of this intervention on other levels of influence.

In the following sections, we will review existing forms of psychosocial intervention for women with breast cancer and present a novel, comprehensive model of African American and white breast cancer disparities. In addition, we will propose an intervention that is based on the model.

Existing Frameworks of Psychosocial Intervention

Breast cancer interventions typically fall into two categories, those for the purpose of breast cancer prevention and those aimed at supporting women already diagnosed with the disease. Preventive and therapeutic interventions have focused on programs that would reduce health risk behaviors such as alcohol and substance abuse or smoking, or increase health promoting behaviors, such as exercise and following a healthy diet. There are other clinical intervention methods such as mammography screening. This is the "gold standard" method for early screening (Fowler, Rodney, Roberts, & Broadus, 2005). In spite of early detection efforts however, African American women still lag behind white women in mammography screening, and the gap widens when SES factors are considered, according to Centers for Disease Control and Prevention. Other interventions have focused at facilitating effective coping with the disease among women who have already been diagnosed with the disease.

Once someone has been diagnosed with cancer, there are supportive mechanisms available to help individuals deal with the situation (e.g., psychosocial interventions). Psychosocial interventions allow the caregivers to activate the unique internal or psychological resources possessed by the individual to facilitate behavior change. Nurses, counselors, and community health workers deliver culturally tailored health information in order to increase patients' knowledge for self-care, decrease barriers to access, and improve providers' cultural competence (Fisher, Burnet, Huang, Chin, & Cagney, 2007).

Psychotherapeutic Approaches

Psychotherapeutic approaches to intervention with women with breast cancer often focus on helping women to cope with a breast cancer diagnosis. Outcomes of interest for this type of intervention range from increased quality of life, improved coping skills, decreased symptoms of depression and anxiety, and even decreased rates of mortality from breast cancer. A recent example of a psychotherapeutic intervention that evaluated improved survival outcomes is a successful clinical trial by Andersen et al. (2008). In this study, 227 women who were surgically treated for regional breast cancer were randomized to either a year-long psychological intervention to increase coping skills or an assessment only condition. The group that received the intervention had a significantly lower risk of breast cancer recurrence and death from breast cancer than the group that did not. Further, the treatment group experienced significantly increased levels of overall health and decreased levels of distress (Anderson et al., 2007).

Another example of a psychotherapeutic intervention comes from the work of Spiegel, Bloom, Kraemer, and Gottheil (1989) and Spiegel et al. (2007), in which they tested the effectiveness of a supportive group therapy approach on breast cancer survival. Supportive Expressive Group Therapy is a group psychotherapeutic model in which patients are encouraged to build relationships, confront problems, and find enhanced meaning in their lives. Treatment is provided weekly over the course of 1 year. In the original study done in the 1980s, Spiegel et al. noted a significant increase in survival for the intervention group; however, a recent attempt to replicate this study by Spiegel et al. found no significant overall effect of treatment in a group of 125 women with confirmed metastatic or locally recurrent breast cancer. Although survival outcomes were not replicated in the overall sample, significant reduction in distress and improvement in emotion regulation was found for the treatment group (Classen et al., 2001; Spiegel et al.). Additionally, there was a significant increase in survival for women with ER negative breast tumors, suggesting a need for research that examines effectiveness among subtypes of women with breast cancer. In light of the disparities associated with breast cancer subtypes in race and age noted above, exploring this difference may in fact be critical for understanding effective psychotherapeutic interventions among younger, African American women.

Although results from these studies are promising, there are critical limitations in our knowledge about how interventions tested primarily among white women generalize to use among African American women. The sample used by Andersen et al. (2008), for example, was 90% white, with a mean education level of 14.75 years and a mean family income of $68,000 per year. Clearly, this sample is not representative of African American women and reflects only the effects of this intervention on a group of well-educated, middle to upper SES white women. Of further concern is that 68% of the sample was both ER and PR positive, meaning that the subtype of breast cancer experienced by women in this study is not reflective of the subtype exhibited by most African American women. Spiegel et al.'s sample (2007) included 92.2% white women in its experimental group, with a mean education of 16.1 years. Only 21.9% of the treatment group earned less than $39,999 per year. Again, 79% of the women were ER positive, meaning that, although there was a significant effect of treatment for those who were ER negative, the group was very small and generalization of these results are limited. Both treatment groups in these studies met in clinical settings that were far removed from the natural social environment, raising important issues about access to care for those with transportation issues and relevance of care outside of the clinical setting.

Traditional Support Groups and Patient Advocacy

Health clinics, community centers, and inpatient units around the nation host and facilitate support groups and advocacy campaigns for women with breast cancer. These groups are at times led by professionals, but are also sometimes led by community members who are either survivors or advocates for the cause. Support groups have proved to increase levels of social support and increase quality of life for participants; however, there are concerns about whether such groups adequately address the needs of minority populations (Michalec, 2005). In a recent study by Michalec, a large sample of breast cancer survivors was drawn from the Eastern North Carolina Tumor Registry, which is a tumor registry that tracks all cases of breast cancer occurring in this region, as mandated by state law. Participants of the study were asked interview questions about psychosocial outcomes, including dependent variables such as quality of life, social support, and life satisfaction with the independent variable being participation in breast cancer support groups. These interview data were linked with tumor registry data for age and stage of diagnosis. Although the majority of the sample had never participated in a support group (82%), those who did participate reported higher social and overall quality of life. Despite these benefits, it must be noted that women in the sample who participated in support groups tended to have high levels of income, education, and employment. Because the majority of women who participated in support groups had these characteristics, we are left wondering about the efficacy of these groups among minority populations that do not share these economic advantages.

Breast cancer advocacy groups and campaigns such as a campaign in Boston called Pink and Black do suggest an avenue for providing support and encouragement for African American women at risk for breast cancer. Volunteers in the Pink and Black campaign provide education, often using personal stories of African American survivors, and encourage those in attendance to be screened and practice good breast health. Ambassadors associated with this program travel to various locations and speak to groups of women about risk and prevention, increasing breast cancer awareness among minority populations (Pidgeon, 2010).

Patient Navigation Approaches

Another form of intervention aimed at individuals is patient navigation. Patient navigator interventions have proved successful in improving breast cancer outcomes among underserved women. Variously referred to as navigators, *promotoras*, *comadres*, Ambassadors, lay health workers, or community health workers, these individuals usually are clinic based and help women with breast cancer and their families to overcome barriers within the health care system. In a meta-analysis of 16 published reports of patient navigator programs, Wells et al. (2008) found evidence of efficacy in increasing participation in cancer screening and diagnostic follow-up care, but less evidence of efficacy in reducing late-stage cancer diagnosis, delays in the initiation of treatment, or improving outcomes during survivorship. The group found methodological limitations in the efficacy studies they reviewed, including lack of control groups, small sample sizes, and contamination with other interventions. Further, this approach to intervention is limited to the health care setting, and fails to help women navigate more complex social systems.

With this said, Wells et al. (2008) advocate for a research agenda that further explores the efficacy of patient navigators with greater scientific rigor. The patient navigation intervention holds some promise in reaching underserved populations, but much is left unknown about its efficacy, given the methodological limitations listed above. Keeping these beneficial and promising results in mind, research in this area remains incomplete, leaving gaping holes in our knowledge about how to best intervene with African American women with breast cancer.

In summary, it is clear that existing interventions fall short of fully addressing the needs of African American women with breast cancer. In light of the myriad psychosocial obstacles faced by African American women, including poverty, systematic racism, and the aggressive nature of the disease in this population, these models, although promising, do not fully address the health disparities of this group of women. The model presented in the following pages of this chapter moves beyond existing models to provide a more holistic, comprehensive approach. The remainder of this chapter will focus on the work at the Center for Interdisciplinary Health Disparities Research, and the innovative proposed model of intervention for African American women with breast cancer that specifically addresses the psychosocial context that has led to the existence of these disparities.

The Center for Interdisciplinary Health Disparities Research

The Center for Interdisciplinary Health Disparities Research (CIHDR) addresses a single question shared across its team of social, biological, and behavioral scientists, namely why, despite the fact that white women are more likely to develop breast cancer than are African American women, African American women are more likely to die from the disease. Faced with the fact that African American women are 37% more likely to die from breast cancer than their white counter parts (Ries et al., 2008), investigators at the CIHDR are faced with a looming question: What makes breast cancer mortality rates higher and 5-year survival rates lower in African American women?

According to the CIHDR team, cancer develops, according to studies, after a complex genetic and environment interaction (McClintock, Conzen, Gehlert, Masi, & Olopade, 2005). The period at which cancer "gets under the skin" to influence the development of breast cancer is fundamentally unknown. What is empirically known is that 70–80% of breast cancer is due to sporadic or acquired rather than inherited breast cancer genes (Gehlert et al., 2008).

CIHDR investigators, for example, have found that socially isolated rodents develop larger mammary gland tumors (analogous to human breast cancer tumors) than do their group housed peers (Hermes et al., 2010). Also, isolated rodents have increased stress hormone response to an acute stressor (Williams et al., 2009). Consequently, these researchers have found increased stress hormone receptors in more invasive tumors among more vulnerable women with breast cancer (S. Gehlert, personal communication, December 8, 2009). Consistent with the hypothesis of a stress-biology link, the team has found that 69% of invasive cancers were positive for glucocorticoid (stress hormone) receptors compared to only 29% of ductal carcinoma in situ (DCIS) cases ($p < 0.03$). Other research experiments with monkeys as well as humans show that chronic stress can overwhelm and erode the body's defense mechanisms (Herbert & Cohen, 1993). Like gunning the engine of a car, constant activation of the stress response wears down the body's system, resulting in higher rates of disease and early death (Geronimus, Hicken, Keene, & Bound, 2006).

Health disparities among minority populations have been one of the two major foci of the federal Healthy People 2010 initiative (U.S. Department of Health and Human Services, 2010). Recent effort in the reduction of disparity has focused on the importance of level of education as major contributors to health outcomes (Meara, Richards, & Cutler, 2008). Based on this and other knowledge, initiatives like the Centers of Excellence in Cancer Communication Research (CECCR), funded by the National Cancer Institute, have launched efforts to shape health communications to decrease health disparities (National Cancer Institute, 2008).

Chin et al. (2007) argue that the current racial/ethnic differences in cancer episodes are primarily due to interventions that have been misguided causes, by virtue of focusing on inappropriate determinants of disparities. They point to an overemphasis on breast cancer screening to decrease African American and white mortality differences. They observe that a diagnosis of breast cancer must consider multifactorial determinants. Successful efforts to address African American and white breast cancer disparities must be holistic and based on fundamental realities facing African American women. After an extensive meta-analysis of more than 200 journal articles that addressed race and ethnic disparities in diseases such as depression, breast cancer, cardiovascular diseases, and diabetes, Chin et al. found that only a few of the interventions yielded significant reductions in disease disparity. It is evident that there is a need for a comprehensive approach to intervention.

The CIHDR Model and Disparities in Breast Cancer

This is a model that recognizes inherent stressors at the societal, community, and neighborhood levels, starting with poverty, disruption, and neighborhood crime that disproportionately affect African Americans in the USA (see Fig. 11.1). These stressors cumulatively lead to social isolation

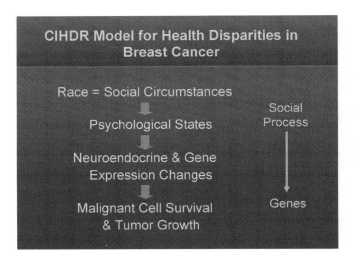

and its associated felt loneliness acquired vigilance, and depression (Gehlert et al. 2008). These psychosocial sequella disrupt stress and metabolic hormone dynamics, ultimately leading to a failure of the programmed death of malignant cancer cells and the growth of malignant tumors. Donald Campbell (1974) is credited with his theory of downward causation in describing how organizational levels influence lower levels in hierarchically organized biological systems, as cited in Gehlert et al.. According to Campbell, every process at the lower and intermediate levels in the hierarchy is restrained and acts in conformity dictated by the laws of the higher levels. This process is used to describe the interrelationship between social, behavioral, and biological factors as they impact health outcomes. The CIHDR model of downward causation from social environmental conditions to psychosocial factors identified stress hormone (glucocorticoid) receptors which are activated by social isolation. This situation activates biochemical pathways that bind with stress hormone receptor complex that create a perfect "soil" in which cancer grows (Gehlert et al.). Although imperfect, because it fails to take into account the effect of "downstream" factors on those that occur "upstream" from them, the metaphor nonetheless is compelling.

Community/Neighborhood and Social Ecology

The nature and quality of the physical environment are important, and often overlooked, determinants of health outcomes. Empirical studies have documented an association between neighborhood characteristics and health conditions such as low birth weight, depression, cancer, and cardiovascular disease (Yen & Kaplan, 1999). A comparison of two indigenous groups illustrates how biology can interact with physical environment to produce group differences.

The Pima Indians live in Arizona and in the Sierra Madre mountains of Mexico. The two are genetically quite similar, based on a shared history and confirmed by genetic testing. Yet, the rate of type 2 diabetes among the Pima of Arizona is five times that of the Pima of Mexico (Schulz et al., 2006). Diabetes was virtually unknown among the Pima people a century ago, so it would seem that the Pima of Arizona have experienced the greatest change in rates of diabetes. The authors convincingly attribute the variation among the two Pima subgroups to differing environmental circumstances. While the Pima in Mexico maintain their traditional rural environment, the Arizona Pima now live in a markedly changed, Westernized environment, which has produced fewer opportunities for physical activity. Consequently, they have higher rates of obesity than their Mexican cousins.

The quality of neighborhoods reflected in buildings, open spaces, and the overall appearances of a community have profound effect on health outcomes. When neighborhoods are faced with a deteriorated infrastructure, there is a high propensity for anomie and decay (Sampson, Raudenbush, & Earls, 1997). The conclusion of this study was that people living in a low social environment, with fewer signs of occupation and proliferated with graffiti, had a 58% increased odds of dying compared with people who lived in a high social environment after adjusting for all other covariates factors (1997). There are cues that are reflected in existing neighborhoods, blocks or building that might signal criminal behavior (Cohen et al., 2003). The authors observe that when buildings have more than 50 apartments, residents treat each other as strangers and would be less likely to challenge or confront criminal activities. Houses are also more likely to be burglarized if they are in areas of higher speed limits, fewer fences, or other barriers (Rand, 1984). Such situations create a state of individual alienation and could cause residents to retreat into their homes and as a consequence, their interactions become limited, increasing feelings of loneliness (Gehlert et al., 2008).

Based on empirical evidence linking inflammatory responses to cancer incidence, CIHDR investigators have evaluated EBNA, a component of Epstein Barr Virus (EBV). This in part was based on evidence suggesting that EBV, a member of the herpes virus family and related to several specific carcinomas (Baumforth, Young, Flavell, Constandinou, & Murray, 1999), may also be related to breast cancer (Glaser, Hsu, & Gulley, 2004). In preliminary analyses, CIHDR investigators were able to predict levels of EBNA among African American women with breast cancer using data on crimes (i.e., aggravated assaults and robberies) geocoded to women's addresses and psychosocial functioning (e.g., felt loneliness and perceived stress), with education, income, and age included in the model ($R^2 = 0.26$; $p = 0.05$). A one unit increase in felt loneliness was associated with a statistically significant increase in EBNA ($b = 8.215$; $p < 0.05$). The same trend was observed for perceived stress ($b = 1.475$; $p < 0.05$). This evidence is critical in understanding how neighborhood factors affect biology, which leads to the need to address vulnerable populations at the neighborhood and community level.

Toward a New Intervention Approach: The Neighborhood and Community Level

Neighborhood and community interventions have the unique advantage of being able to address many of the contingencies of being African American in the USA. This is true for women newly diagnosed with breast cancer. The team of CIHDR investigator proposes a neighborhood support coordinator (NSC) intervention, based on their novel model of African American and white breast cancer disparities that is designed to work with women in the context of their communities. The NSC has some of the features of a patient navigator, that is to say, her goal is to help women overcome systemic barriers, but there are two critical differences. First, rather than being clinic based, this intervention focuses on engaging the women in the neighborhood and community in which they live. Secondly, the NSC helps the women to navigate overlapping systems rather than limiting the scope to the health care system only.

African American women with breast cancer face a myriad of psychosocial problems, which can exacerbate the disease situation. There are women for whom finding safe and affordable housing for themselves and their children is a constant struggle. Situations where women cannot maintain their prescribed chemotherapeutic or radiation therapy regiments are not uncommon. Barrett et al. (2008) examined the impact of change in upward socioeconomic status in a neighborhood on probability of distant metastasis at diagnosis of cancer among women. They found that level of the neighborhood affluence gravely affects the disadvantaged group and can have strong relations to distant metastasis. These researchers postulated that poor women with breast cancer who reside in improved neighborhoods can be "left out" even after the neighborhoods have improved. Consequently, they may experience a disruption of customary patterns of interaction, lack of social networks and access to healthcare services because of a lack of transportation. This creates a situation of isolation, decreased social support resulting from neighborhood change (Barrett et al.).

For these and other reasons, the NSC will first assess each woman in the experimental condition for social and psychological needs, with an instrument designed by the academic and community partners that uses the social and psychosocial problems listed in DSM-IV (Axis IV) as its starting point. The NSC will then work with each woman and local service providers to address these identified needs. A strength of the CIHDR approach is the active participation of partners who use neighborhood resources daily and are aware of their intricacies. In this model, women receive weekly phone calls from the NSC and meet weekly with her in a space designated by CIHDR for such meetings. In addition, the women meet weekly as a group within their own neighborhood for two purposes. One reason is for networking and the second is to learn and practice group problem-solving skills for addressing complex systems, such as navigating public and private agencies for needed resources. Rather than assuming a deficit of skills among the women in the study, the group problem solving approach assumes that the maze of social service agencies in a large metropolitan area (e.g., agencies that provide Section 8 housing), would be difficult for anyone to negotiate. Arguably, it would be more difficult for a woman newly diagnosed with a major disease. This is a strengths-based approach, meeting the women within the context of their own communities, and working with them to build support and navigate a difficult and often confusing system.

To accomplish good health for individuals, a comprehensive approach is needed through policy to address sources of social and health problems. The trauma facing poor communities in the USA can no longer be ignored. The quality of individuals' life as this chapter demonstrates is an amalgam of many integral units. Any area in the human ecosystem that is deficient or unstructured, including living in debased neighborhoods can overwhelm the system and shred the health fabric of the individual.

Conclusion and Recommendations

In the late 1990s, breast cancer mortality rates had declined for white women; however, they remained stable for older and African American women (Greenlee, Murray, Bolden, & Wingo, 2000). A number of factors were attributed to this scenario, among them low social economic status, advanced stage at diagnosis, delays in diagnosis and treatment, biological factors and treatment differences (Greenlee et al.). Interventions in the form of psychotherapeutic process, support groups, and patient navigators have been helpful in providing opportunity for women to share cancer experiences, gain access to the health care system, improve sharing and the exploration of treatment options. For minority patients however, such opportunities for emotional and psychological assistance are less likely compared to white patients (Barg & Gullatte, 2001).

As has been noted, African American women are diagnosed less frequently with breast cancer as whites. They also continue to have a greater number with late stage disease and greater mortality from breast cancer. In spite of existing interventions, studies show that African American breast cancer cases are still disproportionally high. Although more outreach programs are still needed to arrest this problem, there are environmental and social factors that must be considered in addressing the problem. This handbook recommends inclusive intervention approaches that understand the mechanisms of cell biology as well as the impact of environmental factors on cell biology. It is critical to address these glaring health disparities in the context of a holistic, community environment in order to ultimately affect change in the lives of African American women.

References

Albain, K. S., Unger, J. M., Crowley, J. J., Coltman, C. C., & Hershman, M. D. (2009). Racial disparities in cancer survival among randomized clinical trials of the Southwest Oncology Group. *Journal of the National Cancer Institute, 101*(14), 984–992.

American Cancer Society. (2009). *Cancer facts and figures 2009.* Retrieved November 13, 2009, from http://www.cancer.org/downloads/STT/CAFF2007PWSecured.pdf

Anders, C., & Carey, L. A. (2008). Understanding and treating triple-negative breast cancer. *Oncology, 22*(11), 1233–1239.

Andersen, B. L., Farrar, W. B., Golden-Kreutz, D., Emery, C. F., Glaser, R., Crespin, T., et al. (2007). Distress reduction from a psychological intervention contributes to improved health for cancer patients. *Brain, behavior, and immunity, 21*(7), 953–61. doi: 10.1016/j.bbi.2007.03.005.

Andersen, B. L., Kiecolt-Glaser, J. K., & Glaser, R. (1994). A biobehavioral model of cancer stress and diseases course. *The American Psychologist, 49*(5), 389–404.

Andersen, B. L., Yang, H. C., Farrer, W. B., Golden-Kreutz, D. M., Emery, C. F., Thornton, L. M., et al. (2008). Psychological intervention improves survival for breast cancer patients. *Cancer, 113*(12), 3450–3458.

Avis, N. E., Crawford, S., & Manuel, J. (2005). Quality of life among young women with breast cancer. *Journal of Clinical Oncology, 23*(15), 3322–3330.

Barg, F. K., & Gullatte, M. M. (2001). Cancer support groups: Meeting the needs of African Americans with cancer. *Seminars in Oncology Nursing, 17*(3), 171–178.

Barrett, R. E., Cho, Y. I., Weaver, K. E., Ryu, K., Campbell, R. T., Dolecek, T. A., et al. (2008). Neighborhood change and distant metastasis at diagnosis of breast cancer. *Annals of Epidemiology, 18*(1), 43–47.

Baumforth, K. R. N., Young, L. S., Flavell, K. J., Constandinou, C., & Murray, P. G. (1999). The Epstein Barr virus carcinogenesis. *Journal of Clinical Pathology: Molecular Pathology, 52,* 307–322.

Bell, R., LeRoy, J., & Stephenson, J. (1982). Evaluating the mediating effects of social support upon life events and depressive symptoms. *Journal of Community Psychology, 10,* 325–340.

Burgess, C., Cornelius, V., Love, S., Graham, J., Richards, M., & Ramirez, A. (2005). Depression and anxiety in women with early breast cancer: Five year observational cohort study. *British Medical Journal.* doi:10.1136/bmj.38343.670868.D3.

Cacioppo, J. T., Ernst, J. M., Burleson, M. H., McClintock, M. K., Malarkey, W. B., Hawkley, L. C., et al. (2000). Lonely traits and concomitant physiological processes: The Macarthur social neuroscience studies. *International Journal of Psychophysiology, 35,* 143–154.

Campbell, D.T. (1974). 'Downward causation' in hierarchically organized biological systems. In F.J. Ayala, & T. Dobzhansky (Eds.), Studies in the philosophy of biology (179-186). Berkeley: University of California Press.

Carey, L. A., Perou, C. M., Livasy, C. A., Dressler, L. G., Cowan, D., Conway, K., et al. (2006). Race, breast cancer subtypes, and survival in the Carolina breast cancer study. *Journal of the American Medical Association, 295*(21), 2492–2502.

Chida, Y., & Hamer, M. (2009). Chronic psychosocial factors and acute physiological responses to laboratory induced stress in the healthy populations: A quantitative review of 30 years of investigations. *Psychological Bulletin, 134*(6), 829–885.

Chin, M., Walters, A. E., & Cook, S. C. (2007). Interventions to reduce racial and ethnic disparities in health care. *Medical Care Research and Review, 64*(5 Suppl), 7S–28S.

Classen, C., Butler, L. D., Koopman, C., Miller, E., DiMiceli, S., Giese-Davis, S., et al. (2001). Supportive-expressive group therapy and distress in patients with metastatic breast cancer: A randomized clinical intervention. *Archives of General Psychiatry, 58,* 494–501.

Cohen, D. A., Mason, K., Bedimo, A., Scribner, R., Basok, V., & Farley, T. A. (2003). Neighborhood physical conditions and health. *American Journal of Public Health, 93*(3), 467–471.

Cohen, S., Underwood, L. G., & Gottlieb, B. H. (2000). *Social support measurement and intervention.* New York: Oxford University Press.

Datta, G., Colditz, G. A., Kawachi, I., Subramanian, S. V., Palmer, J. R., & Rosenberg, L. (2006). Individual, neighborhood, and state-level socioeconomic predictors of cervical carcinoma screening among U.S. black women. *Cancer, 106*(3), 664–669.

Eley, J. W., Hill, H. A., Chen, V. S., Austin, D. F., Wesley, M. N., Muss, H. B., et al. (1994). Racial differences in survival from breast cancer. Results of the National Cancer Institute Black/White Cancer Survival Study. *Journal of the American Medical Association, 272,* 947–954.

Fisher, T. L., Burnet, D. L., Huang, E. S., Chin, M. H., & Cagney, K. A. (2007). Cultural leverage: Interventions using culture to narrow racial disparities in health care. *Medical Care Research and Review, 64,* 243S–282S.

Fowler, B. A., Rodney, M., Roberts, S., & Broadus, L. (2005). Collaborative breast health intervention for African American women of lower socioeconomic status. *Oncology Nursing Forum, 32,* 1207–1216.

Freeman, H. P., & Chu, K. C. (2005). Determinants of cancer disparities: Barriers to cancer screening, diagnosis, and treatment. *Surgical Oncology Clinics of North America, 14*, 655–669.

Ganz, P. A., Greendale, G. A., Peterson, L., Kahn, B., & Bower, J. E. (2003). Breast cancer in younger women: Reproductive and late health effects of treatment. *Journal of Clinical Oncology, 21*(22), 4184–4193.

Gehlert, S., Sohmer, D., Sacks, T., Mininger, C., McClintock, M., & Olopade, O. (2008). Targeting health disparities: A model for linking upstream determinants of downstream interventions. *Health Affairs, 27*, 339–349.

Gerend, M. A., & Pai, M. (2008). Social determinants of black-white disparities in breast cancer mortality: A review. *Cancer Epidemiology, Biomarkers, & Preview, 17*(11), 2913–2923.

Geronimus, A. T., Hicken, M., Keene, D., & Bound, J. (2006). "Weathering" and age patterns of allostatic load scores among blacks and whites in the United States. *American Journal of Public Health, 96*(5), 826–833.

Glaser, S. L., Hsu, J. L., & Gulley, M. I. (2004). Epstein-barr virus and breast cancer: States of the evidence for viral carcinogenesis. *Cancer Epidemiology, Biomarkers & Prevention, 13*, 688–697.

Goldhirsch, J. H., Glick, R. D., Gelber, A. S., Coates, B., Thurlimann, H., Sennet, J., et al. (2005). Meeting highlights: International expert consensus on the primary therapy of early breast cancer. *Annals of Oncology, 16*, 1569–1583.

Gorin, S. S., Heck, J. E., Cheng, B., & Smith, S. J. (2006). Delays in breast cancer diagnosis and treatment by racial/ethnic group. *Archives of Internal Medicine, 166*, 2244–2252.

Greenlee, R. T., Murray, T., Bolden, S., & Wingo, P. A. (2000). Cancer statistics, 2000. *CA: A Cancer Journal for Clinicians, 50*(1), 7–33. Cancer Research Treatment, 8.

Gwyn, K., Bondy, M. L., Cohen, D. S., Lund, M. J., Liff, J. M., Flagg, E. W., et al. (2004). Racial differences in diagnosis, treatment, and clinical delays in a population-based study of patients with newly diagnosed breast carcinoma. *Cancer, 100*, 1595–1604.

Härter, M., Reuter, K., Aschenbrenner, A., Schretzmann, N., Marschner, N., Hasenburg, A., et al. (2001). Psychiatric disorders and associated factors in cancer: Results of an interview study with patients in inpatient, rehabilitation and outpatients treatment. *European Journal of Cancer, 37*(11), 1385–1393.

Herbert, T. B., & Cohen, S. (1993). Stress and immunity in humans: A meta-analytic review. *Psychosomatic Medicine, 55*, 364–379.

Hermes, G. L., Delgado, B., Tretiakova, M., Cavigelli, S. A., Krausz, T., Conzen, S. D., & McClintock, M. K. (2010). Social isolation dysregulates endocrine and behavioral stress while increasing malignant burden of spontaneous mammary tumors. *Proceedings of the National Academy of Sciences* [Preprint version]. Retrieved from http://www.pnas.org/cgi/10.1073/pnas.0910753106

Huo, D., Ikpatt, F., Khramtsov, A., Dangou, J. M., Nanda, R., Digman, J., et al. (2009). Population differences in breast cancer: Survey in indigenous African women reveals over-representation of triple-negative breast cancer. *Journal of Clinical Oncology, 20*(27), 4515–4521.

Li, C. I., Malone, K. E., & Darling, J. R. (2003). Differences in breast cancer stage, treatment and survival by race and ethnicity. *Archives of Internal Medicine, 163*, 49–56.

Martinez, M. E., Nielson, C. M., Nagle, R., Lopez, A. M., Kim, C., & Thompson, P. (2007). Breast cancer among Hispanic and non-Hispanic white women in Arizona. *Journal of Health Care for the Poor and Underserved, 18*, 130–145.

McClintock, M., Conzen, S., Gehlert, S., Masi, C., & Olopade, O. (2005). Mammary cancer and social interactions: Identifying multiple environments that regulate gene expression throughout the life span. *Journal of Gerontology, 60*(Special Issue I), 32–41.

McEwen, B. S. (2008). Central effects of stress hormones in health and disease: Understanding the protective and damaging effects of stress and stress mediators. *European Journal of Pharmacology, 583*(2–3), 174–185.

McEwen, B. S. (1998). Protective and damaging effects of stress mediators. *The New England Journal of Medicine, 338*(3), 171–179.

McGregor, B. A., & Antoni, M. H. (2009). Psychological intervention and health outcomes among women treated for breast cancer: A review of stress pathways and biological mediators. *Brain, Behavior, and Immunity, 23*(2), 159–166.

Meara, E. R., Richards, S., & Cutler, D. M. (2008). The gap gets bigger: Changes in mortality and life expectancy, by education, 1981–2000. *Health Affairs, 27*(2), 350–360.

Michalec, B. (2005). Exploring the multidimensional benefits of breast cancer support groups. *Journal of Psychosocial Oncology, 23*(2/3), 159–179.

Miller, P., & Ingram, J. G. (1979). Reflections on the life events to illness link with some preliminary findings. In I. G. Sarason & C. D. Spielberger (Eds.), Stress and anxiety (Vol. 6, pp. 313–336). New York: Hemisphere.

Morris, G. J., Naidu, S., Topham, A. K., Guiles, F., Xu, Y., McCue, P., et al. (2007). Differences in breast carcinoma characteristics in newly diagnosed African-American and Caucasian patients: a single-institution compilation compared with the National Cancer Institute's Surveillance, Epidemiology, and End Results database. *Cancer, 110*(4), 876–84. doi: 10.1002/cncr.22836.

National Cancer Institute. (2009). *Cancer in women*. Retrieved November 4, 2009, from http://www.cancer.gov/cancertopics/types/breast

National Cancer Institute. (2007). Triple-negative breast cancer disproportionately affects African American and Hispanic women. *National Cancer Institute Cancer Bulletin, 4*(22).

National Cancer Institute. (2008, December 15). *NCI centers of excellence in cancer communication research.* Retrieved from http://dccps.nci.nih.gov/hcirb/ceccr/

Newman, L. A. (2005). Breast cancer in African American women. *The Oncologist, 10*(1), 1–14.

O'Connor, D. B., Jobes, F., Conner, M., McMillan, B., & Ferguson, E. (2008). Effects of daily hassles and eating behavior. *Health Psychology, 27*(1 suppl), 20–31.

Orsi, J. M., Margellos-Anast, H., & Whitman, S. (2010). Black–White health disparities in the United States and Chicago: A 15-year progress analysis. *American Journal of Public Health, 100*(2), 349–356.

Pidgeon, N. (2010). *Boston public health commission Pink and Black Campaign.* Retrieved from http://www.bphc.org/programs/cib/civicengagement/outreach/pinkandblack/Pages/Home

Porter, P. L., Lund, M. J., Lin, M. G., Yuan, X., Liff, J. M., Flagg, E. W., et al. (2004). Racial differences in the expression of cell cycle-regulatory proteins in breast carcinoma. *Cancer, 100*, 2533–2542.

Rand, G. (1984). Crime and environment. A review of the literature and its implications for urban architecture and planning. *Journal of Architecture and Planning Research, 1*, 3–19.

Reich, M., Lesur, A., & Perdrizet-Chevallier, C. (2008). Depression, quality of life and breast cancer: A review of the literature. *Breast Cancer Research and Treatment, 110*, 9–17.

Ries, L. A. G., Melbert, D., Krapcho, M., Stinchcomb, D. G., Howlader, N., Horner. M. J., et al. (2008). *SEER cancer statistics review, 1975–2005.* Bethesda, MD: National Cancer Institute. Retrieved from http://seer.cancer.gov/csr/1975_2005/

Sarker, M., Jatoi, I., & Becher, H. (2007). Racial differences in breast cancer survival in women under age 60. *Breast Cancer Research and Treatment, 106*, 135–141.

Sampson, R. J., Raudenbush, S. W., & Earls, F. (1997). Neighborhoods and violent crime: A multilevel study of collective efficacy. *Science, 277*(5328), 918–924.

Schulz, L. O., Bennett, P. H., Ravussin, E., Kidd, J. R., Kidd, K. K., Esparza, J., et al. (2006). Effects of traditional and western environments on prevalence of type 2 diabetes in Pima Indians in Mexico and the U.S. *Diabetes Care, 29*(8), 1866–1871.

Schneider, B. P., Winer, E. P., Foulkes, W. D., Garber, J., Perou, C. M., Richardson, A., et al. (2008). Triple-negative breast cancer: Risk factors to potential targets. *Clinical Cancer Research, 14*(24), 8010–8018.

Spiegel, D., Bloom, J. R., Kraemer, H. C., & Gottheil, E. (1989). Effect of psychosocial treatment on survival of patients with metastatic breast cancer. *Lancet, 2*, 888–891.

Spiegel, D., Butler, L., Giese-Davis, J., Koopman, C., Miller, E., DiMiceli, S., et al. (2007). Effects of support-expressive group therapy on survival of patients with metastatic breast cancer: A randomized prospective trial. *Cancer, 110*(5), 1130–1138.

Turner, J., Kelly, B., Swanson, C., Allison, R., & Wetzig, N. (2005). Psychosocial impact of newly diagnosed advanced breast cancer. *Psychooncology, 14*, 396–407.

Underwood, S. M. (2006). Breast cancer in African American women: Nursing essentials. *Journal of the Association of Black Nursing Faculty, 17*(1), 3–14.

U.S. Department of Health and Human Services. (2010). *African American profile.* Retrieved February 13, 2009, from http://minorityhealth.hhs.gov/templates/browse.aspx?lvl=2&lvlID=51

Vona-Davis, L., Rose, D. P., Hazard, H., Howard-McNatt, M., Adkins, F., Partin, J., et al. (2008). Triple-negative breast cancer and obesity in a rural Appalachian population. *Cancer epidemiology, biomarkers & prevention: A publication of the American Association for Cancer Research, cosponsored by the American Society of Preventive Oncology, 17*(12), 3319–24. doi: 10.1158/1055-9965.EPI-08-0544.

Vona-Davis, L., & Rose, D. P. (2009). The influence of socioeconomic disparities on breast cancer tumor biology and prognosis: A review. *Journal of Women's Health, 18*(6), 883–893.

Watlington, A. T., Byers, T., Mouchawar, J., Sauaia, A., & Ellis, J. (2007). Does having insurance affect differences in clinical presentation between Hispanic and non-Hispanic white women with breast cancer? *Cancer, 109*(10), 2093–2099.

Wells, K. J., Battaglia, T. A., Dudley, D. J., Garcia, R., Greene, A., Calhoun, E., et al. (2008). Patient navigation: State of the art or is it science? *Cancer, 113*, 1999–2010.

Williams, J. B., Pang, D., Delgado, B., Kocherginsky, M., Tretiakova, M., Krausz, R., et al. (2009). A model of gene-environment interaction reveals altered gene expression and increased tumor growth following social isolation. *Cancer Prevention Research, 2*(10), 850–861.

Wong-Kim, E., & Bloom, J. (2005). Depression experienced by young women newly diagnosed with breast cancer. *Psychooncology, 14*, 564–573.

Yen, I. H., & Kaplan, G. A. (1999). Neighborhood social environment and risk of death: Multilevel evidence from the alameda county study. *American Journal of Epidemiology, 149*, 898–907.

Zebrack, B. J., Mills, J., & Weitzman, T. S. (2007). Health and supportive care needs of young adult cancer patients and survivors. *Journal of Cancer Survivorship, 1*, 137–145.

Chapter 12
Prevention of Risky Sexual Behaviors Among African American Men

Benjamin P. Bowser

Introduction

Twenty years is a long time in the life of a preventable epidemic. In 1990 when HIV was infecting and AIDS was killing white gay and bisexual men and threatening the general public, there was public concern about the disease and federal research and prevention dollars flowed. It was well established that HIV was spread primarily through sexual intercourse without barrier protection such as condoms. "Risky sex" occurred between men and between men and women. By 2000, HIV infection rates and deaths due to AIDS were in decline among White men in AIDS epi-centers, but continued among African Americans. The HIV/AIDS epidemic has not only continued its course among Blacks but also concentrated among black men and in black communities and has become yet another affliction among Blacks. At the very same time, public attention and urgency to the AIDS epidemic has waned and prevention dollars have been largely replaced by funding of clinical trials of new drugs. If you are Black and poor, there are now, in fact, more incentives to get infected with HIV to get social support through a clinical trial then to avoid getting infected in the first place. Public and government indifference to disease among Blacks but a willingness at the same time to use them in research are precisely the same reactions to disproportionate rates of yellow fever, typhus, syphilis, and tuberculosis among Blacks during Jim Crow segregation in the early twentieth century (McBride, 1991).

Given public indifference and federal neglect of HIV among Blacks, how does one write in 2010 about preventing risky sex among black men and between black men and women? This review could compare the few existing efforts to prevent risky sex among and by black men with what is needed to ameliorate HIV/AIDS among Blacks. What if the Obama or some future federal administration was willing to suddenly make sufficient funds available to do effective HIV prevention among Blacks? To attempt such an undertaking, we would have to know enough about preventing HIV infections among black men to mount more effective national and local prevention efforts. In effect, does the research literature show that enough field research and program evaluations have been done with sufficient scientific rigor to show (1) the principles of effective prevention of HIV among black men; (2) what actions work in successful prevention program efforts; and (3) what are best practices? Perhaps, the past decades of indifference to HIV among Blacks have also not impacted research. In which case, additional years will not have to be spent learning what we should have acquired over the past 20 years. Let us review this literature and see what the answers are to these questions.

B.P. Bowser (✉)
Department of Sociology and Social Services, California State University,
East Bay, San Francisco, CA, USA
e-mail: benjamin.bowser@csueastbay.edu

A.J. Lemelle et al. (eds.), *Handbook of African American Health: Social and Behavioral Interventions*,
DOI 10.1007/978-1-4419-9616-9_12, © Springer Science+Business Media, LLC 2011

Method

From September to November, 2009, key journal articles were identified by using the California State University Libraries' search engines for Health Science, Nursing and Psychology journals that combines article databases from PubMed, CINAHL (1,160 journals), PsycINFO, SocioFile, Academic Search Premier, and the Cochrane Database of Systematic Reviews (approximately 5,600 peer-review journals). The key terms used were risky sex, HIV prevention, AIDS prevention, interventions, programs, black men, and African American men. Another search with the same key terms was repeated using The University of California Libraries' MELVYL system, and WorldCat (8,000 journals). One hundred and twenty-five journal articles were identified with 70% overlap between CSU and UC library search systems; all of the articles were downloaded into an ENDNOTE bibliographic database. The article abstracts were reviewed and 75 articles were found directly relevant. The full texts of these articles were downloaded; 60 were found directly useful.

Presentation: The 60 relevant articles in the database reflect use of cross-sectional and cohort research methods; there were national and state random samples; systematic, snowball and convenience local samples; records reviews based upon random samples of agency client files; focus groups and ethnographic observations; and program evaluations. These articles were published from 1992 to 2009. It was decided that the way to highlight the knowledge and gaps in knowledge reflected in these articles was to present their findings and insights in four sections. The first section identifies patterns or the specific behaviors that constituted "risky sex." The second section identifies the correlates to risky behaviors; these are the factors that condition whether or not the risky behavior occurs and have a high probability of leading to HIV infection. The third section lists any explanations or theories that suggest some complex interrelationships between variables that can predict risky sexual behaviors. The final section outlines actually fielded prevention efforts specifically aimed at reducing risky sexual behaviors among black men described in the research literature. Were these applications of scientific knowledge regarding risky sex among black men evaluated for their effectiveness and are they replicable? In effect, we want to show the risky behaviors, the factors conditioning these behaviors, any theories that could predict these behaviors, and then any effective application of this knowledge. Effective prevention would require precisely such background science if there was a change in political will and a willingness to prevent risky sex among black men. But before we begin the sectional review, the issue of sexual identity must be addressed.

Issue of Sexual Identity: In reviewing the research literature on risky sex among black men, sexual identity complicates the research which is divided into two populations (1) "men who have sex with men" (MSM) which includes men who may or may not self-identify as gay or bisexual; and (2) men who self-identify as or are assumed to be heterosexual. A problem that all of this research faces is that behaviorally this division between men is not so neat. Because homophobia is so extensive among Blacks and Hispanics, an unknown proportion of Black and Hispanic men refuse to identify as gay or bisexual and remain hidden among heterosexual men. These men have sex with men and/or women. Ironically, many of these men are strongly homophobic. It is assumed that if their racial subculture was more tolerant of homosexuality, most of these hidden MSMs would be more open about their homosexuality and bisexuality. So what appears as mutually distinct sexual identities in public (heterosexual vs. gay or bisexual) is, in fact, a sexual continuum in private. There are self-identified heterosexual men at one end, self-identified gay or bisexual men at the other, and men who have sex with men and/or women bridging the two ends of the continuum. This means that the HIV epidemic among Black and Hispanic gay and bisexual men is not separate from the HIV epidemic among heterosexual men and women in Black and Hispanic communities. The two epidemics are linked by an unknown number of men who have sex with men and women. Here, sexual social identity collides with HIV/AIDs where HIV prevention cannot be effectively addressed without also addressing sexual identity (Phillips, 2005). In the next section, we will focus on only ways in which risky sex occurs.

Section 1: Patterns of Risky Sexual Behavior

Gay and bisexual men: Historically, the initial research on HIV risk that led to the earliest effective prevention among gay and bisexual men was conducted in San Francisco in the 1990s. In one sense, research on gay and bisexual men in San Francisco was unique. San Francisco had the largest politically active and openly gay communities in the USA. San Francisco's "Castro" district, along with perhaps Greenwich Village in New York City, is a cultural center of gay community life and self-identification. But the initial research on HIV risks among gay and bisexual men in San Francisco focused on White men. When a study of HIV risk among black gay men in San Francisco, Oakland, and Berkeley was finally done, it showed that 50% of the sample had engaged in unprotected anal intercourse in the 6 months prior to their interview (Peterson et al., 1992). This is a considerably higher rate than was found among White gay and bisexual men in San Francisco through 1988 and 1989.

One study compared various MSM partner patterns (men-to-men, men-to-women, and men-to-men-and-women) and suggested that there may be distinctly different risk levels by partner pattern (Mimiaga et al., 2009). That is self-identified gay and bisexual men may take significantly fewer sexual risks of becoming HIV infected than hidden MSMs. The surprise is that there are not more studies that explore differences between self-identified gay and bisexual men and hidden MSMs. A review of the literature on black men who are hidden MSMs and who have sex with women ("on the down-low") suggests that they engage in a lower prevalence of HIV risks than black MSM who do disclose their sexual preference for men. Black men who are currently bisexually active account for a very small proportion (2%) of the overall population of black men (Millett, Malebranche, Mason, & Spikes, 2005). It might be important in prevention efforts to know if any difference is made by self-identification and engagement in gay culture and community. Instead, what one finds in many studies is that self-identified gay and bisexual men are routinely combined with hidden MSMs.

Men Who have Sex with Men (MSMs): Virtually all studies since 1990 use the U.S. Centers for Disease Control and Prevention definition of MSMs that combines self-identified gay and bisexual men with other men who have sex with men – those who otherwise still identify as heterosexual men. So, in the descriptions to follow it is impossible to know whether the behaviors described are driven more so by one subgroup or the other; an exception is Flores, et al. (2009). In study after study, MSMs engage in varying rates of unprotected anal intercourse for 1–6 months prior to their interview. It also appears that rates of anal intercourse without condoms and of HIV infections were lower in random samples of respondents in State and in multisite studies (i.e., Harawa et al., 2004; Xia et al., 2006) when compared to respondents drawn from community-based systematic and convenience samples (i.e. Hart & Peterson, 2004; Mimiaga et al., 2009).

MSMs who meet anonymous partners and have sex in public venues use condoms less often than MSMs who meet and have sex in more personal settings (Koblin et al., 2007). MSMs who use websites to find sex partners engage in higher levels of unprotected anal sex as well (Klein, 2008). Focus groups suggest that there is another pattern by which MSMs might engage in risky sex. Sex may be had "at the spur of the moment" or spontaneously where there is little prior planning or preparation; these are risky occasions if condoms are not immediately available, remembered, wanted, and then used (Peterson, Bakeman, Blackshear, & Stokes, 2003). Finally, black MSMs in historically black colleges and universities were found to have more sex partners and to use condoms less frequently than their heterosexual peers (Browne, Clubb, Wang, & Wagner, 2009).

Heterosexual men: In studies using sample and community surveys, sexually active African American and Hispanic heterosexual teens consistently have higher HIV sexual risk levels than their white peers. They report using birth control (in particular, condoms) less often and having more sex partners (Bartlett, Buck, & Shattell, 2008; DiIorio, Hartwell, & Hansen, 2002). Adolescent males returning from jail engage in sex without condoms more often than their peers who did not go to jail (Daniels, Crum, Ramaswamy, & Freudenberg, 2009). The same is true for adult black men released from incarceration (Khan et al., 2008). Black men who have been incarcerated are 8–10 times more likely to be HIV positive than their peers who have not been to jail. But most were infected prior to their incarceration (Inciardi et al., 2007).

Black men who may not use illicit drugs or who have not been incarcerated have varying attitudes toward condom use. Some of these men use condoms primarily as a means of birth control with their main partner, but do not use them with their casual partners. Others use condoms with casual partners, but not with their main partner. Still others refuse to use condoms with either. All three patterns risk giving and acquiring STDs and HIV from either partner in different ways. A topic of research has been to figure out the HIV risks associated with each pattern and how does one get men who take each type of risk to use condoms consistently. There is research which suggests that there are informational and personality differences between college men who intend to use condoms and college men who have no intention of using them (Winfield & Whaley, 2005). There are also attitudinal and personality differences between men who use condoms consistently, taking few HIV risk, and those who are inconsistent in their condom use (Johnson, Hinkle, Gilbert, & Gant, 1992). Finally, some older black men engage in risky sex (Jackson, Early, Schim, & Penprase, 2005). There are older men with steady retirement incomes who seek out and are sought by women who realize that they are a steady source of money for sex – "pension day sex." Many of these older men lack knowledge about HIV risks; are reluctant to use condoms in transactional sex and end-up acquiring STD and HIV infections.

Section 2: *Correlations to Risky Sex*

What conditions must be present for the fore-mentioned sex risks to occur and risk HIV infection? Are any conditioning factors the same for different risks and for different subgroups? For all three sub-groups (gay and bisexual, MSMs, and heterosexual men), *alcohol and drug use* are consistently found as correlates to HIV sexual risk taking. It has been found that self-identified black gay and bisexual men are most likely to engage in anal sex without condoms if they used recreational drugs before sex or drank heavily alcoholic beverages before and during sex (Wilton, 2008). Among heterosexual men alcohol and drugs before or during sex results in less consistent condom use even if condoms are available and there is an intent to use them (Johnson et al., 1992). *Sex with multiple partners* is another consistent covariate of HIV infection for all three subgroups. There is a particularly high association between *crack cocaine use* and engaging in risky sex and HIV infection (Edlin et al., 1994). The economy of crack cocaine dealing partly takes place through *transactional sex –* drugs for sex and/or money (Caetano & Hines, 1995). Dealing crack cocaine is virtually synonymous with transactional sex. The sexual risks taken for money and/or drugs links high rates of HIV among those who have been incarcerated since the majority of black men who go to jail are there for drug-related crimes (Lichtenstein, 2009). Then, whether or not one's peers have a *condom, social norm* regarding condom we are also very important. Risk-takers whose social groups have a condom use norm use condoms more consistently than those who do not. The development of a condom use social norm was primarily responsible for reducing HIV infections in the first generation of gay and bisexual AIDS victims.

In recent research, early childhood experiences are increasingly prominent as sources of correlates to adult risky HIV behaviors. The *early onset of sexual activity* in one's pre-adolescence is associated with engaging in riskier sexual behavior as an adolescent and adult for all identities of black men, especially if they were abused as children (Browne et al., 2009; Welles et al., 2009). Respondents to a telephone survey who reported having child sex experiences (CSE) were separated from those who did not (non-CSE). Those with CSE were further divided by those who considered their *early sexual experience as not abusive* (nondefiners) from those who did (definers). Of the three groups of respondents, those who reported having child sexual experiences that they believed were not abusive (nondefiners) were significantly more risky in their sexual behaviors than those who reported not having any child sexual experiences (non-CSE). They also took more risk than those who had CSE and viewed their experiences as abusive (definers). Nondefiners reported having sex under the influence of drug and alcohol more often and they had more sexual partners, more STDs and had more post-traumatic stress. Significantly more gay men were among those who reported having early child sexual experiences (Holmes, 2008).

For heterosexual respondents, there is a high correlation between having been *treated for a sexually transmitted disease* (STD), using more drugs in one's life-time, *frequent HIV testing*, and acquiring HIV (Feist-Price, Logan, Leukefeld, Moore, & Ebreo, 2003). In contrast, MSMs with a history of sexual transmitted disease infections, especially gonorrhea, were more likely to be HIV infected than those without based upon health clinic facility records (Do, Hanson, Dworkin, & Jones, 2001). Other correlates suggest that social class factors play some role in the extent to which one engages in risky sex and the likelihood of acquiring HIV. *Not completing high school*, being *homeless*, *unemployed*, working a difficult job, and not having health insurance have been associated with more frequent risky sex (Garofalo, Deleon, Osmer, Doll, & Harper, 2006; Raj, Reed, Welles, Santana, & Silverman, 2008). Young adults, who attend school regularly and who have part-time work, have lower rates of risky sex than their peers who have dropped out and are unemployed. *Socializing with risky peers* and *having fathered a child as a young adult* is also associated with risky sex while frequent engagement with family and high religiosity are protective (Kogan et al., 2008). Other research has pointed out that having *less social support* for low risk HIV behavior, having a *perception being at high risk* of HIV infection, and ever having been *paid for sex* increases the likelihood of being HIV infected through risky sex (Peterson et al., 2003).

One of the longest ongoing attempts to understand the differences between low and high HIV risk-takers is through psychosocial factors. Differences have been found between black, white, and other respondents. Generally, study response sizes of black participants have not been large enough to compare black low risk-takers with high risk-takers. In one of the few studies to look specifically at black men and psychosocial factors, the major findings were that high psychological distress, being HIV-negative, older age, low socioeconomic status (SES), and being gay were the best predictors of more frequent sexual risk-taking (Myers, 2003). High distress and anxiety are functions of the chaotic and unpredictable life-style of those associated with street-life, the drug-culture, and transactional and commercial sex. MSMs who perceive their sexual behaviors as risking HIV infection were compared with those who did not. Those who perceived that they were at HIV risk had lower rates of sex without condoms compared to those who perceived little risk (Peterson et al., 1992). If there was more research on the association between psychosocial factors and HIV risks, high levels of depression among high risk-takers might be another consistent finding.

The patterns of risky sex outlined by subgroup above have an array of correlates described in this section. Table 12.1 lists correlates by findings among subgroups.

The horizontal axis of Table 12.1 lists black men by sexual identities (gay/bisexual, gay/bisexual, and MSM and heterosexuals). The vertical axis lists all of the identified correlates to HIV infection. The asterisks represent finding of specific correlations by sexual identity in at least one of the 60 relevant studies. In cells without asterisks, the specific HIV risk correlate was not found for that sexual group in these studies. For example, factors associated with social class impact levels of risky sex among heterosexuals are SES, homelessness, not completing high school, and unemployment. The research that explores this question among gay and bisexual men and MSMs is partial and incomplete (Hart & Peterson, 2004; Peterson et al., 1992). Certainly, there may be intragenerational and perhaps even intergenerational social class differences among these men. But this work remains to be done. Full social class differences among these men may have some impact on exposure to HIV and engagement in risky behaviors. Self-identified black gay and bisexual men may be predominantly middle class and free enough from black community antihomosexual attitudes to self-identify. Underclass black MSMs may not have the freedom to go against convention and

Table 12.1 Black sexual identities by HIV risk factors

Risk factors	Gay/bisexual (G&B)	G&B + MSM	Heterosexuals
Alcohol use	*	*	*
Crack cocaine			*
Other illicit drugs			
Transactional sex		*	*
Condom use norm	*		*
Multiple sex partners	*	*	*
Pre-teen sexual activity	*	*	*
Child-sex victims			
STD treatment		*	*
Freq. HIV testing			*
Socioeconomic status		*	*
Homelessness			*
Less high school grad.			*
Unemployed			*
Socialize w/risky peers			*
Fathered child as teen			*
Less social support			*
Perception at high HIV risk		*	
Total identified risks	4	7	15

self-identify as gay or bisexual and must remain hidden. In which case, their higher HIV risks are conditioned by more intensely oppressive social class and gender circumstances than their middle class peers.

This table points to gaps in the research as of November 2009. Each gap (where there are no asterisks) does not suggest that a risk factor is nonexistent for a sexual identity. Table 12.1 shows the extent to which the little research that has been conducted on HIV sexual risk among black men has focused on heterosexuals. Half as much attention has been given to MSMs and half again attention has been given to self-identified gay and bisexual men. Perhaps MSMs get more attention because they are hidden and are viewed as a threat to the heterosexual majority because they have sex with women as well. This emphasis on heterosexuals in the research is the reverse of infection rates. Black G&B + MSMs have considerably higher HIV infection rates than black heterosexuals. The point is: there is not enough research on HIV among black men period and what exist privileges heterosexuals who have comparatively lower HIV infection rates. It appears that the production of HIV research on black men matches gender bias both in mainstream society and in black communities.

Table 12.1 sets the stage for the next section. A listing of all the individual correlates of risky sex by risk group begs the question of the extent to which we know what combinations of covariates might predict varying levels of risky sexual behavior. There is multivariate analysis that explores disparities between black and white men who have sex with men (Millett, Flores, Peterson, & Bakeman, 2007). But there is no comparable multivariate analysis that explains disparities in HIV risk among all sexual identities of black men using the above correlates.

Section 3: Explanations of Risky Sexual Behavior

Are there explanations of HIV sexual risks derived from this research that suggests interrelationships between correlates? In effect, are there any theories that can predict risky sexual behaviors among black men? In reviewing the 60 articles that constitute current research on risky sexual behavior among black men, as of the year 2009, there are no theories directly derived from this research.

Theories have been used to assess the dynamics of individual sexual HIV risk-taking. They include the health belief model, the AIDS risk reduction model, trans-theoretical model, the social cognitive theory, the theory of reasoned action, the theory of planned behavior, and the information–motivation–behavior skills model (Fisher & Fisher, 2000). Some of these constructs have been used in HIV prevention research on homosexuals (Ross & Kelly, 2000). But wherever these theories have been used in research on HIV sexual risk among black men, they are used as background and are not central to the findings and conclusions. In effect, none of these theories have been advanced with black men as subjects nor has our understanding of black men's HIV sexual risks been advanced by any of these theories. Patrick Wilson (2008) comes close by defining a dynamic ecology model that explains identity formation and conflict among bisexually behaving African American men. But this model has yet to be tested as a predictor of HIV sexual risk-taking for all three sexual identities of black men. Research on black men is primarily descriptive in mission and outcome. In which case, there is no systemic theoretical development or modeling that has advanced this work to the level of inference or prediction. The atheoretical nature of this research is in no way unique to the study of black men. The same point can be made about a good deal of the HIV/AIDS and drug abuse prevention research.

Despite the general lack of theory, a number of researchers have offered explanations of risky sex among black men. Bakeman and Peterson suggest that the presence or absence of a condom use norm might explain much more HIV risky sex than other factors (2007). A good start is Millett et al., critical review of the literature on men who have sex with men (2006). They critique 12 hypotheses about greater HIV prevalence among Black MSMs, and suggest the following hypothesis as the most promising: the higher rate of past and current STDs among black MSMs the more likely they will acquire HIV. Of all the covariates discussed above, this is the most promising relative to the others. A second promising hypothesis is that higher HIV rates among black MSMs are due to fewer of these men knowing their HIV status and getting tested. In effect, they continue to be sexually active and to spread HIV long after they are unknowingly infected. In which case, there are higher rates of unrecognized HIV infections among black MSMs than other ethnic groups of MSMs. The same point has been made by others (Do et al., 2001). Millett et al. point out that the relative strength of one or the other covariate and hypothesis in explaining high rates of HIV among MSMs is dependent upon future research. I would add that such research has to move beyond description as it has been done for MSMs (Millett & Peterson, 2007; Peterson & Jones, 2009) and move more toward inference and theory to explain HIV rates among all black men.

Other researchers have also made explanative suggestions. An objective of qualitative research is to identify new risk factors and relations between factors which might later be proven to predict HIV sexual risk-taking. In focus groups with MSMs, prolonged and repeated abuse as a child by a close male relative comes up repeatedly as a factor that might impact not only sexual identity but also sexual HIV risk-taking as adults (Fields, Malebranche, & Feist-Price, 2008). It has been suggested that childhood sexual abuse might be more prevalent than we realize (DiIorio et al., 2002). With heterosexual men, it was repeatedly found across a series of nine focus groups of men that knowingly engage in irrational sexual behaviors. It was explained in several unrelated focus groups that some will do anything to get the attention of an attractive woman or do anything if they are "in love." Another important point made is that condoms are rejected if they are thought to reduce pleasure or compromise one's sexual performance. Also, it was reported that one can be so "carried away" in sex that condoms can get broken, rubbed off, and ultimately just become a nuisance. It was also suggested that younger men may differ in the extent to which they believe and are influenced by older black men's anticondom attitudes (Thompson-Robinson et al., 2007). None of these insights have been confirmed in quantitative research.

Does any of this help us to understand how we might effectively prevent HIV infections across all sexual identities of black men and ultimately slow the continuing AIDS epidemic among Blacks? Perhaps the answer to this question is in the next section on prevention interventions.

Section 4: HIV Prevention Efforts

What is the record of fielded prevention efforts specifically aimed at reducing risky sexual behaviors among black men based upon the research literature outlined above? Darbes et al. (2002) found in the literature 52 theory-based interventions aimed at reducing HIV risk among African Americans published between 1985 and 2000. Only four of these interventions were successful, theoretically-based and explicitly aimed at reducing HIV sexual risk among men who were not injection drug users (Kalichman & Cherry, 1999; Kalichman, Cherry, & Browne-Sperling, 1999; Malow, West, Corrigan, Pena, & Cunningham, 1994). Of this subset of studies, only one focused on MSMs by evaluating an intervention based upon the AIDS Risk Reduction Model (Peterson et al., 1996).

In this 60 article review of the literature since 2000, 12 new theory-based studies of HIV prevention intervention efforts among African Americans were found. Only two focused specifically on HIV prevention among black men; seven focused on men and women and three were specifically on women. Both of the two studies of prevention among men, ironically, focused on prison-based populations of presumably heterosexuals. There was no prevention effort found that focused specifically on MSMs. The first of these two prevention studies was based upon social learning theory. Its objective was to change the attitudes of soon to be released prison inmates toward HIV risk-taking and improve their self-efficacy toward condom use and other prevention behaviors. The program was only partly successful; it improved intent to use condoms and participants' willingness to participate in follow-up activities (Bryan, 2006). The second study was the Returning Educated African American and Latino Men to Enriched Neighborhoods (REAL MEN) program, a jail and community-based program to reduce drug use, HIV risks and re-arrest. The program was based upon helping young ex-offenders examine alternative paths to manhood and to consider racial/ethnic pride as a source of strength (Griffin, 2005). Neither of these studies was a breakthrough in prevention or the application of theory. They show that in terms of effectiveness we have a long way to go.

Translation of research to prevention: Even if there was adequate research, there is a related problem that must be addressed. The translation of research findings into "field-able" interventions is a formidable barrier to effective prevention interventions, in general (Valdiserri, 2000), and for African Americans in particular. When investigators find that African Americans differ in some way in their behaviors from Whites, it is now a virtual ritual to say that these behaviors must be addressed in culturally appropriate ways. In effect, the research findings are left to someone else to figure out how to implement cultural relevance. The problem with this recommendation is that it calls for sensitivity to only one party in the process of translating research into programs, the risk-takers. Those in Black communities who must translate the researchers' counsel and implement interventions are not considered. For example, when young black men attending historically black colleges and universities (HBCUs) were found to engage in sexual high risk-taking, it was recommended that the colleges and universities need to conduct HIV/STD educational and prevention education (Browne et al., 2009). The problem is health services and counseling programs at HBCUs already have programs to address HIV and STD risks among their students (Walker & Bragg, 2005). This counsel does not address the more precise problem "on the ground." There is a disconnection between students and the colleges as to where and when they engage in risky sex and who should offer an intervention based upon research findings. Solving this disconnect is as important to figure out as was finding the HIV high risk. A prevention education effort and intervention in some other venue than the colleges might be more effective.

There is another example. Black men returning from prison engage in much more risky sex than their nonprison peers in the community. Therefore, it would seem reasonable to have a program for ex-offenders while they are in prison and after release when they are so sexually active (Khan et al., 2008). Such a recommendation assumes that the most effective place and time to mount prevention is in the community in which inmates are released and right after release. But it might be too late to most effectively address risky sex after release from jail. The most effective point of intervention might be before they go to jail when they are most likely to have become HIV infected (Lichtenstein, 2009). Black men who have been through drug treatment have high relapse rates to crack and the sexual risk associated with crack use and dealing. A direct implication of such a finding is to recommend that programs are needed that will address the special clinical psychological needs of men returning to their home environment (Cavazos-Rehg et al., 2009). But a clinical effort in a low-income community to keep former treatment clients from relapsing to crack may be ineffective in itself. Such an effort must also address clients' other unmet needs – security, resolution of arrest warrants, lack of identification and drivers license, need for job training, lack of jobs, housing, sufficient income, childcare, and healthcare. Perhaps, if these other needs were met, clients would not have such a high need for clinical assistance.

The point is there is no direct translation of basic behavioral and attitudinal research findings into prevention interventions. Implementation of research findings requires a great deal more than cultural sensitivity. The program design, administration, mode, and location of delivery all have to be conceptualized and planned. Funding has to be obtained. The mix of skills, backgrounds, and personalities of staff has to be decided. Then whatever program is started must come together as an organization and go through a period of refinement based upon its initial experiences in the field. This will require some change of staff, refinement of program objectives, perhaps new field sites, alternative funding and even additional office locations. Then once the program is running, it must be evaluated, whatever short-comings must be addressed and then the program must be re-evaluated and refined continuously. The current research literature on HIV risky sex among black men offers no clues as to how such programs should be implemented to actualize research findings and recommendations.

The irony is that there are hundreds, if not more, community-based efforts to prevent HIV infections among black men in African American communities. Most now do HIV prevention as an adjunct to addressing other critical needs and are doing HIV prevention without funding. Each effort approaches HIV/AIDS prevention based upon the philosophy, experience, and insight of the founders such as in the REAL MEN program described above. The problem is that the research community and federal agencies responsible for HIV prevention efforts do not interface with or perhaps even know about most of these grass-roots efforts. All of the programs that might have effective HIV interventions for black men are not reported in the research literature – only three until 2002 and two since 2009. In effect, the very audience and people who need the prevention research to create interventions are ignored and the outcome is that researchers publish and "talk" primarily to themselves about black men in journals.

Conclusion

It should be clear by this point that if there was sudden federal interest in mounting a serious effort to prevent HIV infections among black men, that effort as a scientific undertaking would have to start anew. The withdrawal of public and federal government attention and funding from HIV/AIDS prevention among Blacks during the 2000s is reflected in the current state of the research as well. What research exists is insufficient in scope relative to the problem. If preventing AIDS among Blacks was considered important, there should easily be well over 100 rather than just 60 research articles. In addition, there is an under-representation of research on gay and bisexual men and MSMs in the work that has been done. We know virtually nothing about the differences between gay and bisexual men and MSMs who still identify as heterosexuals – an important point for HIV prevention. Existing research is clearly insufficient to address the prevention needs of black self-identified gay men who are estimated to be 1–2.5% of the general population of men in the USA or of men who have bisexuals experiences, estimated to be as high as 35% of all men (Wikipedia, 2009). Finally, the gaps in existing research are clear evidence of just how extreme is the inadequacy in current efforts. But even if there was sufficient research, the critically important issue of transferring research findings to actual prevention interventions has been missed in reference to black men.

A generation of investigators has worked largely independent of one another and without major support to identify correlates associated with patterns of risky sex. It is no coincidence that only two of the published research reports since 2000 were based upon multisite research; all of the rest were based upon community samples derived from local efforts and funding. What has been identified is critical to future efforts, but more rigorous science remains to be done. It is problematic that current research on risky sex among black men is primarily descriptive. Multisite community-based studies with large enough samples are now needed to test the efficiency of the identified correlates and to isolate new ones – to fill in the gaps. Then analysis needs to move to modeling to identify relations between groups of correlates that predict specific risky sexual behaviors. This is when description will move to inference and theory. Why is this needed? Rigorous science can provide a blueprint for effective prevention or what is done on the ground will only be as effective as the science that informs it. The problem warrants our best rather than least efforts.

If sufficient attention and funding materialized, the research of the past two decades provides its own testimony for a need to approach prevention in a different way than in the years since 2000. Effective prevention cannot come about if the scientific community doing the research is separate from the people who do the prevention. A step in the right direction is the CDC/NIH requirement of participatory research with community-based organizations for all intervention studies. But we are still learning the specifics of what makes for successful collaborations and how some research findings can and cannot be implemented in community settings. The off-hand presumption that virtually any research findings have direct implications for prevention is clearly erroneous. Research findings that do not functionally work or make sense at the level of implementation are not helpful even in community collaborations. People who know and work with at risk groups must be fully engaged in formulating hypotheses, executing the research, and making sense of the findings well before the research gets underway (Bowser, Mishra, Reback, & Lemp, 2004). This is not a call for replacing "top down" research for equally problematic "bottom-up" research. Research done in community-based agencies is not better than "downtown" research done through university and organizational community field-sites. Researchers and practitioners must genuinely work together to merge the best of what they both have to offer (Bowser, Quimby, & Singer, 2007). The scientific method must be merged with knowledge and insights of the subgroup in question in their social context. Then, the outcome of the research will be rigorous, make sense and be useful toward effective prevention interventions. There will be no need to call for cultural-sensitivity after the fact or for community collaboration to try to make untenable theory and research tenable.

There is an opportunity that should not be missed in the hundreds of community-based efforts to prevent HIV infections among African Americans. Some subset of these programs may be effective. We may be able to fast-track our knowledge of HIV prevention among black men by identifying effective programs and then find out specifically what they do to get their results. Through such an effort we can find out in what way their interventions impact known correlates of HIV risk patterns. CDC/NIH funding of "translation projects" needs to be greatly expanded. So, instead of trying to build effective prevention based directly on risk-takers behavior and then trying to figure out how to implement the findings in communities, we can build our knowledge of prevention out of the trial and error of programs' actual experiences. We may find that effective interventions have points in common and that there are best practices that can be replicated across many different program settings. But here again this would require close collaborative working relationships between researchers and people in community-based prevention efforts in both defining and executing the research.

Finally, we may have to completely reconceptualize sexual risk and the factors associated with it (Martin, 2006). The behavioral definition of risky-sex and its correlates may ultimately be inadequate to understand why people are willing to take HIV risks in the first place. The focus groups of black men spoke to the limits of behaviorism by identifying the circumstances under which they were willing to do unreasonable and sexually risky things. There is an emotional side to risky sex and other human adventures that cannot be completely reduced to behavior or psychology. The emotions of risky sex may have their own rules that we need to learn. People are willing to engage in a complex calculus whether it is risky sex, knowing consumption of unhealthy foods, drug use, driving too fast, or gambling. If the circumstances are right, they are willing to take extraordinary risks to seemingly transcend their ordinary lives and to experience "a little piece of heaven" however, they might define it. Some may be more highly motivated than others to take chances; sexuality is where they take risks. In which case, our research has given us only half the story. There is a whole other missing side to HIV sexual risk or other influences on "behaviors" awaiting discovery.

Acknowledgements I would like to acknowledge the substantive assistance of John Peterson and Anthony Lemelle.

References

Bakeman, R., & Peterson, J. L. (2007). Do beliefs about HIV treatments affect peer norms and risky sexual behaviour among African American men who have sex with men? *International Journal of STD & AIDS, 18*(2), 105–108.

Bartlett, R., Buck, R., & Shattell, M. M. (2008). Risk and protection for HIV/AIDS in African American, Hispanic, and White adolescents. *Journal of National Black Nurses' Association, 19*(1), 19–25.

Bowser, B. P., Mishra, S., Reback, C., & Lemp, G. (Eds.). (2004). *Preventing AIDS: Community–science collaboration*. Binghamton, NY: Haworth.

Bowser, B. P., Quimby, E., & Singer, M. (Eds.). (2007). *When communities assess their AIDS epidemics: Results of rapid assessment of HIV/AIDS in eleven U.S. cities*. Lanham: Lexington Books.

Browne, D. C., Clubb, P. A., Wang, Y., & Wagner, F. (2009). Drug use and high-risk sexual behaviors among African American men who have sex with men and men who have sex with women. *American Journal of Public Health, 99*(6), 1062–1066.

Bryan, A. (2006). Effectiveness of an HIV prevention intervention in prison among African Americans, Hispanics, and Caucasians. *Health Education & Behavior, 33*(2), 154–177.

Caetano, R., & Hines, A. M. (1995). Alcohol, sexual practices, and risk of AIDS among Blacks, Hispanics, and Whites. *Journal of Acquired Immune Deficiency Syndromes and Human Retrovirology, 10*(5), 554–561.

Cavazos-Rehg, P. A., Spitznagel, E. L., Schootman, M., Strickland, J. R., Afful, S. E., Cottler, L. B., et al. (2009). Risky sexual behaviors and sexually transmitted diseases: A comparison study of cocaine-dependent individuals in treatment versus a community-matched sample. *AIDS Patient Care and STDs, 23*(9), 727–734.

Daniels, J., Crum, M., Ramaswamy, M., & Freudenberg, N. (2009). Creating REAL MEN: Description of an intervention to reduce drug use, HIV risk, and rearrest among young men returning to urban communities from jail. *Health Promotion Practice, 12*(1), 44–54.

Darbes, L. A., Kennedy, G. E., Zohrabyan, G. P. L., & Rutherford, G. W. (2002). Systematic review of HIV behavioral prevention research in African Americans. *HIV insite knowledge base chapter*. Retrieved January 5, 2010, from http://hivinsite.ucsf.edu/InSite?page=kb-07-04-09.

DiIorio, C., Hartwell, T., & Hansen, N. (2002). Childhood sexual abuse and risk behaviors among men at high risk for HIV infection. *American Journal of Public Health, 92*(2), 214–219.

Do, A. N., Hanson, D. L., Dworkin, M. S., & Jones, J. L. (2001). Risk factors for and trends in gonorrhea incidence among persons infected with HIV in the United States. *AIDS, 15*(9), 1149–1155.

Edlin, B., Irwin, K., Faruque, S., McCoy, C., Word, C., Serrano, Y., et al. (1994). Intersecting epidemics – crack cocaine use and HIV infection among inner-city young adults. *The New England Journal of Medicine, 331*, 1422–1427.

Feist-Price, S., Logan, T. K., Leukefeld, C., Moore, C. L., & Ebreo, A. (2003). Targeting HIV prevention on African American crack and injection drug users. *Substance Use & Misuse, 38*(9), 1259–1284.

Fields, S. D., Malebranche, D., & Feist-Price, S. (2008). Childhood sexual abuse in black men who have sex with men: Results from three qualitative studies. *Cultural Diversity & Ethnic Minority Psychology, 14*(4), 385–390.

Fisher, J., & Fisher, W. (2000). Theoretical approaches to individual-level change in HIV risk behavior. In J. L. Peterson & R. DiClemente (Eds.), *Handbook of HIV prevention* (pp. 3–55). New York: Plenum.

Flores, S. A., Bakeman, R., Millett, G. A., & Peterson, J. L. (2009). HIV risk among bisexually and homosexually active racially diverse young men. *Sexually Transmitted Diseases, 36*(5), 325–329.

Garofalo, R., Deleon, J., Osmer, E., Doll, M., & Harper, G. W. (2006). Overlooked, misunderstood and at-risk: Exploring the lives and HIV risk of ethnic minority male-to-female transgender youth. *The Journal of Adolescent Health, 38*(3), 230–236.

Griffin, J. P. (2005). Building resiliency and vocational excellence (BRAVE) program: A violence-prevention and role model program for young, African American males. *Journal of Health Care for the Poor and Underserved, 16*(4), 78–88.

Harawa, N. T., Greenland, S., Bingham, T. A., Johnson, D. F., Cochran, S. D., Cunningham, W. E., et al. (2004). Associations of race/ethnicity with HIV prevalence and HIV-related behaviors among young men who have sex with men in 7 urban centers in the United States. *Journal of Acquired Immune Deficiency Syndromes, 35*(5), 526–536.

Hart, T., & Peterson, J. L. (2004). Predictors of risky sexual behavior among young African American men who have sex with men. *American Journal of Public Health, 94*(7), 1122–1123.

Holmes, W. C. (2008). Men's self-definitions of abusive childhood sexual experiences, and potentially related risky behavioral and psychiatric outcomes. *Child Abuse & Neglect, 32*(1), 83–97.

Inciardi, J., Surratt, H., Martin, S., O'Connell, D., Salandy, A., & Beard, R. (2007). Developing a multimedia HIV and hepatitis intervention for drug-involved offenders reentering the community. *The Prison Journal, 87*(1), 111–142.

Jackson, F., Early, K., Schim, S. M., & Penprase, B. (2005). HIV knowledge, perceived seriousness and susceptibility, and risk behaviors of older African Americans. *Journal of Multicultural Nursing & Health, 11*(1), 56–62.

Johnson, E. H., Hinkle, Y., Gilbert, D., & Gant, L. M. (1992). Black males who always use condoms: Their attitudes, knowledge about AIDS, and sexual behavior. *Journal of the National Medical Association, 84*(4), 341–352.

Kalichman, S., & Cherry, C. (1999). Male polyurethane condoms do not enhance brief HIV-STD risk reduction interventions for heterosexually active men: Results from a randomized test of concept. *International Journal of STD & AIDS, 10*(8), 548–553.

Kalichman, S., Cherry, C., & Browne-Sperling, F. (1999). Effectiveness of a video-based motivational skills-building HIV risk-reduction intervention for inner-city African American men. *Journal of Consulting and Clinical Psychology, 67*(6), 959–966.

Khan, M. R., Wohl, D. A., Weir, S. S., Adimora, A. A., Moseley, C., Norcott, K., et al. (2008). Incarceration and risky sexual partnerships in a southern US city. *Journal of Urban Health, 85*(1), 100–113.

Klein, H. (2008). HIV risk practices sought by men who have sex with other men, and who use internet websites to identify potential sexual partners. *Sexual Health, 5*(3), 243–250.

Koblin, B. A., Murrill, C., Camacho, M., Xu, G., Liu, K.-I., Raj-Singh, S., et al. (2007). Amphetamine use and sexual risk among men who have sex with men: Results from the National HIV Behavioral Surveillance Study – New York City. *Substance Use & Misuse, 42*(10), 1613–1628.

Kogan, S., Brody, G., Gibbons, F., Murry, V., Cutrona, C., Simons, R., et al. (2008). The influence of role status on risky sexual behavior among African Americans during the transition to adulthood. *Journal of Black Psychology, 34*(3), 399–420.

Lichtenstein, B. (2009). Drugs, incarceration, and HIV/AIDS among African American men: A critical literature review and call to action. *American Journal of Men's Health, 3*(3), 252–264.

Malow, R., West, J., Corrigan, S., Pena, J., & Cunningham, S. (1994). Outcome of psychoeducation for HIV risk reduction. *AIDS Education and Prevention, 6*(2), 113–125.

Martin, J. (2006). Transcendence among gay men: Implications for HIV prevention. *Sexualities, 9*(2), 214–235.

McBride, D. (1991). *From TB to AIDS: Epidemics among urban Blacks since 1900.* Albany: State University of New York Press.

Millett, G., Malebranche, D., Mason, B., & Spikes, P. (2005). Focusing "down low": Bisexual black men, HIV risk and heterosexual transmission. *Journal of the National Medical Association, 97*(7 Suppl), 52S–59S.

Millett, G. A., Flores, S. A., Peterson, J. L., & Bakeman, R. (2007). Explaining disparities in HIV infection among black and white men who have sex with men: A meta-analysis of HIV risk behaviors. *AIDS, 21,* 2083–2091.

Millett, G. A., & Peterson, J. L. (2007). The known hidden epidemic: HIV/AIDS among black men who have sex with men in the United States. *American Journal of Preventive Medicine, 32*(4S), S31–S33.

Millett, G. A., Wolitski, R. J., Stall, R., & Peterson, J. L. (2006). Greater risk for HIV infection of Black men who have sex with men: A critical literature review. *American Journal of Public Health, 96*(6), 1007–1019.

Mimiaga, M. J., Reisner, S. L., Cranston, K., Isenberg, D., Bright, D., Daffin, G., et al. (2009). Sexual mixing patterns and partner characteristics of Black MSM in Massachusetts at increased risk for HIV infection and transmission. *Journal of Urban Health, 86*(4), 602–623.

Myers, H. (2003). Psychosocial predictors of risky sexual behaviors in African American men: Implications for prevention. *Sage Family Studies Abstracts, 25*(4).

Peterson, J. L., Bakeman, R., Blackshear, J. H., & Stokes, J. P. (2003). Perceptions of condom use among African American men who have sex with men. *Culture, Health & Sexuality, 5*(5), 409–424.

Peterson, J. L., Coates, T. J., Catania, J. A., Hauck, W., Acree, M., Daigle, D., et al. (1996). Evaluation of an HIV risk reduction intervention among African American homosexual and bisexual men. *AIDS, 10*, 319–325.

Peterson, J. L., Coates, T. J., Catania, J. A., Middleton, L., Hilliard, B., & Hearst, N. (1992). High-risk sexual behavior and condom use among gay and bisexual African American men. *American Journal of Public Health, 82*(11), 1490–1494.

Peterson, J. L., & Jones, K. (2009). HIV prevention for black men who have sex with men in the United States. *American Journal of Public Health, 99*(6), 976–980.

Phillips, L. L. (2005). Deconstructing "Down Low" discourse: The politics of sexuality, gender, race, AIDS, and anxiety source. *Journal of African American Men, 9*(2), 3–15.

Raj, A., Reed, E., Welles, S. L., Santana, M. C., & Silverman, J. G. (2008). Intimate partner violence perpetration, risky sexual behavior, and STI/HIV diagnosis among heterosexual African American men. *American Journal of Men's Health, 2*(3), 291–295.

Ross, M., & Kelly, J. (2000). Interventions to reduce HIV transmission in homosexual men. In J. L. Peterson & R. DiClemente (Eds.), *Handbook of HIV prevention* (pp. 201–216). New York: Plenum.

Thompson-Robinson, M., Weaver, M., Shegog, M., Richter, D., Usdan, S., & Saunders, R. (2007). Perceptions of heterosexual African American males' high-risk sex behaviors. *International Journal of Men's Health, 6*(2), 156–166.

Valdiserri, R. (2000). Technology transfer: Achieving the promise of HIV prevention. In J. L. Peterson & R. DiClemente (Eds.), *Handbook of HIV Prevention* (pp. 267–285). New York: Plenum.

Walker, E. A., & Bragg, R. (2005). Racial disparities in health outcomes: Research and intervention perspectives. *Journal of Health Care for the Poor and Underserved, 16*(4, Suppl A), v–xii.

Welles, S. L., Baker, A. C., Miner, M. H., Brennan, D. J., Jacoby, S., & Rosser, B. R. (2009). History of childhood sexual abuse and unsafe anal intercourse in a 6-city study of HIV-positive men who have sex with men. *American Journal of Public Health, 99*(6), 1079–1086.

Wikipedia. (2009). *Demographics of sexual orientation*. Retrieved January 7, 2010, from http://en.wikipedia.org/w/index.php?title=Demographics_of_sexual_orientation&oldid=333830570.

Wilson, P. (2008). A dynamic-ecological model of identity formation and conflict among bisexually-behaving African American men. *Archives of Sexual Behaviors, 37*(5), 794–809.

Wilton, L. (2008). Correlates of substance use in relation to sexual behavior in Black gay and bisexual men: Implications for HIV prevention. *Journal of Black Psychology, 34*(1), 70–93.

Winfield, E., & Whaley, A. (2005). Relationship status, psychological orientation, and sexual risk taking in a heterosexual African American college sample. *Journal of Black Psychology, 31*(2), 189–204.

Xia, Q., Osmond, D. H., Tholandi, M., Pollack, L. M., Zhou, W., Ruiz, J. D., et al. (2006). HIV prevalence and sexual risk behaviors among men who have sex with men results from a statewide population-based survey in California. *Journal of Acquired Immune Deficiency Syndromes, 41*(2), 238–245.

Chapter 13
Post-prison Community Reentry and African American Males: Implications for Family Therapy and Health

Armon R. Perry, Michael A. Robinson, Rudolph Alexander Jr., and Sharon E. Moore

Literature Review

The criminal justice field has shown considerable academic and professional interest in reentry of prisoners into their communities, noting that mental health, social factors, and adjustment issues may impede the success of persons not returning to prisons. Reentry is defined as the process of juvenile and adult offenders returning, hopefully successfully, to schools, families, communities, and society at large (Mears & Travis, 2004). Visher, Kachnowski, La Vigne, and Travis (2004) defined reentry as any processes designed to facilitate individuals' transition from incarceration in prisons, jails, federal institutions, or juvenile facilities to freedom. As such, reentry processes may begin while a person is incarcerated and continue after his release into the community.

Reentry has emerged with such importance that the Office of Justice Programs within the US Department of Justice has created a specialized division within its system and has provided grants and conferences for professionals to gather. According to Massoglia and Hartmann (2006), over 600,000 individuals, who are mostly minorities, are released into the community yearly. This interest has involved both juvenile offenders (Mears & Travis, 2004) and adult offenders. However, all ex-offenders, regardless of age, experience considerable barriers to reentry into the community after their release.

Formal barriers to successful reentry for former prisoners involve not being allowed to work in certain occupations, such as security positions, child care and being barred from any federal programs, such as public assistance, subsidized housing, and federal school loans. In addition to the formal barriers, there are also informal barriers. Incarceration may weaken family ties, alter negatively social networks, and distance ex-offenders from the formal labor market (Weiman, Stoll, & Bushway, 2007). As indicated by Weiman et al. "these combined challenges do not prevent released prisoners from 'going straight,' but they do diminish their odds. In other words, they increase the likelihood that released prisoners will commit a technical parole violation, misdemeanor, or more serious felony offense, and so wind up back in prison. A more extended prison spell or additional prison spells can in transform the marginal offender into a more serious one, who has accumulated a lengthier rap sheet but also has become more deeply enmeshed in illegal rather than legal social network" (pp. 55–56).

S.E. Moore (✉)
Raymond A. Kent School of Social Work, University of Louisville,
Louisville, KY, USA
e-mail: semoor02@louisville.edu

A.J. Lemelle et al. (eds.), *Handbook of African American Health: Social and Behavioral Interventions*,
DOI 10.1007/978-1-4419-9616-9_13, © Springer Science+Business Media, LLC 2011

In their discussions, Weiman et al. (2007) noted the negative impact of mass incarceration and control by the justice system of young, uneducated African American males. Given that African Americans are overrepresented in prisons, they are also overrepresented in the reentry processes. However, specific attention to the problems and issues of African American prisoners has been scant, although African Americans make up a large proportion of persons under the control of the criminal justice systems (i.e., prisons, parole, probation, and halfway houses). Normally, data regarding African American prisoners are reported as a race variable among numerous other variables. For instance, James and Glaze (2006) reported the mental health problems of prison and jail inmates, and they reported that 55% of African Americans in state prisons had mental health problems, 46% of African Americans in federal prisons, and 63% of African Americans in jails had mental health problems.

One reason that the literature one African American prisoners is limited is that few researchers study just African Americans' issues surrounding reentry. This is so because few corrections departments would allow or permit studies to focus on one race when other prisoners, Whites and other minorities, are also faced with reentry issues as well. In fact, Massoglia and Hartmann (2006) contended that being White is not a privilege when it comes to difficulties upon leaving prisons. Contrarily, Pager (2003) has found that Whites leaving prison purportedly with a felony conviction for drugs have an easier time getting jobs than African Americans without any criminal record. Further, empirical evidence supports that African Americans leaving prison encounter racial stereotypes and discrimination that make it more difficult to secure employment in the labor market (Bushway, Stoll, & Weiman, 2007; Pager, 2007).

However, a few researchers have become interested in the problems of African American males in the reentry process. Demonstrating one of the difficulties of reentry, Pager (2007) conducted an experiment to learn the impact of race and criminal records across three different contexts. As in her previous works (Pager, 2003), she sent African American and White testers to apply for entry level positions (i.e., requiring a high school education) in the Milwaukee, Wisconsin area. One tester for each race had a fictitious criminal record for a drug conviction. Employers with advertised job announcements were randomly assigned to testers. The contexts were city versus suburban, restaurant versus nonrestaurant jobs, and personal contact versus no personal contact. The dependent variable was whether the employer called the tester back after the applications were completed. For Whites, where there were no personal contacts, 28% who had no criminal record received callbacks and 9% with criminal records received call backs. For Whites, where there were personal contacts, 53% with no criminal records received call backs and 42% with criminal records received call backs. For African Americans, where there were no personal contacts, 7% with no record received call backs and 4% with criminal records received call backs. For African Americans where there were personal contacts, 36% with no record received call backs and 6% with criminal records received call backs.

Comparing the city and suburb, Pager found that for Whites in the city, 23% with no record received call backs and 7% with criminal records received call backs. In the suburbs, 40% of Whites with no record received call backs and 22% with a criminal record received call backs. In the city, 11% of African Americans with no record received call backs and 6% of African Americans in the city with criminal records received call backs. For African Americans in the suburbs, 16% with no criminal records received call backs and 3% of African Americans with criminal records received call backs. For Whites in nonrestaurant jobs, 32% of them with no records received call backs and 15% with criminal records received call backs. For restaurant jobs, 40% of Whites with no records received call backs and 23 of Whites with criminal records received call backs. For African Americans, 16% of them in nonrestaurant jobs with no criminal records received call backs and 6% of them with a criminal records received call backs. For restaurant jobs, 7% of African Americans with no records received call backs and 2% of African Americans with criminal records received call backs.

Pager, interpreting her findings, concludes that African American ex-offenders are the least favorable group in the labor market. African Americans have the least chance of securing jobs in the restaurant industry though the restaurant industry appears open to White ex-offenders. Pager states that "exploring the interaction between race and criminal record in three contexts, we detect the ways in which black ex-offenders face an intensification of stigma, above and beyond the simple additive effects of either characteristic alone" (Pager, 2007, p. 168).

Although little specific attention has been given to African Americans' reentry into the community, additional problems of African Americans can also be inferred from the literature. Dumond (2000) noted that sexual assaults within the prison population remain a significant problem. Sexual assault in prison had become so problematic that Congress passed legislation (Prison Rape Elimination Act of 2003, P.L. 108–179) aimed at addressing this problem. Wolff, Blitz, and Shi (2007) studied the rates of prisoners with and without mental disorders and whether they were sexually assaulted in prison. A number of professionals have documented serious mental illnesses of prisoners who may have come into the system with serious mental illness or develop them in prisons and thus return to the community needing mental health care (Black et al., 2007; Hartwell 2003a, 2003b; Henderson, Schaeffer, & Brown, 1998; James & Glaze, 2006; Primm, Osher, & Gomez, 2005; Trestman, Ford, Zhang, & Wiesbrock, 2007; Young & Reviere, 2001). Related to serious mental illness, HIV infection is highest among prisoners with mental disorders (Baillargeon et al., 2003; Rosen et al., 2009). All these issues present problems for African Americans' reentry into their communities after serving time in prisons and jails.

Hoping to ascertain factors associated with successful reentry, Visher et al. (2004) conducted a longitudinal study of reentry in four states, which was replicated somewhat several years later in Texas and reentry there (Shollenberger, 2009). An earlier phase of Visher et al.'s study involved prisoners returning to Baltimore, Maryland. The Baltimore sample consisted of 83% African Americans, 8% Whites, 3% Latinos, and the remaining sample was other minorities. Among the key findings and policy implications were (1) families and intimate partners are a critical foundation for successful prisoners' reentry. They provide housing, emotional support, financial resources, and overall stability. (2) Released prisoners who found employment were able to secure employment due to personal connections such as family, friends, and former employers; (3) released prisoners who found jobs were more likely to have participated in prison work-release programs than released prisoners who had not found jobs; (4) younger prisoners with family members with substance abuse problems and friends who sold drugs were more likely to use drugs upon release into the community; (5) released prisoners who participated in drug treatment while incarcerated were less likely to use drugs in the community; (6) about one-third of prisoners were rearrested within 6 months and these prisoners tended to be younger, had a more extensive criminal history, and were more likely to use drugs prior to incarceration; (7) released prisoners reported physical and mental health problems more than the general public; (8) most released prisoners were optimistic about their futures. As a result, Visher et al. recommended strengthening the ties between prisoners and their families, friends, and intimate partners; Visher et al.'s findings about the importance of family and friends support what Alexander (2001) wrote, who served almost 8 years in prison and had the unqualified support of family and friends upon his release.

Visher et al. elaborated upon released prisoners' mental health issues. According to them:

In terms of mental health treatment, exactly half of all respondents indicated a desire for help obtaining counseling following their release from prison, and 30% wanted help acquiring mental health treatment. Less than 10% of the respondents interviewed after release believed they suffered from mental illness, although about one-quarter of respondents reported experiencing serious anxiety and depression. About one in five respondents reported experiencing symptoms associated with post-traumatic stress disorder (PTSD) in the 1–3 months after their release, including feeling upset when reminded of prison, avoiding thinking or talking about prison and having repeated, disturbing memories, thoughts, or images of prison (2004, p. 11).

In sum, African American males are disproportionately represented in the criminal justice system. Therefore, they are disproportionately affected by the problems associated with being incarcerated. This is exacerbated by the fact that even upon release, African American males are further isolated and marginalized due to stigma and civic alienation associated with being an ex-offender. As a result, African American males face significant barriers in their attempts to successfully negotiate reentering their home communities after a period of confinement. The remainder of this chapter is dedicated to a discussion of how incarceration and reentry can contribute to increased levels of anxiety among African American males, a potential treatment model that may be employed to utilize ex-offenders' individual and environmental strengths to address the anxiety brought on by facing the challenges associated with reentry, the implications of developing and incorporating culturally sensitive, strength-based treatment models into mainstream reentry services and program, and recommendations for practitioners working with African American males with a history of incarceration.

Incarceration, Reentry, and Anxiety

It has been well established that contact with the juvenile and criminal justice systems is associated with many deleterious social and economic outcomes that severely truncate ex-offenders' attempts to successfully reenter their home communities. For African American males, contact with the criminal justice system has been associated with future criminal behavior (Sampson & Laub, 1990), decreased income (Kerley, Benson, Lee, & Cullen, 2004; Western, 2002), labor market instability (Clayton & Moore, 2003; Lewis, Garfinkel, & Qin, 2007; Roy & Dyson, 2005; Tonry & Petersilia, 1999), family disruption (Arditti, Smock, & Parkman, 2005; Day, Acock, Bahr, & Arditti, 2005; Hairston, 1989, 1995), and a reduced likelihood of marriage (Huebner, 2007). Perhaps, most damaging is the negative influence of past incarceration on the ex-offenders' mental health (London & Myers, 2006). In addition to dealing with the depression associated with feelings of loss, grief, and hopelessness while incarcerated (Domalanta, Risser, Roberts, & Hisser, 2003; Gaylord-Harden, Ragsdale, Mandara, Richards, & Petersen, 2007), African American male ex-offenders must also cope with anxiety that is often related to their impending release. Research has found that recently released or soon to be released ex-offenders have significant concerns with regard to matters as practical as whether or not they will be able to secure housing (Rhine, Matthews, Sampson, & Daley, 2003) to more complex issues such as if and how they will be able to reestablish connections with their families (Nurse, 2002; Tripp, 2001).

Community Reentry

Social service providers, community practitioners, and faith-based organizations have acknowledged these concerns and are attempting to help ex-offenders make the transition back into the community as smooth as possible through reentry programs. In recent years, policymakers have begun to understand the important role that reentry programs play in helping ex-offenders make successful transitions from institutionalization to positive contributor to society (Rhine et al., 2003). In doing so, these programs and services attempt to address the ex-offenders' employment, education, familial, mental health, substance abuse, housing, social, and spiritual concerns (Rhine et al.). A number of researchers have found that when ex-offenders are involved with reentry programs prior to their release or shortly thereafter, there are oftentimes positive economic and social outcomes (King, 1999; Travis, 2007). In addition to providing direct services, another benefit that ex-offenders receive from participating in reentry programs is through the connection to informal networks of social capital that can promote economic and social well-being. Unfortunately, there are barriers to reentry programs that keep some ex-offenders from reaping the full extent of the programs' benefits. In particular, maintaining negative peer relationships, living in an unstable home environment, and returning to an economically disadvantaged neighborhood have all been shown to thwart the positive impact of reentry programs (Caldwell, Sturges, & Silver, 2007; Kubrin & Stewart, 2006). Although these structural and contextual barriers can be powerful forms of adversity, perhaps no barrier looms as large for ex-offenders making the transition back into the community as the pressure, fear, and overall anxiety that accompanies the perception or reality that they will not be able to "make it" on the outside (McGarrell, Hipple, & Banks, 2003).

Therapeutic Intervention

Reintegration and readjustment into society after serving a prison sentence can be a source of anxiety for many former inmates and their families as well. Anxiety is a feeling brought on by stressful events which are a result of psychological, economic, social, and physical occurrences (World Health Organization, 2001). Oftentimes, families are destroyed by the direct or indirect actions of former inmates. This highlights the need for healing to take place in order to repair the tear in the fabric of their lives. There are a number of treatments which can be used to manage this experience, but psychotherapy or talk treatments are the most useful (WHO, 2001). Family therapy is an approach that treats the family unit, not the individual or an individual problem. The primary focus of this intervention is *what* is happening not *why* it is happening (Becvar & Becvar, 2003). Therefore, in order to treat an ex-offender for anxiety we need to treat the family unit as a whole and not focus on the illness. This is important with regard to reentry in that ex-offenders are not released in a vacuum. Rather, they are released back into their home communities where they will need access to a system of social, emotional, and oftentimes financial support to successfully reenter the community. For many ex-offenders, the immediate, extended, and fictive kin networks play a prominent role in their ability to provide much needed support.

Afrocentric Perspective

The authors propose an Afrocentric approach to family therapy as a therapeutic model for dealing with families that have an ex-offender who suffers from anxiety and is seeking to reunite with his/her family and society. The Afrocentric movement in therapy has been around since the 1960s and was developed by Molefi Kete Asante (Moore, Madsen-Coleman, & Moore, 2003). Central to the Afrocentric movement are the notions of togetherness and a sense of community coupled with making a stand against all systems that ignore the African worldview and deny the African achievement (Asante, 2007). Asante (1980) contends that all cultures have a history and a focal point from which they develop as a people, based on their historical origins and future prospects, and African Americans are no different. Afrocentricity, according to Mazama (2003), postulates that the main problem African Americans encounter is their readiness to adopt the Western worldview and subscribe to mainstream perspectives and conceptual frameworks.

The Afrocentric movement distinguishes itself from mainstream psychotherapy by incorporating African principles of wellness (Asante, 1980; Boyd-Franklin, 2003). The therapist must realize that coming to therapy is a new experience for many people but particularly for African Americans, and historically therapists have been accused of prying into family business (Boyd-Franklin, 2003). If this experience is to be successful, the therapist must understand the historical plight of African Americans in general, and males in particular.

Family Structure

We live in a class-stratified multifaceted society and individuals and families are impacted by this dynamic. The therapist must be able to understand how the family makes sense of the construct of social class. Moreover, the therapist must be able to recognize how family members' lives are influenced by changing class structures, because the family is seen as one system that exists as a subset of a larger system. Likewise, in order to effectively treat the African American family, the therapist must explore his/her own perception of class, family, family values, and the roles that each family member plays as well. Typically, the family structure varies with African American families which are oftentimes headed by the mother or grandmother. In addition, there is a relationship with *fictive kin* that has to be considered in the family context. Fictive kin are people who participate and play an important role within the family such as neighbors, play mother [a term of endearment given to a woman who is treated the same as a biological mother] (Hall, 2008), family friends, and church members who are intimately involved in significant life events and are usually given the title of aunt or uncle. Moreover, there are people who are highly respected by the family – this may include ministers, coaches, teachers, friends, social service workers, and others who take an interest in the wellbeing of the family. These relationships deemed fictive kin may be a part of all families, but they are crucial in the African American family and must be considered as part of the therapeutic process and the therapist should invite them into the session. According to McCollum (1997):

> The strength of the *African* American family is tied to the ways in which its members perform, based on the needs within the family itself. In accordance with these needs, the family develops its own personality, which revolves around several aspects of socialization including family communication, role development, and family structure (p. 219).

The family unit has a personality that is unique in that it is developed by amalgamating the individual perspectives and contextual nuances of each of the members.

Joining

The therapist must harness all of these concepts in order to facilitate change within the family. According to Minuchin (1974) the therapist must *join* the family, which is establishing rapport with members of the family if he/she is going to be accepted by the family unit. Communication is paramount and *African Americans* and their White counterparts tend to assign dissimilar meanings to verbal and nonverbal behaviors. Therefore, if the therapist is not African American, he/she must first understand how African Americans communicate, verbally and nonverbally (Kochman, 1983).

Familial Subsystems

The structural approach to family therapy has been selected as a viable therapeutic approach for dealing with African Americans largely because this approach was originally developed for use with

African American families. Structural family therapy has been primarily attributed to Salvador Minuchin; however, Harry Aponte, Charles Fishman, Steven Greenstein, Jay Haley, Braulio Montalvo, Bernice Rosman, and Marianne Walters contributed to its development as well. Structural family therapy has three basic key constructs: structure, subsystem, and boundary. The structure of the family consists of patterns of interaction which help to organize the family system. There are three subsystems – the spousal, the parental, and the sibling (Becvar & Becvar, 2003).

In the African American family, these subsystems oftentimes are arranged in a nontraditional format. The parental subsystem may include mother, grandmother, aunt, uncle, and fictive kin. The African Proverb "it takes a village to raise a child" is central to how African Americans have functioned historically. Therefore, the parental subsystem takes on new members and the therapist must accept this configuration. In addition, the spousal subsystem may include a biological parent in a relationship with someone else. One method a therapist may use to assess the family and explore its makeup is with a cultural, spiritual genogram which is a multigenerational map of family members' religious and spiritual affiliations, events, and conflicts (Frame, 2000; Moore et al., 2003).

The African American Church

The church is a crucial entity in the lives of many African Americans and has been documented in numerous scholarly works (Chatters & Taylor, 2005; Marks & Chaney, 2006). According to Barnes (2005), "The Black Church has long been considered a bulwark in the Black community and research supports its religious, economic, sociocultural, and political dimension" (p. 967). According to Chaney (2008) the church provides spiritual, emotional, and material assistance to many African Americans. The phrase "let me pray on it" is a common sentiment in many African American families, and therapists should be aware of the power in this statement.

Throughout history, the African American church has been a significant support network to its members through fellowship and assistance in times of need. These churches are indigenous community resources and they provide a sense of comfort for its members through spiritual and moral guidance (Caldwell, Greene, & Billingsley, 1992; Taylor & Chatters, 1989). The church should be used as an ally to the therapeutic process and generally, the minister is the representative of the church and if possible should be included in the session if deemed important by the family.

Boundaries

Each of these relationships is defined by their boundaries, which are an invisible set of rules that stipulate who participates and to what extent in each family subsystem. In addition, boundaries also exist between the family and subsystems that the family and family members interact with in the larger community (Becvar & Becvar, 2003; Minuchin, 1974). Figure 13.1 illustrates the conceptual normal boundaries continuum.

The optimal position for any family on this continuum would be clear or normal boundaries and according to Boyd-Franklin (2003), most US families fall within this range; however, many African American families typically have enmeshed boundaries. Therapists need to move the family toward a clear or normal range. A clear range is one that there are open lines of communication between family members as well as between the family and the community at large. Oftentimes boundaries are not clear and must be defined and generally after one or two sessions, the therapist knows where the boundaries lie on the continuum. Enmeshed boundaries occur when there is no privacy and everyone knows everything about everyone in the family. Family support is readily available and

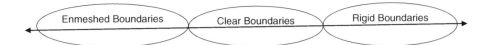

Fig. 13.1 Boundary relationships continuum

given even when it is unwanted. Rigid boundaries are the extreme opposite of enmeshed boundaries and arise when family members are disengaged from one another and also isolated from the community that surrounds the family and can be considered very dysfunctional (Becvar & Becvar, 2003; Minuchin, 1974).

Engagement

Once the therapist has joined the family, assumed a leadership role, defined the boundaries and understands the family structure, healing can begin. The therapist must understand the family structure because this will inform the therapist of who is held in high esteem in the family and thus determines which family member's opinion is sought first. Once opinions are stated, the therapist must reframe and transform the opinion to reflect the overall goal of the therapeutic process. For instance, the mother states, "I would like to see Joe get his lazy butt out of bed, get a job, and stop hanging around on the corner with those good for nothing thugs." The therapist may reframe this request by saying, "…so Mom, what you want is for Joe to get a job and choose his friends more wisely." The therapist has to reframe constantly if varying points of views are to be heard and discussed. The ex-offender is also asked what he wants from the family and together a common goal related to the ex-offender's successful re-integration into the family and community is forged. In addition, the therapist must realign boundaries, help family members to change the way in which they relate to one another, and help members who are disengaged from the family to increase the frequency of their contact (Becvar & Becvar, 2003). The process works if the therapist supports, respects, and understands the family members. The therapist must make challenges to each and every one of the family members to improve their relationships within the family unit. The challenges can be paradoxical in nature. For example, the therapist may suggest to the family that they may not be strong enough at this time to overcome the problem and perhaps they should wait, or work on smaller, less important issues. This paradoxical challenge may spark a sense of family pride, and dominant family members may rise to the challenge and thus help them to evolve the current family structure, one that moves the family closer to a place of healing. Madsen (1999) states:

> Therapy proceeds better when both microcultures (helper and family) are on the same wavelength (i.e., hold similar beliefs about what the problem is, what should be done about it, and who should do what when addressing the problem or are aware and respectful of differences in those beliefs) (p. 97).

Moreover, the therapeutic plan must have an accountability measure where the family members and the therapist are held accountable for the actions each agree to do (Madsen, 1999). This coupled with the family's commitment to change should yield positive results. Remember, a successful family is one that can make adaptive changes to its structure when adverse consequences occur within the family unit as well as when negative outside influences, such as involvement with the criminal justice system and the marginalization that accompanies having a criminal history, bear down on the family.

Estimates with Other Populations

While there is only scant literature on efforts to facilitate the successful reentry of African American males and most of it addresses adults, reentry can also be a daunting task for other population segments within the African American community. Thus, more attention should be paid to the challenges faced by adolescent African American males and African American males entering into late adulthood. These two distinct stages in the life course bring with them unique circumstances and concerns that must be considered, addressed, and incorporated into reentry efforts targeting these specific population segments. The following section provides a brief overview of the ways in which African American males' current position in the life course may influence their reentry-related anxiety and important considerations for practitioners working with these populations.

Life Course Considerations

Consistent with the approach of understanding the structural and contextual influences on African American males' attempts to successfully reenter their communities after a period of confinement and the anxiety that often accompanies it, the males' position in the life course and level of psychosocial development must be considered. The life course has been defined as "pathways through the age differentiated lifespan where age differentiation is manifested in expectations and options that impinge on decision processes and the course of events that give shape to life stages, transitions, and turning points" (Elder, 1985, p. 7). Salient to the life course perspective are the concepts of trajectories and transitions. Trajectories represent one's line of development over the life span (e.g., work, parenting) and transitions are the specific life events (e.g., arrest, incarceration) that occur and heavily influence his or her trajectory. While the life course perspective provides a broad or panoramic view of a person's development over time, psychosocial theory provides a lens through which various stages of the life course may be examined in detail. With its emphasis on age-specific benchmarks of social and psychological development, psychosocial theory provides clear criteria for assessing African American males' successful matriculation through the life span. Specifically, the organizing concepts of psychosocial theory are the developmental tasks (skills that contribute to one mastering his environment), psychosocial crisis (psychological efforts to adjust to the demands of one's social environment), and central process (the mechanism through which the psychosocial crisis is resolved) of each stage of development (Newman & Newman, 1999).

African American Males in Early Adolescence

Research has established that like adults, adolescent African American males are at an increased risk for contact with the criminal justice system (Roberts, 2004). Reasons for this increased risk include, but are not limited to, economic disadvantages (Kubrin & Stewart, 2006; Wilson, 1987) and the impact of early exposure to the criminal justice system that results from the mass incarceration of adult African American males (Clayton & Moore, 2003). In fact, many researchers argue that in some communities, so many adult African American males are currently or have been incarcerated that younger males begin to perceive incarceration as an inevitable rite of passage (Roberts). Therefore, recidivism prevention is a priority in the development of effective reentry programs for adolescent African American males and is also crucial to the progression of the communities where these young men return after being incarcerated. In addition to infusing Afrocentric perspective into family therapy approaches, practitioners working with adolescent African American males in reentry programs should also consider the specific developmental challenges characteristic of this stage in the life course.

Consistent with psychosocial theory, adolescence is a period of time that encompasses ages 12–18 and is accompanied by growth and development in physical maturation, emotional development, sexual relationships, and peer group membership. Further, the psychosocial crisis is group identity, allying oneself with a group that provides a sense of belonging versus alienation, an absence of social support or meaningful connections to others (Newman & Newman, 1999). Combining Afrocentric perspective with family therapy is a conceptually appropriate treatment approach for African American males at this stage in the life course because of the emphasis on working with the family as a collective unit and the rejection of strict adherence to mainstream norms and values. In an attempt to resolve the psychosocial crisis of their stage of development and achieve a sense of belonging with members of the peer group, many adolescent African American males fall victim to negative influences (e.g., gangs and individuals involved in criminal activity). These adolescents are also bombarded with numerous reports from media, popular culture, and local authorities that devalue African American males and stereotype them as nonproductive members of society (Smith, Allen, & Danley, 2007). Through the rejection of the degrading portrayals and placing an emphasis on ethnic socialization, Afrocentric perspective works to instill a sense of pride in young African American males about who they are and what they can become. Ethnic socialization has also been found to serve as a protective factor against anxiety among adolescent African Americans (Gaylord-Harden et al., 2007). Moreover, in the context of family therapy, working collaboratively with the family unit and fostering a sense of familial togetherness is likely to promote positive peer group membership choices.

African American Males in Late Adulthood

While the literature on reentry for adolescents tends to focus on reducing recidivism, this is less of a concern with African American male ex-offenders in late adulthood because crime declines with age (Sampson & Laub, 2003) and only a small proportion of the prison population can be categorized as life course persistent (Moffitt, 1993). Continued criminal activity is especially unlikely when the ex-offender has strong familial and labor market ties (Sampson & Laub, 1990). Despite these facts, very little is known about reentry among African American males in late adulthood. This is surprising, considering that African American males are more likely than other groups to be faced with reentry related anxiety during late adulthood because they continue to receive disproportionately long prison sentences (Coker, 2003; Shelden, 2004; Tonry & Melewski, 2008).

Similarly to working with adolescents, practitioners working in reentry programs should consider how to best blend Afrocentric perspective, family therapy, and psychosocial theory to address the unique developmental concerns of African American males in late adulthood. Late adulthood ranges from 60 to 75 years of age and is characterized by developmental tasks such as redirecting energy to new roles, accepting one's life, and developing a point of view about death. At this stage of the life course, the psychosocial crisis is integrity, being content with the results of one's life versus despair, the realization that one's most cherished hopes and dreams cannot and will not be accomplished within one's lifetime (Newman & Newman, 1999). As with adolescents, taking an Afrocentric approach to family therapy is also conceptually appropriate with African American males in late adulthood. Central to the conceptual fit of Afrocentric family therapy approaches with African American males in late adulthood is the importance of working with family unit, which consists of blood and marital relatives, as well as fictive kin. While with adolescents, working with the family unit serves the purpose of providing a source of ethnic socialization and a buffer against negative peer group affiliations, for males in late adulthood, the family unit offers a mechanism through which men can find value and meaning in their lives. In many African American families, the elder members are often held in high esteem for the knowledge, experience, and wisdom that they possess and impart upon younger members of the family unit (Taylor, 2002). With regard to the psychosocial crisis, integrity may be achieved as males in late adulthood come to understand that although their ability to achieve many of their individual goals was truncated by their period of confinement, they can take solace in knowing that they are functioning and contributing members of the family. Thus, utilizing the communal orientation of an Afrocentric family therapy approach, males in this population segment can look introspectively and be content with the totality of their lives as opposed to being preoccupied with despair based on the "what ifs" of their past.

In a general sense, the reentry needs of adolescent African American males differ from those of African American males in late adulthood. Because they are at different points in the life course, their reentry-related anxiety stems from very distinct antecedents. Focusing on the future, adolescent African American male ex-offenders are concerned with whether or not they are going to "make it" in terms of being a productive member of society who will be able to make meaningful contributions to his family and community (McGarrell et al., 2003). On the other hand, African American male ex-offenders in late adulthood are often oriented toward the past with concerns over whether or not they have "made it" in terms of accomplishing their goals, significantly contributing to the upcoming generation's development, and overall, being content with the results of their lives.

Implications

Implications for the Health of African American Males

The physical and mental health and well-being of an individual is perhaps his or her most important and valuable asset. Ashford, LeCroy, and Lortie (2006) define well-being as "a person's emotional and psychological capacity to cope with demands across time, circumstance, and setting" (p. 530). The physical, spiritual, and social healths of the person are also included in this concept. A number of factors affect a person's well-being among which includes anxiety producing life circumstances such as imprisonment. As has been earlier discussed in this chapter, many African American males have been subjected to a plethora of negative experiences as a result of their often traumatic involvement with the criminal justice system. These experiences include police harassment and brutality, arrest, financial burdens as a result of legal fees, overt hostility, and discrimination by unfair judicial officials, and having to overcome further marginalization and civic alienation upon release. In part, as a result of inherent racism within the US society and not having the economic resources to obtain proper legal representation, numerous African American males find themselves incarcerated.

To say that prisons are dangerous and nefarious places is an understatement. While incarcerated they are likely to have experienced the violence and victimization that are intrinsic in the despotic nature of these institutions. For instance, they have been isolated from intimate contact with family, friends, and their community, subjected to or witnessed criminal acts of violence (such as rape and murder) by other inmates and may have endured beating by some prison officials (Wolff et al., 2007). Coupled with pre-incarceration variables such as possibly having a history of being physically and sexually abused as children, substance abuse and other deleterious health issues, poor education and work histories which, because they do not have the necessary credentials to compete in the legitimate employment sector, limit their employment opportunities and their ability to provide for themselves and their families upon release, once released many African American men reenter society with feelings of overwhelm, poor self-esteem, disempowerment, devaluation, and with a range of mental health issues including anxiety (Oliver & Hairston, 2008; Rich, 2001).

Implications for the Health of African American Families

Reentering the lives of family members and reestablishing the relationship with his spouse or girl-friend and children can be a daunting task for a former inmate. Family dynamics change drastically when a man is incarcerated. Upon his incarceration, his family immediately suffers from the loss of "the good provider role" (Miller, Browning, & Spruance, 2001, p. 4). They bear the burden of the loss of his income. This may in turn have a direct affect on his family's ability to maintain their place of residence, provide for the education of his children, and have the necessary income for activities of daily living. As a result of this loss, in an effort to maintain family stability, his wife or girlfriend often assumes the breadwinner responsibility and becomes the sole financial supporter for the family. That his female counterpart is now the family provider has serious implications for the economic stability of the family because African American female headed households with children are 2.4 times more likely to be impoverished than their White counterparts (Snyder, McLaughlin, & Findeis, 2006).

Hence, finding employment and living accommodations are two major tasks facing him upon release. These assignments are compounded by his likelihood of experiencing job discrimination by potential employers who may be unforgiving of his criminal record and by mates who have become economically independent, self-sufficient and assertive (Boyd, 2007). Perhaps she has furthered her education, gotten a new and better job or moved to a new area. Her assertiveness and independence coupled with their lost opportunity for intimacy, which affects the couples level of closeness, some-times creates conflict, such as domestic violence, within their relationship. Additionally, she may have replaced him with someone new. All of these factors together or any one alone can lead to the dissolution of the couple's relationship (Miller et al., 2001; Oliver & Hairston, 2008).

Over 1.5 million American children have an incarcerated parent (Miller et al., 2001). Once free, establishing a relationship with his children can be equally as difficult as establishing a relationship with his wife or girlfriend. While imprisoned, the relationship between the inmate and his children was affected by a number of factors that include (1) the quality of the relationship that he had with the children's mother, (2) the frequency of visits that he and his children had, and (3) the social and emo-tional consequences experienced by his offspring as a result of his incarceration. If the relationship with his children's mother deteriorated while he was imprisoned, so likely would the relationship between him and his children, if they are minors and were dependent upon her to bring them for visitation. Perhaps their visits decreased due to the financial hardship of visitation particularly if he was incarcer-ated out of their state of residence or in state at a distance from them. If she is angry with him for her feelings of desertion and loneliness, she may speak unfavorably about him to their children which can affect their feelings toward him. Often children bear the stigma, shame, and guilt of his being involved with the criminal justice system, internalize those feeling and subsequently externalize them in a num-ber of negative behavioral ways, one of which may be to distance themselves from him.

Sometimes the parents and other family members of the incarcerated man assumed the financial burden of obtaining his lawyer and paying other fees involved in his case. They, too, may be angry at him for having been incarcerated and the financial strain that this caused them; therefore, may be unwilling to have close association with him once he returns to the community. Restoration of fam-ily relationships, although sometimes difficult, is not necessarily impossible. This will be a key and primary initial goal of family therapy.

Implications for the Health of the African American Community

The health of African American males is crucial because their overall health is tied to their ability to be viable husbands, fathers, financial and emotional supporter of their family; equally important community role models, leaders, and mentors. There are 840,000 African American males behind bars who represent almost half of the two million people who are in US custody (Boyd, 2007). Once removed from citizenry and the day-to-day activity of his environment, the African American community looses political power via the absence of his vote. This has implications for policy development and implementation. While incarcerated his voice in the polity of his community through the power of his vote is absent. It is not uncommon for entities that operate outside of the community to assume that they know what is best for African American people and to then develop programs that they deem viable for the community (Connerly, 2002). As part of his reentry into society it becomes imperative for him to explore voter registration restoration. His input into the political activity of the community may have a direct impact on programs that may be well thought out and planned by others but may not be viewed by members of the African American community as being in their best interest.

The need for positive African American male role models is great and his role modeling cannot be underscored. In fact, he is a role model to other African American males whether or not he intends it. There are those who silently and without his knowledge watch his actions, listen to his conversation and are influenced by both. He can make constructive use of self, for instance, through volunteer activities at youth activities and by participating in church and other community forums where he can share his experience with the law in an effort to deter other males from becoming involved with the legal system. There are also innumerable mentoring opportunities within the African American community. "Strong," trusting relations with mentees facilitate the use of "solution-focused measures" designed to "change problem behavior by teaching life skills, promoting active learning, personal responsibility and self-discipline and encouraging independence" (Marbley, 2006; Odih, 2002, p. 4). Under his mentorship others may see that positive life changes are possible and can be inspired to achieve dreams and goals. He may also have valuable hidden abilities such as technological, math or writing skills that can be utilized in mentoring programs. Although he was once incarcerated, his life is far from over and his potential contributions to the African American community and at-large society should never be underestimated.

Implications for Human Service Professionals

African American males are often reluctant to participate in mental health and counseling services. More than White men, they are likely to be involuntarily committed to psychiatric institutions and present themselves at later stages of disease processes (Dhooper & Moore, 2000; Thorn & Sarata, 1998). Several explanations have been given to clarify this. One is that most American counselors have been trained using Eurocentric grounded practice approaches that are "person-centered." This therapeutic method stresses independence from family and individualism both of which are opposite of the Afrocentric tradition (Asante, 1980; Okonji, Ososkie, & Pulos, 1996). Secondly, historically African Americans have not been welcomed or viewed favorably by social scientists and members of the counseling professions. They have often been labeled as unmotivated for treatment, disengaged, dangerous, and unconcerned about their health (Gary & Leashore, 1982; Johnson, 2006; Rosenthal, 2004). To this end, the degree of counselor cultural sensitivity to this population has implications for mental health service utilization by African American males.

Counselors who are culturally competent, meaning that they are familiar with and knowledgeable of African American culture and are skilled in basic counseling skills and attending behaviors are more likely to be successful with African American male clients (Dhooper & Moore, 2000; Fuertes, Mueller, & Chauhan, 2002; Kendrick, Moore, Thomas, Matlock, & Flaskerud, 2009; Plowden, John, Vasquez, & Kimani, 2006). Thirdly, it has been found that the rate of client termination of services is higher among African American clients who are highly mistrustful when the therapist is White versus when the therapist is also African American. The White counselor may be viewed as an extension or representation of the racist and oppressive system that so impacts their everyday lives. Additionally, African American clients tend to gravitate to same race therapists (Okonji et al., 1996).

The following are recommendations for encouraging African American males who have been released from prison to seek treatment when mental health and family therapy services are warranted:

1. *Counselors must become culturally competent* – The USA is an amalgamation of a plethora of ethnicities. The U.S. Census Bureau identified 6,133,326 persons who indicated that their racial composition consisted of two or more races. Of those individuals, 4.0% were African Americans (U.S. Census Bureau, 2008). African Americans are not now nor have ever been a homogenous group, as they are often spoken of, but represent and demonstrate a wide range of diversity. For instance, often when referenced, "the African American church" is described as if it were a singular institution. However, the African American church represents seven major denominations and a host of minor denominations between and among which are differences in religious practices and theology (Lincoln & Mamiya, 1990).

    Before a therapist can offer effective counseling to African American males he/she must be skilled at providing culturally competent service. Becoming a culturally competent service provider involves far more than sporadically attending diversity courses, conferences, or seminars. Rather, the authors suggest that developing cultural competence is a life-long process that includes cultural emersion as well as continuous personal and professional development. Albeit, there is no shortage of forums from which helping professional can learn about the richness of African American culture. Inclusive of these are the African American church, HBCUs (historically Black colleges and universities), Black fraternities and sororities, funeral directors, African American libraries, the N.A.A.C.P., and the National Urban League. Demonstrating a genuine understanding and appreciation for African American culture can go a long way toward encouraging African American males to participate in counseling services.

2. *Seek clients from indigenous community places* – Churches, barbershops, laundromats, sports events, and areas such as basketball courts, and sports bars are just a few places where African American men feel safe and welcome. During the process of distributing agency flyers, pamphlets and other African American male focused material (brochures with pictures of African American males on the cover, etc.) through these outlets, helping professionals should make purposeful efforts to build rapport with men who frequent these establishments in an effort to gain trust and communicate good will.

3. *Tailor the treatment approach to the cultural needs of the client* – Once in family therapy, the African American male needs to see himself represented in the literature that is used during treatment, spoken to and about from a strength rather than a pathos perspective, valued and respected as a man, and encouraged to reach his potential for greatness, all tenants of the Afrocentric worldview (Todisco & Salomone, 1991).

Conclusion

As has been discussed, the reentry of African American men into society has far reaching implications. It can be a time for reconnecting with former relationships, strengthening existing ones and creating new interpersonal opportunities. It can be a period of personal development through educational attainment. Instead of being marginalized, in so many ways men can participate in the advancement of the African American community while self-actualizing and fulfilling their divinely created destiny. First, by focusing on becoming and remaining as healthy as they are able so that they will have the strength to be active participants in all that is involved with living. Second, by taking their proper place within the family and doing what they can to ensure its health and thrive ability. Finally, by "giving back" to their community in such a way that their life energy encourages and promotes the positive development of all African Americans throughout the Black Diaspora. Regardless of one's stage in life course, reentry programs represent an opportunity to help African American males successfully reestablish familial and community connections, as well as reduce reentry-related anxiety. Specifically, making use of the communal nature of Afrocentric perspective to guide family therapy approaches offers a culturally responsive alternative to traditional or mainstream approaches. As the literature yields, the propositions consistent with Afrocentricity such as togetherness, participation in one's community, and ethnic socialization can provide a unifying framework from which practitioners can facilitate the successful transition back into the community for adolescent, adult, and elder African American males.

References

Alexander, R., Jr. (2001). *To ascend into the shining world again*. Westerville, OH: Theroe Enterprises.

Arditti, J. A., Smock, S. A., & Parkman, T. S. (2005). "Its been hard to be a father": A qualitative exploration of incarcerated fatherhood. *Fathering, 3*, 267–288.

Asante, M. K. (2007). *An afrocentric manifesto*. Malden, MA: Polity.

Asante, M. K. (1980). *Afrocentricity*. Buffalo, NY: Amulefi.

Ashford, J., LeCroy, C. W., & Lortie, K. L. (2006). *Human behavior in the social environment: Multidimensional perspective* (3rd ed.). Belmont, CA: Thompson.

Baillargeon, J., Ducate, S., Pulvino, J., Bradshaw, P., Murray, O., & Olvera, R. (2003). The association of psychiatric disorders and HIV infection in the correctional setting. *Annals of Epidemiology, 13*(9), 606–612.

Barnes, S. L. (2005). The church culture and community action. *Social Forces, 84*(2), 967–994.

Becvar, D. S., & Becvar, R. (2003). *Family therapy: A systemic integration* (5th ed.). Boston: Allyn and Bacon.

Black, D. W., Gunter, T., Allen, J., Blum, N., Arndt, S., Wenman, G., et al. (2007). Borderline personality disorder in male and female offenders newly committed to prison. *Comprehensive Psychiatry, 48*(5), 400–405.

Boyd-Franklin, N. (2003). *Black families in therapy* (2nd ed.). New York: Guilford.

Boyd, H. (2007). It's hard out here for a black man! *The Black Scholar, 37*(3), 2–9.

Bushway, S., Stoll, M. A., & Weiman, D. F. (2007). Introduction. In S. Bushway, M. A. Stoll, & D. F. Weiman (Eds.), *Barriers to reentry: The labor market for released prisoners in post industrial America* (pp. 1–25). New York: Russell Sage.

Caldwell, C. H., Greene, A. D., & Billingsley, A. (1992). The Black church as a family support system: Instrumental and expressive functions. *National Journal of Sociology, 6*, 21–40.

Caldwell, R. M., Sturges, S. M., & Silver, N. C. (2007). Home versus school environments and their influences on the affective and behavioral states of African American, Hispanic, and Caucasian juvenile offenders. *Journal of Child and Family Studies, 16*, 119–132.

Chaney, C. (2008). The benefit of church involvement for African Americans. *Journal of Religion and Society, 10*, 1–23.

Chatters, L. M., & Taylor, R. J. (2005). Religion and families. In V. Bengtson, A. Acock, K. Allen, P. Dillworth-Anderson, & D. Klein (Eds.), *Sourcebook of family theory and research* (pp. 517–522). Thousand Oaks, CA: Sage.

Clayton, D., & Moore, J. (2003). The effects of crime and imprisonment on family formation (pp. 84–102). In O. Clayton, R. Mincy, & D. Blankenhorn (Eds.), *Black fathers in contemporary society: Strengths, weaknesses, and strategies for change*. New York: Russell Sage.

Coker, D. (2003). Supreme Court review: Addressing the real world of racial injustice in the criminal justice system. *The Journal of Criminal Law and Criminology, 93*(4), 827–879.

Connerly, C. E. (2002). From racial zoning to community empowerment: The interstate highway system and the African American community in Birmingham, Alabama. *Journal of Planning Education & Research, 22*(2), 99–114.

Day, R. D., Acock, A. C., Bahr, S. J., & Arditti, J. A. (2005). Incarcerated fathers returning home to children and families: Introduction to the special issue and a primer on doing research with men in prison. *Fathering, 3*, 183–200.

Dhooper, S. S., & Moore, S. E. (2000). *Social work practice with culturally diverse people*. Thousand Oaks, CA: Sage.

Domalanta, D., Risser, W. L., Roberts, R. E., & Hisser, J. M. (2003). Prevalence of depression and other psychiatric disorders among incarcerated youths. *Journal of the American Academy of Child and Adolescent Psychiatry, 42,* 477–484.

Dumond, R. W. (2000). Inmate sexual assault: The plague that persists. *Prison Journal, 80*(4), 407–414.

Elder, G. H. (1985). Perspectives on the life course. In G. Elder (Ed.), *Life course dynamics* (pp. 23–49). Ithaca, NY: Cornell University Press.

Frame, M. W. (2000). The spiritual genogram in family therapy. *Journal of Marital and Family Therapy, 26*(2), 211–216.

Fuertes, J. N., Mueller, L. N., & Chauhan, R. V. (2002). An Investigation of European American Therapists' Approach to Counseling African American Clients. *Counseling Psychologist, 30*(5), 763–788.

Gary, L. E., & Leashore, B. R. (1982). High-risk status of black men. *Social Work, 27*(1), 54–58.

Gaylord-Harden, N. K., Ragsdale, B. L., Mandara, J., Richards, M. H., & Petersen, A. C. (2007). Perceived support and internalizing symptoms in African American adolescents: Self esteem and ethnic identity as mediators. *Journal of Youth & Adolescence, 36,* 77–88.

Hairston, C. F. (1995). Fathers in prison. In K. Gabel & D. Johnston (Eds.), *Children of incarcerated parents* (pp. 31–40). New York: Lexington Books.

Hairston, C. F. (1989). Men in prison: Family characteristics and parenting views. *Journal of Offender Counseling, Services, and Rehabilitation, 14,* 23–30.

Hall, C. (2008). The impact of kin and fictive kin relationships on the mental health of Black adult children of alcoholics. *Health & Social Work, 33*(4), 259–266.

Hartwell, S. (2003a). Prison, hospital or community: Community re-entry and mentally ill offenders. *Research in Community and Mental Health, 12,* 199–220.

Hartwell, S. (2003b). Short-term outcomes for offenders with mental illness released from incarceration. *International Journal of Offender Therapy and Comparative Criminology, 47*(2), 145–158.

Henderson, D., Schaeffer, J., & Brown, L. (1998). Gender-appropriate mental health services for incarcerated women: Issues and challenges. *Family & Community Health, 21*(3), 42–53.

Huebner, B. M. (2007). Racial and ethnic differences in the likelihood of marriage: The effect of incarceration. *Justice Quarterly, 24,* 156–183.

James, D. J., & Glaze, L. E. (2006). *Mental health problems of prison and jail inmates.* Washington, DC: Bureau of Justice Statistics.

Johnson, P. D. (2006). Counseling African American men: A contextualized humanistic perspective. *Counseling and Values, 50,* 187–196.

Kendrick, L., Moore, B., Thomas, C., Matlock, J., & Flaskerud, J. H. (2009). African American men and mental health: Is the climate changing? *Issues in Mental Health Nursing, 30*(9), 587–588.

Kerley, K. R., Benson, M. L., Lee, M. R., & Cullen, F. T. (2004). Race, criminal justice contact, and adult position in the social stratification system. *Social Problems, 51,* 549–568.

King, A. (1999). Working with incarcerated African American males and their families. In L. Davis (Ed.), *Working with African American males* (pp. 219–228). Thousand Oaks, CA: Sage.

Kochman, T. (1983). *Black and White cultural styles in conflict.* Urbana: University of Illinois Press.

Kubrin, C. E., & Stewart, E. A. (2006). Predicting who reoffends: The neglected role of neighborhood context in recidivism studies. *Criminology, 44,* 165–197.

Lewis, C. E., Garfinkel, I., & Qin, G. (2007). Incarceration and unwed fathers in fragile families. *Journal of Sociology and Social Welfare, 34,* 77–94.

Lincoln, C. E., & Mamiya, L. H. (1990). *The Black church in the African American experience.* Durham, NC: Duke University Press.

London, A. S., & Myers, N. A. (2006). Race, incarceration, and health: A life course perspective. *Research on Aging, 28,* 409–422.

Madsen, W. C. (1999). *Collaborative therapy with multi-stressed families: From old problems to new futures.* New York: Guilford.

Marbley, A. (2006). Indigenous Systems – 100 Black Men: Celebrating the empowerment and resiliency in the African American community. *Black History Bulletin, 69*(1), 9–16.

Marks, L. D., & Chaney, C. (2006). Faith communities and African American families: A qualitative look at why the Black church matters. In S. D. Ambrose (Ed.), *Religion and psychology: New research* (pp. 277–294). Hauppauge, NY: Nova Science.

Massoglia, M. A., & Hartmann, D. (2006, November 1). *Race and the impact on midlife mental health: Where whiteness is not a privilege.* Paper presented at the annual meeting of the American Society of Criminology, Los Angeles, CA.

Mazama, A. (Ed.). (2003). *The Afrocentric paradigm.* Trenton, NJ: Africa World Press.

McCollum, V. J. C. (1997). Evolution of the African American family personality: Considerations for family therapy. *Journal of Multicultural Counseling & Development, 25*(3), 219–229.

McGarrell, E. F., Hipple, N., & Banks, D. (2003). *Applying problem solving approaches to issues of inmate reentry: The Indianapolis pilot project*. Indianapolis, IN: Hudson Institute.

Mears, D. P., & Travis, J. (2004). Youth development and reentry. *Youth Violence and Juvenile Justice, 2*(1), 3–20.

Miller, R. R., Browning, S. L., & Spruance, L. M. (2001). An introduction and brief review of the impacts of incarceration on the African American family. *Journal of African American Men, 6*(1), 3–12.

Minuchin, S. (1974). *Families and family therapy*. Cambridge, MA: Harvard University Press.

Moffitt, T. E. (1993). Adolescence-limited and life course persistent anti-social behavior: A developmental taxonomy. *Psychological Review, 100*, 674–701.

Moore, S. E., Madsen-Coleman, O., & Moore, J. L. (2003). An Afrocentric approach to substance abuse treatment with adolescent African American males: Two case examples. *The Western Journal of Black Studies, 27*(4), 219–230.

Newman, B. M., & Newman, P. R. (1999). *Development through life: A psychosocial approach*. Belmont, CA: Wadsworth.

Nurse, A. (2002). *Fatherhood arrested: Parenting from within the juvenile justice system*. Nashville, TN: Vanderbilt University Press.

Odih, P. (2002). Mentors and role models: masculinity and the educational 'underachievement' of young Afro-Caribbean males. *Race Ethnicity and Education, 5*(1), 91–105.

Okonji, J. M., Ososkie, J., & Pulos, S. (1996). Preferred style and ethnicity of counseling by African American males. *Journal of Black Psychology, 22*(3), 329–339.

Oliver, W., & Hairston, C. F. (2008). Intimate partner violence during the transition from prison to the community: Perspectives of incarcerated African American men. *Journal of Aggression, 16*(3), 258–276.

Pager, D. (2003). The mark of a criminal record. *The American Journal of Sociology, 108*(5), 937–975.

Pager, D. (2007). Two strikes and you're out: The intensification of racial and criminal stigma. In S. Bushway, M. A. Stoll, & D. F. Weiman (Eds.), *Barriers to reentry: The labor market for released prisoners in post industrial American* (pp. 151–173). New York: Russell Sage.

Plowden, K. O., John, W., Vasquez, E., & Kimani, J. (2006). Reaching African American men: A qualitative analysis. *Journal of Community Health Nursing, 23*(3), 147–158.

Primm, A. B., Osher, F. C., & Gomez, M. B. (2005). Race and ethnicity, mental health services and cultural competence in the criminal justice system: Are we ready to change? *Community Mental Health Journal, 41*(5), 557–569.

Prison Rape Elimination Act of 2003, Public Law 108–79, 108th Congress.

Rich, J. A. (2001). Primary care for young African American men. *Emerging Issus in College Health Practice, 49*, 183–186.

Rhine, E., Matthews, J. R., Sampson, L. A., & Daley, H. (2003). Citizens circles: Community collaboration in reentry. *Corrections Today, 65*, 52–55.

Roberts, D. (2004). The social and moral cost of mass incarceration in African American communities. *Stanford Law Review, 56*, 1271–1305.

Rosen, D. L., Schoenbach, V. J., Wohl, D. A., White, B. L., Stewart, P. W., & Golin, C. E. (2009). Characteristics and behaviors associated with HIV infection among inmates in the North Carolina prison system. *American Journal of Public Health, 99*(6), 1123–1130.

Rosenthal, D. A. (2004). Effects of client race on clinical judgment of practicing European American vocational rehabilitation counselors. *Rehabilitation Counseling Bulletin, 47*(3), 131–141.

Roy, K. M., & Dyson, O. L. (2005). Gate keeping in context: Baby mama drama and the involvement of incarcerated fathers. *Fathering, 3*, 289–310.

Sampson, R. J., & Laub, J. H. (1990). Crime and deviance over the life course: The salience of adult social bonds. *American Sociological Review, 55*, 609–627.

Sampson, R. J., & Laub, J. H. (2003). Life course desisters? Trajectories of crime among delinquent boys followed to age 70. *Criminology, 41*, 555–592.

Shelden, R. G. (2004). The imprisonment crisis in America. *Review of Policy Research, 21*(1), 5–12.

Shollenberger, T. (2009). *Family and reentry: The impact of incarceration and reentry on family members of returning prisoners in Texas*. Paper presented at the annual meeting of the American Society of Criminology, Atlanta Marriott Marquis, Atlanta, GA. Retrieved May 24, 2009 from http://www.allacademic.com/meta/p201978_index.html

Smith, W. A., Allen, W. R., & Danley, L. (2007). "Assume the position...you fit the description": Psychosocial experiences and racial battle fatigue among African American male college students. *American Behavioral Scientists, 51*, 551–578.

Snyder, A., McLaughlin, D. K., & Findeis, J. (2006). Household composition and poverty among female-headed households with children: Differences by race and residence. *Rural Sociology, 71*(4), 597–624.

Taylor, R. (2002). *Minority families in the United States: A multicultural perspective* (3rd ed.). Upper Saddle River, NJ: Prentice Hall.

Taylor, R. J., & Chatters, L. M. (1989). Family, friend, and church support networks of Black Americans. In R. L. Jones (Ed.), *Black adult development and aging* (pp. 310–320). Berkeley: Cobb and Henry.

Thorn, G. R., & Sarata, B. P. (1998). Psycotherapy with African American men: What we know and what we need to know. *Journal of Mulitcultural Counseling & Development, 26*(4), 240–254.

Todisco, M., & Salomone, P. R. (1991). Facilitating effective cross-cultural relationships: The White counselor and the Black client. *Journal of Multicultural Counseling & Development, 19*(4), 146–157.

Tonry, M., & Petersilia, J. (1999). Prison research at the beginning of the 21st century. In M. Tonry & J. Petersilia (Eds.), *Prisons* (pp. 1–16). Chicago, IL: University of Chicago Press.

Tonry, M., & Melewski, M. (2008). The malign effects of drug and crime control policies on Black Americans. In M. Tonry (Ed.), *Crime and justice: A review of research* (pp. 1–44). Chicago: University of Chicago Press.

Travis, J. (2007). Reflections on the reentry movement. *Federal Sentencing Reporter, 20*, 84–87.

Trestman, R. L., Ford, J., Zhang, W., & Wiesbrock, V. (2007). Current and lifetime psychiatric illness among inmates not identified as acutely mentally ill at intake in Connecticut's jails. *The Journal of the American Academy of Psychiatry and the Law, 35*(4), 490–500.

Tripp, B. (2001). Incarcerated African American fathers: Exploring changes in family relationships and the father identity. *Journal of African American Men, 6*(1), !3–30.

U.S. Census Bureau. (2008). *ACS demographic and housing estimates: 2005–2007* [Data file]. Retrieved from http://factfinder.census.gov/servlet/ADPTable

Visher, C., Kachnowski, V., La Vigne, N. G., & Travis, J. (2004). *Baltimore prisoners' experiences returning home.* Washington, DC: Urban Institute.

Weiman, D. F., Stoll, M. A., & Bushway, S. (2007). The regime of mass incarceration: A labor-market perspective. In S. Bushway, M. A. Stoll, & D. F. Weiman (Eds.), *Barriers to reentry: The labor market for released prisoners in post industrial American* (pp. 29–79). New York: Russell Sage.

Western, B. (2002). The impact of incarceration on wage mobility and inequity. *American Sociological Review, 67*, 526–546.

Wilson, W. J. (1987). *The truly disadvantaged: The inner city, the underclass, and public policy.* Chicago, IL: University of Chicago Press.

Wolff, N., Blitz, C., & Shi, J. (2007). Rates of sexual victimization in prison for inmates with and without mental disorders. *Psychiatric Services, 58*(8), 1087–1094.

World Health Organization. (2001). *Mental health and its problems.* Retrieved August 9, 2009 from http://www.emro.who.int/mnh/whd/PublicInformation-Part6.htm

Young, V. D., & Reviere, R. (2001). Meeting the health care needs of the new woman inmate: A national survey of prison practices. *Journal of Offender Rehabilitation, 34*(2), 31–48.

Chapter 14
Beyond the Myth: Addressing Suicide Among African American Males

Michael A. Robinson, Armon R. Perry, Sharon E. Moore, and Rudolph Alexander Jr.

Introduction

Suicide is the act of killing oneself intentionally. Approximately 30,000 people per year commit suicide in the USA and nearly 500,000 people per year commit suicide worldwide (Joiner, 2005). Although it is rare, suicide ranks as the ninth leading cause of death in the USA, ahead of liver and kidney disease (Maris, Berman, & Silverman, 2000). Despite not being well developed (Joiner), there is general agreement in the suicide literature that in the USA males have a higher suicide mortality than females despite the fact that females are more likely to attempt suicide or be admitted to the hospital as a result of a suicide attempt (Maris et al.). Males experience more fatalities from suicide attempts than females because they are more likely to use lethal methods (e.g., firearms), they are more likely to use impulsive violence, they are more likely to abuse substances, and are less likely to seek help for physical or mental health problems (Cantor, 2000). Among US males, White males are disproportionately represented in suicide mortality, committing more than four times the number of suicides of African American males (Joiner). Researchers have concluded that African American males commit suicide less often than their White counterparts because they are more likely to be religious and receive high levels of social support from friends and family (Joiner; Maris et al.). However, in recent years, there has been a dramatic increase in the number of suicides committed by African American males (Joiner). Since suicide is highly stigmatized, it is often misunderstood as an act of selfish and narcissistic anger (Joiner, 2010). Moreover, the increase in suicide among African American males has not yet received the attention it deserves as a major public health concern. Therefore, the purpose of this chapter is to fill a gap in the literature by advancing the discourse related to suicide by providing an overview of the literature on suicide among African American males, presenting viable intervention and prevention models, as well as discussing their implications for African American males, their families, and their communities.

S.E. Moore (✉)
Raymond A. Kent School of Social Work, University of Louisville, Louisville, KY, USA
e-mail: semoor02@louisville.edu

A.J. Lemelle et al. (eds.), *Handbook of African American Health: Social and Behavioral Interventions*, DOI 10.1007/978-1-4419-9616-9_14, © Springer Science+Business Media, LLC 2011

Literature Review

Suicide by African American males takes many forms. Bell (2007) stated that some Africans committed suicide on the slave ships during slavery and during escape attempts when they were in jail waiting to be returned to cruel plantations. Typically, suicides occur when an African American shoots himself, but other circumstances have occurred leading to death. For example, the 18-year-old son of the former Super Bowl winning coach of the Indianapolis Colts, Tony Dungy, committed suicide by taking drugs (Montgomery & Altman, 2005). A 19-year-old African American commit- ted suicide by taking an overdose of prescription drugs while connected to a chat room (Alston, 2008). Then an 11-year-old African American boy hanged himself due to repeated bullying at school (Plaisance & Johnson, 2009). Also, suicides may occur after an African American male has killed his wife or girlfriend and then takes his life either in remorse or to avoid jail. For example, 47-year-old Marvell Greer killed his girlfriend, 36-year-old Lorine Greer, and then killed himself in Kansas City, Missouri (Chief Corwin's Blog, 2010). One African American male, after getting a poor evaluation during a probationary period and subsequently dismissed, shot two supervisors at work and one died (Decker & Gray, 2010). He subsequently killed himself before the police arrived (Decker & Gray). A rather new form of suicide is called "suicide by cop," which occurs when a man wants to die but does not want to kill himself. So, he does something threatening to get a law enforcement officer to kill him (Hutson et al., 1998; Pinizzotto, Davis, & Miller, 2005).

Despite these examples, professionals and researchers agree that suicides by African Americans and particularly African American males, is rarer than are suicides among Whites and that African American males are more likely to commit suicide than African American females (Bernard, Paulozzi, & Wallace, 2007a; Griffin-Fennell & Williams, 2006; Joe, 2006a; U.S. Department of Health and Human Services, 2001). Professionals note that in the last 20 or 30 years the suicide rate for African American males has significantly increased. Suicide research from 1999 to 2003 found that all total, there were 145,846 suicides during this 4-year period (Rockett, Lian, Stack, Ducatman, & Wang, 2009). Of this total, 7,827 (5%) were African Americans (Rockett et al.). By way of com- parison, 1,563 (1%) were African American females (Rockett et al.). Thus, 5,264 African American males committed suicide. In 2006, there were 33,330 suicides within the USA. By sex, there were 26,308 (79%) who were males and 2,149 (21%) were females (Heron et al., 2009). Of the 33,330 suicides, 1,954 (6%) were African Americans. African American males constituted 1,669 (5%) and African American females, 285 or less than 1% (Heron et al.).

The literature does not report the various types of suicides just for African American males. Generally, workplace violence involving suicides are not likely to have information by race. Also, some articles theorized regarding suicidal ideation among African Americans (Cohen, Coleman, Yaffee, & Casimir, 2008; Griffin-Fennell & Williams, 2006) or studied suicidal ideation among African American adolescents (Spann et al., 2006). Empirical information regarding African American males must be teased out from reports and studies involving suicides that have examined race and sex as variables.

The Centers for Disease Control and Prevention (CDC) monitors all deaths within the USA. For adolescents, suicides were the highest for American Indians and Alaska Natives and were less common among African American adolescents compared to White adolescents (Bernard, Paulozzi, & Wallace, 2007b). In addition, the CDC has examined the role of alcohol and race in suicides. In 17 states from 2005 to 2006, the CDC reported that the highest percentage of suicides who were characterized as dependent upon alcohol was American Indian and Native Alaskan (21%) and the lowest was for non-Hispanic African Americans (7%) (Crosby, Espitia-Hardeman, Hill, Ortega, & Clavel-Arcas, 2009). Further, the highest percentage of suicides *tested* for alcohol consumption was non-Hispanic African Americans, 76% (Crosby et al.). Among those tested, 33.2% had alcohol in their blood at the time they committed suicide (Crosby et al.). American Indians and Native

Alaskans, along with Hispanics, were more likely to have alcohol in their systems (Crosby et al.). Karch, Barker, and Strine (2006) were interested in mental diagnosis and substance use at the time of suicides. They found that African Americans were most likely to have been diagnosed with schizophrenia, but African Americans were least likely to have used alcohol at the time of their suicides compared to Whites, Hispanics, or other racial groups.

Similar in topic area, Garlow, Purselle, and Heninger (2005) were interested in studying the role of alcohol and cocaine use by persons who had committed suicide. They examined the coroner's files for Fulton County (Atlanta), Georgia and learned that there were 1,296 suicides from 1989 to 2003. For persons under 19, 62% (49) of those who committed suicide were African Americans. However, for persons 20 and over who committed suicide only 28.5% were African American and 69% were White. Most of those who committed suicides in both age groups were males. For African males under 20 years of age, the rate per 100,000 was 9.73 and for African American females it was 1.34. For all ages, the rate per 100,000 for African American males was 16.37 and for African American females the rate was 2.2. For African Americans teenagers, 82% had no cocaine or alcohol in their systems at the time they committed suicide (Garlow et al.).

Joe (2006b) studied suicide trends among African American males and females. He was interested in examining influences of age, cohort, and period. The ages were grouped in intervals of five from 10–14 to 80–84. Joe reported that the male rate at 25–29 and 20–24 were higher than the 80–84 rate. The highest rate period for suicide for African American males was 25–29, and this rate was 41.05 per 100,000. Joe theorized that the African American higher rate of suicide paralleled deindustrialization (i.e., the economy losing industrial jobs) and increased social deprivation. In an interview, Joe further elaborated about suicides by African American males (Singer, 2010). Joe recommended destigmatizing the topic of suicide and focusing on self-destructive behaviors.

Kubrin and Wadsworth (2009) investigated suicides among African American and White males under the age of 35. Their unit of analysis was cities' suicides, and they studied 179 sites. The predictor variables were at the macrolevel and consisted of poverty, inequality, joblessness, family disruption, and firearms availability. In the model for African Americans, only the amount of disadvantage was a significant predictor. This model for African Americans also had the degree of mobility, African American/White inequality, dissimilarity, Northeast cities, Central cities, and West cities. The data showed, however, that cities with higher levels of African American poverty, male joblessness, single-female headed households, and lower levels of high school graduates had higher levels of suicides among African American males. Kubrin and Wadsworth added firearm availability to the model and found that "although the effect of gun availability is highly significant in both the Black and white models, it is stronger in the Black models. More importantly, for Blacks, the inclusion of gun availability reduces the coefficient for disadvantages by over 40% and attenuates its influence on Black suicide to the point that disadvantage is no longer significant" (p. 1218). They noted that the African American community has always had high levels of poverty but the availability of guns is a relatively recent phenomenon. Commensurate with the increase in gun violence in the African American community, the increase of suicides among African Americans occurred as well.

Using routine activity theory, Stack and Wasserman (2008) studied suicide by Russian Roulette and race. A Russian Roulette suicide is determined by one bullet in the chamber and likely witnesses' testimonies, whereas a suicide by gunshot to the head likely has more bullets in the gun and by evidence. They hypothesized that the increased availability of handguns by African Americans explained suicide by Russian Roulette. Taking a portion of a sample of 1,412 suicides from 1997 to 2005 from the Detroit Metropolitan area that was labeled as Russian Roulette suicides; they matched it with a control sample. They reported among African Americans, 80% of the suicides were Russian Roulette compared to suicides by gunshots to the head, compared to 30.7% who died by gunshot to the head. However, the percentage for gunshots to the head should be 20% and not 30.7%. The researchers used cross-tabulation and had race as the row variable and type of suicide as the column variable. However, they used percentages down the column variable. Type of suicide cannot influence race, but race can influence type of suicide. The independent variable must total 100%. Nonetheless, the 80% is highly significant and appears to be correct. Clearly, suicide among African American males is on the rise and help is warranted for this population.

Intervention-Community Level

Suicide is difficult to prevent because of the absence of reliable means for predicting who will and will not commit suicide (Bryant & Harder, 2008) and because of the finality of suicide, it is prudent to assume that the best intervention is prevention. Mood disorders such as depression increase the risk of suicide in individuals and 60% of African Americans do not acknowledge depression as a mental illness, which makes it unlikely they will seek help for it (Poussaint & Alexander, 2000). According to the American Foundation of Suicide Prevention (2010), there are a multitude of factors that increase the risk of suicide in depressed individuals. Such factors are anxiety, agitation, or enraged behavior, isolation, drug and/or alcohol use or abuse, history of physical or emotional illness, and feelings of hopelessness or desperation.

The 1999 Report of the Surgeon General: Depression and Suicide in Children and Adolescents states "the incidence of suicide attempts reaches a peak during the mid-adolescent years, and mortality from suicide, which increases steadily through the teens, is the third leading cause of death at that age" (CDC, 1999; Hoyert, Kochanek, & Murphy, 1999). According to Bonhomme and Young (2009), suicide is more polarized among African American male adolescents than any other demographic group, and as such the focus of this section is African American male adolescents. Suicide prevention requires a multidimensional approach; we must effect changes in the community and within the individual.

Suicide prevention can be effective at the community level only if the community is a viable entity that has the capacity to sustain its residents. "…African American men's health must be considered a vital aspect of the health of the African American community" (Bonhomme & Young, 2009, p. 75). Communities, according to Chaskin, Brown, Venkatesh, and Vidal (2001), provide their residents with services, housing, jobs, education, and oftentimes, race and social class determine the level of services provided by a community. Therefore, communities without these resources end up in distress. Likewise, distressed communities give rise to problems, which often cause them to suffer and lose the resources that are necessary to sustain its inhabitants. Oftentimes, these conditions can lead to crime, substance abuse, and poor physical and mental health (Chaskin et al.). The vast majority of African American men reside in poor socioeconomically deprived communities in major metropolitan cities (Bryson, 1996). Moreover, these communities have limited civic, economic, and social resources (Menchik, 1993). Therefore, these communities are more likely to experience distress.

Ultimately, community level interventions can begin with building community capacity. This entails helping African American communities sustain themselves by providing adequate and safe housing, employment, and educational opportunities for its inhabitants in addition to promoting community health and resilience. Additionally, neighborhood mental health facilities are needed which can provide culturally sensitive treatment and education about mood disorders.

The African American male can often feel inadequate when he cannot provide his family with the basic necessities of life, such as food and shelter. Policymakers, social service organizations, churches, and neighborhood organizations can support African American communities by supporting projects that focus on revitalizing socioeconomically distressed neighborhoods. Shoring up the infrastructure in these communities requires government intervention. For instance, safety is an issue for many of these communities, so an increased presence in police and fire departments that have been trained to be culturally sensitive to the residents is a must. If the community residents do not trust the police, then safety will remain a barrier to building community capacity. Providing affordable and safe housing is also an issue with these communities. Therefore, privately funded and government programs aimed at encouraging builders to build affordable housing in distressed communities is a must.

Investing in the educational system in distressed neighborhoods is also desperately needed. Approximately, 21.5% of African American men have less than a high school education, 34.8% graduated from high school, and only 16.4% have earned an undergraduate degree (U.S. Census Bureau 2000). Receiving a quality education can help to increase one's socioeconomic standing through higher paying jobs. Moreover, research has shown that income is positively correlated with better health outcomes. Additionally, research shows that health outcomes tend to improve as the level of education increases (Bonhomme & Young, 2009).

Individual Level Intervention

Research has shown that it is important when dealing with African Americans to incorporate African worldviews as a basis for understanding psychological functioning and well being (Bynum, 1999; Kambon, 1998; Nobles, 1991). Therefore, it is our contention that an Afrocentric-based intervention is needed to effectively treat the African American adolescent male who is at risk for suicide. This is not to say that other more traditional therapeutic interventions are not effective. The Afrocentric perspective has been in existence since the 1960s and was developed by Molefi Kete Asante (Moore, Madsen, & Moore, 2003). It is important to remember that traditional African philosophy predates European influences (Harvey & Rauch, 1997). The Afrocentric perspective provides a culturally specific paradigm for serving African Americans and focuses on spirituality and connectiveness (Meyers, 1988).

There is a body of research that promotes cognitive therapy as a successful methodology for treating suicide (Bryant & Harder, 2008; Burns, 1980; NIMH, 2010) we do not dispute this finding. However, we believe that the use of support groups and mentorship in conjunction with cognitive therapy further aids in suicide prevention (Harvey & Rauch, 1997; Utsey, Howard, & Williams, 2003). Support groups should stress involvement of the parents and/or caretakers because support and trust of the caretakers is vital if the support group intervention is to be successful. These groups can be housed in neighborhood churches or community centers, where the family can also receive formal and informal counseling free of charge or for a nominal fee.

In addition, the support should extend to help with homework, drug and alcohol counseling, sex education, and discussions on what it means to be an African American male in today's world. One major component to this preventative program is to assign mentors to the group participants. Role modeling is an important aspect of mentorship, so it helps if the mentors are college graduates with professional jobs. This recommendation is not mandatory for success, but it aids positive role modeling. For instance, a college student or professional mentor with a college degree can offer personal insight to the mentee about the importance of obtaining a college education. Addressing the needs of this high-risk population can lead to providing protection from discrimination. The African American male adolescent is at high risk for dropping out of school, incarceration, and early death. According to Harris (1995), Black masculinity is at stake because many African American males have redefined what it means to be a man. For some, this definition includes promiscuity, toughness, thrill seeking, violence, posturing, certain style of clothes, and a certain type of speech. This mindset can be problematic in that it may prevent meaningful family and church life, educational attainment, and employment. Oftentimes, in pursuit of money, youth drop out of school to obtain fast money. In this instance, a positive African American role model can help dispel the false sense of masculinity, help to redefine what it means to be a man, and instill values more in line with Afrocentricism.

Retention of participants in programs of this kind can be problematic, so group facilitators need to be vigilant when participants disengage. Therefore, follow-up calls are needed or even home visits. For many low-income participants, transportation is a barrier to participation. Thus, program administrators should arrange for transportation by arranging carpools or contracting with public transit when available. The group should also be a clearinghouse of resource and referral information for the clients and their families. For example, facilitators should be able to find help for clients who need the basic necessities such as food, shelter, and clothing, as well as employment and educational opportunities. By providing individual and family services to group participants, group members are more inclined to participate and the group has a better chance at being successful. Overall, an effective preventative measure includes therapy, support groups, and mentorship.

Implications for African American Males

Suicide is a tragic event under any circumstance. According to lifespan developmental theorist Erik Erikson, from birth to death there are skills and competencies to be mastered, reasonably well, at a particular time in life in order for successful personality development to occur (Sneed, Whitbourne, Krauss, & Culang, 2006). From infancy through older adulthood ideally an African American male learns (1) to trust those in his environment to provide for his basic survival needs (food, thirst, comfort); (2) to assert his own behavior, thereby developing a sense of autonomy; (3) the value of exploration and the art of creativity; (4) to focus on what he must learn to be successful in the adult world such as math, reading, writing, and social skills; (5) to develop a sense of identity; (6) to form intimate relationships; (7) to give back to upcoming generations; and finally (8) that the end of life is a period of self-reflection about the life choices, for better or worse, that have been made. In essence, there is so much living to do and so many experiences that germinate from living that a question that begs an answer is why then do African American males, in increasingly larger numbers, choose death instead of life?

The answer may lie, in part, in the overall grim life circumstances that many African American males encounter. Durkheim defines suicide as self-murder and defines it as "any death which is the direct or indirect result of a positive or negative act accomplished by the victim himself" (Durkheim, 1951, p. 42). He suggested that there is a collective force that compels men to kill themselves that gradually impacts them and that the tendency to kill oneself results from the toll that these social forces, such as chronic unemployment, despair, racism-related stress, poverty, incarceration, and low self-esteem, have on the psyche and emotions (Joe, 2006a). In their research on suicidality among African American men, Wingate et al. (2005) considered unemployment as a risk factor for suicide because it was an indicator of a man's ineffectiveness in obtaining much needed material possessions. For instance, being unemployed places men at a disadvantage for providing for their basic daily living needs. Further, their ability to create and sustain healthy families is diminished because they are unable to provide for the basic necessities of life for a family. As a result, many men who find themselves unable to provide for self and others experience depression and other mental health issues which may lead to thoughts of suicide (Meadows, 2009).

Life for many African American males can be considered as ongoing experiences that are often disappointing. The American African American male is in a dubious position. Often portrayed by the media as over-sexed, menacing, lazy, and buffoonish he is at-risk for suicide as a result of one or a combination of several psycho-socioeconomic factors which include having low self-esteem and feelings of alienation. These feelings may result, partially, from his being marginalized and considered by many in society to be an odious being (Moore, 1998).

He may be among the 25% of African Americans who live in poverty and the 43.2% who do not have a spouse (due to widowhood, divorce, or separation) or he may be one of the four in ten Black males who have never married and does not have the buffer from stress and disease that is associated with marriage (U.S. Census Bureau, 2000; Meadows, 2009). At some point in his life he may have been incarcerated. Among the 2,396,140 inmates held in custody in federal or state prisons or local jails in 2008, Black males numbered 846,000 which represents an incarceration rate that is 6.6 times higher than for white males. At the middle of 2008, one in 21 Black males was incarcerated compared to one in 138 white males. Hence, roughly 37% of all male inmates by the middle of 2008 were Black (McCarthy, 2009). Additionally, he may have been a victim of child physical, sexual, and/or psychological abuse that may have had a devastating effect upon his self-esteem.

All people want to be accepted, loved, and appreciated. African American men, like others, want to be praised for who they are, encouraged to know and pursue their potential for greatness and reminded that they have a unique contribution to make in society. Having a positive sense of one's self as a member of one's group is important for psychological health. So powerful is the need to belong that "it can prevent suicide; however, in the absence of social connection the risk for suicide is increased" (Wingate et al. 2005, p. 616).

Implications for African American Families

The African American family is the single most important institution within the African American community. It takes on a variety of forms and is made up of kin, fictive kin, and extended family. In essence, when African Americans refer to family they often include those who are biologically and nonbiologically related to them. Male and female roles are fluid in African American families. The father, although present, is not always the head of the family. Sometimes, the mother, grandparent, or other relatives operate in this capacity. Fathers often take on cooking, cleaning, grooming of children, and household responsibilities that by traditional European standards are usually carried out by females (Hill, 1997).

As new family forms emerge throughout society, there are some who suggest that male figures and specifically fathers are not an essential and necessary component of functional family life. To the contrary, although many women have successfully raised children to be outstanding and productive citizens, the presence of positive men within the family is extremely important to the development of young males and the overall family functioning. These fathers, sons, brothers, uncles, cousins, and friends serve as a source of social support, mentors, and discipline. Suicide among Black males leaves a void in the family that cannot be filled.

Implications for African American Community

When African American males commit self-murder more than just the individual is lost. The entire community looses the benefit of valuable manpower, wages earned through gainful employment, ideas for community development and other contributions that could have been made by them (Banks, 1970). For instance, African American men who loiter, sometimes out of feelings of hopelessness and despair, are often looked down upon, discussed from a pathos perspective and devalued. However, the authors assert that among those who loiter and congregate in public places are potential doctors, lawyers, physician assistants, teachers, policemen, and others who but for different circumstances could benefit the African American community and wider society.

Failure of African American men to seek treatment for depression and other mental health issues that can lead to suicide is a major community issue. The stigma that is often associated with suicide often serves as a deterrent from help-seeking behavior among African American men. Other deterrents to help seeking include the history that African Americans have had with the counseling professions and past medical experiments that have received wide acclaim (Whitaker, 2001). The African American church has historically condemned suicide. African American clergy often define suicide as an unforgivable sin that is not an imaginable solution to life's problems. Alternatively, clergy encourage African Americans to provide social support to each other in times of difficulty and to focus on an afterlife that will be free of present life struggles. A social audit conducted by the Gallup Organization in 1997 found that 92% of African Americans have an affiliation with a religious institution (Holt et al., 2009; Reese & Ahern, 1999). More than one-half of all African Americans attend church on a regular basis and are likely to encounter antisuicide sentiment (Lincoln & Mamiya, 1990).

The social sciences have historically stereotyped African Americans in negative ways and made assertions about their inferiority (Douglass, 1993; Taylor, 1994). These stereotypes portray African Americans as not committed to treatment, psychologically bankrupt, nonexpressive, and unable to productively engage in therapy. These stereotypes have resulted from the lack of help-seeking behavior by African Americans. For centuries, African Americans have unknowingly been used as subjects in scientific and medical experiments by private and governmental organizations (Weasel, 2006). Some believe that they have been injected with toxic substances. Not all of these beliefs are based on assumptions; some of these beliefs are based on fact. These beliefs may be a contributing factor to low client participation in mental health services. Low participation by African American men in these and other services is unfortunate because through treatment they may receive the necessary support and help to address their mental, emotional, physical, social, and spiritual health concerns thereby decreasing or eradicating their desire to terminate their life.

Conclusion

In recent years, suicide rates among African American males have increased. These increases have largely gone unnoticed by the general public because for many years, strong familial and religious ties served as protective factors that buffered many African American males from suicide. However, Joiner (2005) explains, as more African American males interface with mainstream society, they are at an increased risk for acculturative stress (i.e., stress experienced as a result of moving from one cultural framework to another), are more likely to become disengaged from the their faith and their extended family support systems, and are ultimately at an increased risk for suicide. This is particularly true as many African American males from socially and economically disadvantaged communities experience feelings of despair and hopelessness because they have little to no access to other buffers from suicide such as social capital and economic opportunity (Helliwell, 2004). Therefore, attempts to reduce suicides among African American males should aim to enhance their social, emotional, and economic support systems. Then, and only then, will the well-being of African American males be enhanced so that they may reach the point of self-actualization and not only grow and develop successfully as individuals, but also make significant contributions to the growth and development of the their families and communities.

References

American Foundation of Suicide Prevention. (2010). Retrieved May 31, from http://www.afsp.org/
Alston, J. (2008, November 25). Black men and suicide. *Newsweek*. Retrieved May 30, 2009, from http://www.newsweek.com/2008/11/24/Black-men-and-suicide.html
Banks, L. (1970). Black suicide. *Ebony, 25*(7), 76–84.

Bell, R. J. (2007). Suicides by slaves. In J. P. Rodriquez (Ed.). *Encyclopedia of slave resistance and rebellion* (Vol 2). Santa Barbara, CA: Greenwood Press. Retrieved May 26, 2010, from http://aae.greenwood.com.proxy.lib.ohiostate.edu/doc.aspx?i=11&fileID=GR3273&chapterID=GR3273-1113&path=/encyclopedias/greenwood/

Bernard, S. J., Paulozzi, L. J., & Wallace, L. J. D. (2007a). *Fatal injuries among children by race and ethnicity – United States, 1999–2002*. Atlanta, GA: Center for Disease Control.

Bernard, S. J., Paulozzi, L. J., & Wallace, D. L. (2007b). Fatal injuries among children by race and ethnicity – United States, 1999–2002. *MMWR. Surveillance Summaries: Morbidity and Mortality Weekly Report, 56*(5), 1–16.

Bonhomme, J. E., & Young, A. M. W. (2009). The health status of Black men. In R. L. Braithwaite, S. E. Taylor, & H. M. Treadwell (Eds.), *Health issues in the Black community* (pp. 73–94). San Francisco: Jossey Bass.

Bryant, C. E., & Harder, J. (2008). Treating suicidality in African American adolescents with cognitive-behavioral therapy. *Child and Adolescent Social Work Journal, 25*, 1–9.

Bryson, K. (1996). *Household and family characteristics*, March 1995 (Current Population Reports, Series P20-488). Washington, DC: U.S. Government Printing Office. [Available at (12/03): http://www.census.gov/population/www/socdemo/hh-fam.html]

Burns, D. (1980). *Feeling good: The new mood therapy*. New York: William Morrow & Co.

Bynum, E. B. (1999). *The African unconscious*. New York: Teachers College Press.

Cantor, C. H. (2000). Suicide in the Western world. In K. Hawton & K. van Heeringen (Eds.), *The international handbook of suicide and attempted suicide* (pp. 1–9). West Sussex: John Wiley & Sons.

Centers for Disease Control and Prevention. (1999). *Suicide deaths and rates per 100,000* [Electronic version]. Retrieved from http://www.cdc.gov/ncipc/data/us9794/suic.htm

Chaskin, R. J., Brown, P., Venkatesh, S., & Vidal, A. (2001). *Building community capacity*. New York: Aldine De Gruyter.

Chief Corwin's Blog. (2010, April 21). *Victims of murder/suicide identified*. Retrieved May 26, 2010, from http://kcpdchief.blogspot.com/2010/04/victims-of-murder-suicide-identified.html

Cohen, C. I., Coleman, Y., Yaffee, R., & Casimir, G. J. (2008). Racial differences in suicidality in an older urban population. *The Gerontologist, 48*(1), 71–78.

Crosby, A. E., Espitia-Hardeman, V., Hill, H. A., Ortega, L., & Clavel-Arcas, C. (2009). *Alcohol and suicide among racial/ethnic population – 17 states, 2005–2006*. Atlanta, GA: Center for Disease Control.

Decker, T., & Gray, K. L. (2010, March 9). Update: Man who shot two, himself at OSU had been fired. *Columbus Dispatch*. Retrieved May 26, 2010, from http://www.dispatch.com/live/content/local_news/stories/2010/03/09/1-killed-in-tripleshooting-on-osu-campus.html

Douglass, B.C (1993). *Psychotherapy with troubled African American adolescent males: Stereotypes, treatment amenability, and critical issues*. Annual Meeting of the American Psychological Association, Toronto.

Durkheim, E. (1951). *Suicide: A study in sociology*. New York: The Free Press.

Garlow, S. J., Pursell, D. C., & Heninger, M. (2005). Cocaine and alcohol use preceding suicide in African American and White adolescents. *Journal of Psychiatric Research, 41*, 530–536.

Griffin-Fennell, F., & Williams, M. (2006). Examining the complexities of suicidal behavior in the African American community. *Journal of Black Psychology, 32*(3), 303–319.

Harris, S. (1995). Psychosocial development and Black male masculinity: Implications for counseling economically disadvantaged African American male adolescents. *Journal of Counseling & Development, 73*(3), 279–288.

Harvey, A. R., & Rauch, J. B. (1997). A comprehensive Afrocentric rites of passage program for Black male adolescents. *Health & Social Work, 22*(1), 30–38.

Helliwell, J. F. (2004). *Well-being and social capital: Does suicide pose a puzzle?* Working Paper Series, Working Paper 10896. Cambridge, MA: National Bureau of Economic Research Inc.

Heron, M., Hoyert, D. L., Murphy, S. L., Jiaquan, X., Kochanek, K. D., & Tejada-Vera, B. (2009). Deaths: Final data for 2006. *National Vital Statistics Reports, 57*(14).

Hill, R. B. (1997). *The strengths of African American families: Twenty-five years later*. Washington, DC: R & B Publishers.

Holt, C. L., Roberts, C., Scarinci, I., Wiley, S., Eloubeidi, M., Crowther, M., et al. (2009). Development of a spiritually based educational program to increase colorectal cancer screening among African American men and women. *Health Communication, 24*(5), 400–412.

Hoyert, D. L., Kochanek, K. D., & Murphy, S. L. (1999). Deaths: Final data for 1997. *National Vital Statistics Reports, 47*(9).

Hutson, H. R., Yarbrough, A. D., Hardaway, K., Russell, M., Strote, R. M., Canter, M., et al. (1998). Suicide by cop. *Annuals of Emergency Medicine, 32*(6), 665–669.

Joe, S. (2006a). Explaining changes in the patterns of Black suicide in the United States from 1981 to 2002: An age, cohort, and period analysis. *Journal of Black Psychology, 32*(3), 262–284.

Joe, S. (2006b). Implications of national suicide trends for social work practice with Black youth. *Child and Adolescent Social Work Journal, 23*(4), 458–471.

Joiner, T. (2010). *Myths about suicide*. Cambridge, MA: Harvard University Press.

Joiner, T. (2005). *Why people die by suicide*. Cambridge, MA: Harvard University Press.

Kambon, K. K. K. (1998). *African/Black psychology in the American context: An Afro-centered approach*. Tallahassee, Fl.: Nubian Nations.

Karch, D. L., Barker, L., & Strine, T. W. (2006). Race/ethnicity, substance abuse, and mental illness among suicide victims in 13 U. S. States: 2004 data from the National Violent Death Reporting System. *Injury Prevention, 12*(2), 22–27.

Kubrin, C. E., & Wadsworth, T. (2009). Explaining suicide among Blacks and Whites: How socioeconomic factors and gun availability affect race-specific suicide rates. *Social Science Quarterly, 90*(5), 1203–1227.

Lincoln, C. E., & Mamiya, L. H. (1990). *The Black Church in the African American experience*. Durham, NC: Duke University Press.

Maris, R. W., Berman, A. L., & Silverman, M. M. (2000). *Comprehensive textbook of suicidology*. New York, NY: Guilford Press.

McCarthy, K. (2009). *Growth in prison and jail populations slowing*. Washington, DC: Department of Justice, Office of Justice Programs. Retrieved from http://www.ojp.gov/newsroom/pressreleases/2009/BJS090331.htm

Meadows, S. O. (2009). Family structure and fathers' well-being: Trajectories of mental health and self-rated health. *Journal of Health and Social Behavior, 50*(2), 115–131.

Menchik, P. L. (1993). Economic status as a determinant of mortality among non-white and white older males. *Population Studies, 47*, 427–436.

Meyers, L. J. (1988). *Understanding an Afro-centric world view: Introduction to an optimal psychology*. Dubuque, IA: Kendall/Hunt.

Montgomery, B., & Altman, H. (2005, December 23). Friends stunned by suicide of Dungy's son. *NBC Sports*. Retrieved May 30, 2009, from http://nbcsports.msnbc.com/id/10588639//

Moore, S. E. (1998). Review of the book: The assassination of the Black male image. *Black Issues in Higher Education, 15*(1), 41.

Moore, S. E., Madsen, O., & Moore, J. L. (2003). An Afrocentric approach to substance abuse treatment with adolescent African American males: Two case examples. *Western Journal of Black Studies, 27*(4), 219–230.

National Institute of Mental Health. (2010). *Preventing suicide: Individual acts create a public health crisis*. Retrieved May 31, 2010, from http://www.healthyplace.com/depression/nimh/preventing-suicide-individual-acts-create-a-public-health-crisis/menu-id-1406/

Nobles, W. (1991). African philosophy: Foundations of Black psychology. In R. Jones (Ed.), *Black psychology* (pp. 47–64). Berkeley, CA: Cobb & Henry.

Pinizzotto, A. J., Davis, E. F., & Miller III, C. E. (2005, February). Suicide by cop: Defining a devastating dilemma. *FBI Law Enforcement Bulletin, 74*(2), 8–20.

Plaisance, M., & Johnson, P. (2009, May 8). Mom says Springfield boy, 11, who committed suicide was repeatedly bullied at school. *The Republican*. Retrieved June 1, 2020, from http://www.masslive.com/news/index.ssf/2009/04/mom_says_springfield_boy_11_wh.html

Poussaint, A. F., & Alexander, A. (2000). *Lay my burden down: Unraveling suicide and the mental health crisis among African Americans*. Boston, MA: Beacon.

Reese, D. J., & Ahern, R. E. (1999). Hospice access and use by African Americans: Addressing cultural and institutional barriers through participatory action research. *Social Work, 44*(6), 549–560.

Rockett, I. R. H., Lian, Y., Stack, S., Ducatman, A. M., & Wang, S. (2009). Discrepant comorbidity between minority and White suicides: A national multiple cause-of-death analysis. *BMC Psychiatry, 9*(10), 1–10.

Singer, J. B. (Host). (2010, February 21). Suicide and Black American males: An interview with Sean Joe, Ph.D., LMSW [Episode 56]. *Social Work Podcast*. Retrieved May 26, 2010, from http://socialworkpodcast.com/2010/02/suicide-and-Black-ameican-males.html

Sneed, J. R., Whitbourne, S. K., Krauss, S., & Culang, M. E. (2006). Trust identity, and ego integrity: Modeling Erikson's core stages over 34 years. *Journal of Adult Development, 13*(3–4), 148–157.

Spann, M., Molock, S. D., Barksdale, C., Matlin, S., Phil, M., & Puri, R. (2006). Suicide and African American teenagers: Risk factors and coping mechanisms. *Suicide & Life-Threatening Behavior, 36*(5), 553–568.

Stack, S., & Wasserman, I. (2008). Social and racial correlates of Russian roulette. *Suicide & Life-Threatening Behavior, 38*(4), 436–441.

Taylor, R. L. (1994). *Minority families in America: A multicultural perspective*. Englewood Cliffs, NJ: Prentice Hall.

U.S. Census Bureau. (2000). *We the people: Blacks in the United States, Census 2000 Special report*. Retrieved June 20, 2010 from http://www.census.gov/prod/2005pubs/censr-20.pdf

U.S. Department of Health and Human Services. (2001). *Mental health: Culture, race, and ethnicity – a supplement to mental health: A report of the Surgeon General*. Rockville, MD: U.S. Department of Health and Human Services, Substance Abuse and Mental Health Services Administration, Center for Mental Health Services.

Utsey, S. O., Howard, A., & Williams, O., III. (2003). Therapeutic group mentoring with African American male adolescents. *Journal of Mental Health Counseling, 25*(2), 126–140.

Weasel, L. H. (2006). The message beneath the meaning: The role of race in human cloning discourse. *Fireweed, 6*.

Whitaker, C. (2001, April). Why are young Black men killing themselves? *Ebony*, 144–146.

Wingate, L. R., Bobadilla, L., Burns, A., Cukrowicz, K., Hernandez, A., Ketterman, R., et al. (2005). Suicidality in African American Men: The roles of southern residence, religiosity, and social support. *Suicide & Life-Threatening Behavior, 35*(6), 615–629.

Part VII
Clinical Interventions for Healthy Communities

Chapter 15
Increasing Cultural Competency Among Medical Care Providers

Wornie Reed, Ronnie Dunn, and Kay Colby

This chapter describes a video-based approach to assisting physicians and other health workers to become culturally competent in prevention/intervention work with low-income African Americans. This approach is based on the successful Urban Cancer Project, a National Cancer Institute funded collaboration between social scientists, a comprehensive cancer center, and a video-production company (see, Marks et al., 2004).

Culture is often defined in terms of a list of beliefs, values, behaviors, worldview, norms, and attitudes, etc., implying that cultures are static, homogeneous, and passively inherited, often by members of ethnic groups. In this project, culture was defined instead as "shared meanings," a definition derived from interpretive cultural anthropology (Geertz, 1964). In this view, "cancer" is a symbol packed with many meanings that are shared by members of broadly defined groups. These meanings include not only shared beliefs, attitudes, and values, but they also index the political, gender, racial, economic, and power relations experienced by group members. Those with common experiences and information create shared meanings. In this conceptualization, culture is dynamic, historical, complex, and actively created rather than passively inherited. The meanings of any symbol, such as cancer, derive from this process.

Medical anthropologists, trans-cultural nurses, cross-cultural psychologists and psychiatrists, and others have long stressed that cultural beliefs, practices, and meanings can help or hinder health interventions (Chavez, Hubbell, & Mishra, 1999; Friedman et al., 1995; Hahn, 1999; Lannin, Mitchell, Swanson, Swanson, & Edwards, 1998). The following quote from the Institute of Medicine describes this phenomenon:

> Socio-cultural differences between patient and provider influence communication and clinical decision-making. Evidence suggests that provider-patient communication is directly linked to patient satisfaction, adherence, and subsequently, health outcomes. Thus, when socio-cultural differences between patient and provider aren't appreciated, explored, understood, or communicated in the medical encounter, the result is patient dissatisfaction, poor adherence, poorer health outcomes, and racial/ethnic disparities in care. And it is not only the patient's culture that matters; the provider "culture" is equally important (Smedley, Stith, & Nelson, 2003, pp. 200–201).

Figure 15.1 summarizes the importance of appropriate cross-cultural communication – cultural competence – described by the Institute of Medicine.

W. Reed (✉)
Department of Sociology, Virginia Tech,
Blacksburg, VA, USA
e-mail: wornie@vt.edu

A.J. Lemelle et al. (eds.), *Handbook of African American Health: Social and Behavioral Interventions*,
DOI 10.1007/978-1-4419-9616-9_15, © Springer Science+Business Media, LLC 2011

Communication

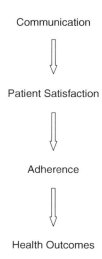

Patient Satisfaction

Adherence

Health Outcomes

Fig. 15.1 Linking communication to outcome

This project was part of a larger project to design and test the effectiveness of a culturally specific video-based campaign to address cancer control for minority patients. In the larger project, our approach was to develop and test methods of educating and training health care providers as well as patients and the broader community. Our objective here was to develop and test a cultural competency training video for cancer medical personnel, using an extended focus group approach.

Methods

Our approach was based on a triad of expertise, including (1) focus groups, (2) media experience, and (3) medical expertise.

Focus Groups

We based the content for our cultural competency video on the qualitative research derived from all aspects of the Urban Cancer Project. This consisted of the following: interviews and experiences documented in interviewing and following the stories of 22 African American cancer patients and their families; telephone interviews conducted with 30 African American cancer patients actively engaged in making treatment decisions; and the 44 focus group sessions conducted with low-income African Americans – residents of public housing in Cleveland, OH. Eight of the 44 focus group meetings were conducted specifically for the purpose of creating the cultural competency video, although data from all 44 meetings were integrated into the final product. The focus group discussions were audio-taped, transcribed, and analyzed with NUD*IST computer software. See Table 15.1 for a description of selected sociodemographic characteristics of the focus group participants; and see Marks et al. (2004), for a more extended description of the focus group process.

Table 15.1 Characteristics of focus group participants ($N = 49$; all were African Americans)

Characteristic	Number	Percent
Age		
40–49	21	43
50–59	14	29
60–69	12	25
≥70	1	2
Education		
<9th grade	3	6
9th to 11th grade	14	29
High school	23	47
>High school	7	15
Gender		
Female	25	51
Male	24	49
Religion		
Protestant	18	37
Muslim	2	4
Christian, no denomination given	24	49
Frequency of religious attendance		
Occasionally	22	45
Once per week	10	20
<Once per week	9	18
Know anyone with cancer		
Yes	39	80
No	10	20

The focus group discussion topics included experiences with physicians and other healthcare providers, cancer causation and prevention, cancer treatments, and coping with cancer, including end of life issues and spirituality. We used concerns, issues, and experiences raised during these discussions to produce the video on cultural competency. We videotaped some of these sessions for use in the video, and we also conducted separate on-camera interviews with participants who had additional comments and experiences to share.

Media Experience

From major themes developed in the analysis of the focus group material, rough cut videos were produced. This production process was iterative, as the draft videos were refined as a result of the critiques of the focus groups and the medical advisors.

A rough version of the cultural competency video that highlighted some of the themes noted above was produced. We then reconvened each of our four focus groups for a final session to screen the draft video. These focus groups commented freely about the video – what they liked, what they did not like, and whether it accurately reflected their views. The video was revised based on their recommendations. The most common suggestions were to insert more about the experiences of low-income people that stem from their financial status and strengthen the section on the importance of faith.

Medical Expertise

Utilizing the triad of expertise, we then showed the revised video to one of our medical advisors – a head and neck surgeon. He, in turn, shared it with a group of ten residents for comments and suggestions. The group suggested valuable feedback; physicians commented that while it was important to learn about the fears and beliefs that many members of this target population share about cancer, the video was too abstract in that it lacked concrete discussions about ways to implement such information. It became clear that we needed to go one step further with the video and tell physicians exactly how to implement this information. We rethought the structure of the video and developed the idea of structuring it with a problem/solution format.

Themes

Using the content analysis of the transcripts of the focus group meetings, we restructured the video around four major themes. We then used these themes, as well as issues we observed in the cases of actual patients, to organize the video into a problem/solution format. The four themes are (1) mistrust of the medical system, (2) ethno-medical beliefs and fears, (3) daily living issues, and (4) spirituality. These themes are the more prominent issues raised in the focus groups: They are listed below with a description of each.

Mistrust of the Medical System

Many low-income African Americans distrust the medical system, seeing it as exploitative of poor people in general, and of blacks in particular. Many believe that cancer(s) can be cured, but that too much money is being made on cancer by physicians and others for them to use these cures or prevent cancer in the first place.

Some low-income African Americans think that doctors give black people diseases deliberately, often through injections, which contributes to a fear of needles, that black people in particular are used as "guinea pigs," that black people are a good supply of cadavers needed for medical students, and that black people's organs are harvested for transplant into white people.

Ethno-Medical Beliefs and Fears

Many persons often have limited understanding of various cancers, human anatomy, or normal or abnormal physiology. They do not understand how cancers spread.

The three major cancer treatments do not make sense to many low-income African Americans. Since some think cancer is a rotting or "eating" process like an infection, they do not understand why antibiotics cannot cure cancer(s) just as they cure other infections. Often, they see complicated cancer treatments as merely money-makers.

(a) Surgery: Though many can understand the rationale for surgery to remove tumors or "knots," since air is thought to be both necessary for growth and also filled with "germs and things," many believe that when a person is opened up and the air hits the cancer, the cancer will spread. Their empirical model is a can of food whose contents remain edible as long as the can is not opened, but which begins to spoil once the can is opened.

(b) Chemotherapy: Many African Americans think that cancer comes from unnatural substances in our "processed" world. "Chemotherapy" connotes chemicals; chemicals are poisons that cause cancer. To them, it is illogical to treat cancer with the very substances that cause it. The side effects are also very frightening.

(c) Radiation: Radiation is known to cause cancer and is to be feared. Again, it makes no sense to treat cancer with its cause. Additionally, radiation is seen as burning the skin or causing it to turn darker or gray.

Daily Living Issues

Physicians need to consider the daily living issues confronted by African American patients: for example, extensive babysitting or actually raising others' children; having to take several buses (often with children) to keep an appointment; or lost wages at work for taking time off for doctor visits. Case managers need to be engaged to help patients with these problems so they can adhere to treatment.

Spirituality

Some African Americans think only God can cure serious diseases, and that having faith in God and learning to accept God's will are most important when coping with a disease. Whereas accepting God's plan for oneself may be viewed negatively and called "fatalism" by some, to many African Americans, such strong faith is a worthy, positive goal.

For each theme, we provided a problem that may arise when physicians do not fully understand or appreciate opinions and perspectives that some low-income African American patients or their families hold about such issues. We then worked with a team of oncologists to devise solutions to such problems that are workable within a clinical setting.

Using this new framework, we developed another version of the video and showed it to our medical advisors. One physician who viewed it suggested providing examples of actual language physicians can use to broach the subject of faith with patients. Again using our iterative process, we compiled a written list of questions for physicians and inserted it into the video. The production process that led to the production of the final video enabled us to develop an approach to cultural competency training that is summarized below.

In an article on patient-provider communication highlighted in the Institute on Medicine's book *Unequal Treatment,* (Cooper and Roter 2003) state: "Cultural competence may be defined as the ability of individuals to establish effective interpersonal and working relationships that supersede cultural differences." Models of interventions to achieve such competence include respecting and addressing deeper, holistic understandings of different audiences' ethno medical ideas and the barriers and facilitators of health-promoting behaviors in local contexts obtained from in-depth formative, often ethnographic, research (e.g., Bailey, Erwin, & Belin, 2000; Loustanunau & Sobo, 2001). It is with this definition of cultural competence and with this model that we approached the creation of our final video. We chose to focus on strategies to assist physicians and other healthcare providers with developing communication skills to help establish effective interpersonal relationships with low-income African American cancer patients. We used an approach that seeks to inform physicians and other healthcare providers about some of the common ethno-medical values, beliefs, and fears held by low-income African Americans regarding cancer and treatment. The goal was to make providers aware of such issues and present them with communication approaches to use if they are pertinent to individual patients. If such values and beliefs are important to a patient, the video then provides sample language that providers can incorporate into treatment discussions in a way that makes patients feel they are being listened to and respected.

The importance of physician/patient communication continues to be an area of growing interest. Two communication strategies that have gained attention are patient centered communication and physician participatory decision-making (PDM) style; both have been shown to have positive emotional and physical effects on patients. Our approach attempts to give physicians some communication tools to conduct more patient centered communication with low-income African Americans by providing strategies for them to acknowledge predispositions and attitudes that may be important to some patients.

Results

The resulting 20-min video was structured around four themes: (1) mistrust of the medical system, (2) ethno-medical beliefs and fears, (3) daily living issues, and (4) spirituality. We were careful in the video and in the presentation of the video to the medical staff to avoid reifying some of the issues raised as always existing among low-income African American patients. Rather, occasionally these problematic issues are present, and consequently appropriate medical care is dependent on addressing them.

The video was tested at a cultural competence seminar during grand rounds in a comprehensive cancer center, using a one-group pretest-posttest design. A total of 49 healthcare providers including nurses, physicians, social workers, and others attended the presentation that was available for continuing medical education (CME) credits.

- 58.3% of the 49 participants in the seminar evaluated the video as "very useful," and another 31.3% judged it as "useful."
- Among the 19 physicians in the test, 52.6% said the video was "very useful," and 26.3% said it was "useful." Thus, nearly 80% of the physicians evaluated it as useful or very useful in their practice.
- Among the 33 physicians and nurses there was a significant increase (at $p=0.07$) in the proportion indicating that physicians should ask probing questions during treatment discussions to discern if their African American patients have strong spiritual beliefs. On no other factor was there a statistically significant change, a function of the small sample size; however, all of the indicators moved toward what might be considered a more culturally competent direction, suggesting an effect of overall positive change toward increased cultural competence.
- In the post-test, 73.7% of physicians said that physicians should ask probing questions about religion, and another 10% said this should occur sometimes. In the pretest only 56.3% of the physicians said this should occur.
- Among physicians and nurses, there was a significant increase (from 77 to 91%) in the proportion indicating that patients should be asked often about their specific fears and concerns about cancer and cancer treatments.
- One physician said for attribution, "I've been in practice 50-odd years and what I learned from this was how much I had missed during all those years."
- Another physician indicated that he had a sense of the need for attention to spiritually among his patients, but he did not have the vocabulary to use in those situations until he viewed our video.

Conclusions

The results indicate that this culturally specific, video-based approach can be used to improve the cultural competence of medical personnel. The results also demonstrate that it is feasible to use a video for cultural competence training.

While the test of this approach presented here was oriented around cancer, the idea of cross-cultural education is not limited to any specific disease. Consequently, this approach should work with other diseases as well.

Acknowledgment This study was funded in part by Grant Number 1R43CA130271 from the National Cancer Institute.

References

Bailey, E. J., Erwin, D. O., & Belin, P. (2000). Using cultural beliefs and patterns to improve mammography utilization among African American women: The witness project. *Journal of the American Medical Association, 92,* 136–142.

Chavez, L. R., Hubbell, F. A., & Mishra, S. I. (1999). Ethnography and breast cancer control among Latinas and Anglo women in Southern California. In R. A. Hahn (Ed.), *Anthropology in public health: Bridging differences in culture and society.* New York: Oxford University Press.

Cooper, L. A., & Roter, D. L. (2003). Patient-centered communication, ratings of care, and concordance of patient and physician race. *Annals of Internal Medicine, 139*(11), 907–915.

Friedman, L. C., Webb, J. A., Weinberg, A. D., Lane, M., Cooper, H. P., & Woodruff, A. (1995). Breast cancer screening: Racial differences in behaviors and beliefs. *Journal of Cancer Education, 10,* 213–216.

Geertz, C. (1964). Ideology as a cultural system. In D. Apter (Ed.), *Ideology and discontent* (pp. 47–56). New York: Free Press.

Hahn, R. A. (1999). *Anthropology in public health: Bridging differences in culture and society.* New York: Oxford University Press.

Lannin, D. R., Mitchell, H. F. J., Swanson, M. S., Swanson, F. H., & Edwards, M. S. (1998). Influence of socioeconomic and cultural factors on racial differences in late-stage presentation of breast cancer. *Journal of the American Medical Association, 279,* 1801–1807.

Loustanunau, M. O., & Sobo, E. J. (2001). *The cultural context of health, illness, and medicine.* Westport, CT: Bergin and Garvey.

Marks, J. P., Reed, W., Colby, K., Dunn, R., Masovel, M., & Ibrahim, S. A. (2004). A culturally competent approach to cancer news and education in an inner city community: Focus groups findings. *Journal of Health Communication, 9*(2), 143–157.

Smedley, B. D., Stith, A. Y., & Nelson, A. R. (Eds.). (2003). *Unequal treatment: Confronting racial and ethnic disparities in health care* (pp. 200–201). Washington, DC: The National Academies Press.

Chapter 16
Tailoring Health Interventions: An Approach for Working with African American Churches to Reduce Cancer Health Disparities

Marlyn Allicock, Marci Kramish Campbell, and Joan Walsh

Introduction

African Americans continue to experience disproportionately high rates of mortality and morbidity due to cancer. Understanding the issues, addressing the causes, and improving survival rates among African Americans will require a composite of strategies. Approaches that address the unique barriers, beliefs, and concerns of African Americans are needed.

The African American church has long been used as a venue for delivering programs and as a key partner in health promotion. Evidence continues to aggregate about how best to work with African American churches regarding key research elements, considerations required, and challenges that remain when tackling health disparities issues among African Americans. The purpose of this chapter is to discuss working with African American churches as a culturally relevant strategy for disease prevention and health promotion, and to reduce health disparities. Specifically, we examine interventions using communications tailored and targeted for cancer prevention and control among African American congregations. We summarize the cancer burden faced by African Americans, outline the importance of working with African American churches for health promotion, and focus, in large part, on using targeting and tailored communication approaches to reduce the cancer health disparity burden facing this population. Though it is widely recognized that other minority populations (e.g., Latinos and Pacific Islanders) also experience cancer disparities, we focus on African Americans and the pivotal institution of the church as a means to address cancer disparities. Studies have suggested that programs aimed at rural whites and low-income Latinos and conducted through faith-based programs also may have the potential to reduce disparities (Bowen et al., 2004; Welsh, Sauaia, Jacobellis, Min, & Byers, 2005; Winett, Anderson, Wojcik, Winett, & Bowen, 2007). The literature pertaining to work with churches in other ethnic populations is sparse compared to that regarding African American churches. This does not necessarily reflect a lesser role of religion in these communities, but rather differences in the health concerns of the population, the feasibility and fit of messages and programs thought to be appropriate, less research conducted, and other factors. The historical and deep-rooted role of the church is unique among African Americans (Eng, Hatch, & Callan, 1985), and as such provides a context for efforts at this level as well as some insights about future endeavors within African American churches.

M.K. Campbell (✉)
Department of Nutrition, Gillings School of Global Public Health,
University of North Carolina, Chapel Hill, NC, USA
e-mail: campbel7@email.unc.edu

A.J. Lemelle et al. (eds.), *Handbook of African American Health: Social and Behavioral Interventions*,
DOI 10.1007/978-1-4419-9616-9_16, © Springer Science+Business Media, LLC 2011

African Americans and the Cancer Burden

Cancer health disparities in the United States have been extensively documented by multiple studies (U.S. Cancer Statistics Working Group, 2006; Clegg, Li, Hankey, Chu, & Edwards, 2002; Chu, Lamar, & Freeman, 2003). Incidence rates for many common cancers vary substantially among racial and ethnic segments of the population. Disparities in incidence among African Americans, Hispanics, and whites for 12 relatively common cancer sites are shown in Fig. 16.1 (U.S. Cancer Statistics Working Group).

Some sites have pronounced racial/ethnic disparities, while others have smaller differences. African Americans have the highest incidence rates for three of the four most common cancers: lung, colorectal, and prostate. Hispanics fare better than others across six sites, but for liver cancer their rates are highest, and for melanoma, lymphoma, stomach, bladder, and ovarian cancer, their rates fall between those of the two other major population groups. Mortality rates offer a starker contrast as shown in Fig. 16.2 (National Cancer Institute, 2006).

For the 12 sites shown in Fig. 16.1 and 16.2, African Americans had higher incidence rates than whites for six sites, but higher mortality rates for eight sites, the two differences being for female breast cancer and uterine cancer. More white women (by rate) are diagnosed with these two cancers annually, but more African American women die, and breast cancer is the most common cancer in women. In addition, for the other three most common cancers, all of which have higher incidence rates for African Americans than for whites, the mortality rate percentage difference is substantially greater than the incidence rate percentage difference: for colorectal, 48% vs. 19%; for lung and bronchus, 11% vs. 2%; for prostate, 138% vs. 51%. These high mortality differences may reflect unequal access to screening, resulting in later diagnoses among African Americans, and/or unequal access to treatment. Other factors affecting both incidence and mortality may include lifestyle factors and tumor biology.

As shown, there appear to be racially- and ethnically related factors involved in the occurrence and lethality of most, if not all, common cancers. While some cancers affect Hispanics or whites more often than African Americans, it is African Americans who have the highest rates of cancer incidence and mortality overall, due to their higher incidence of three of the most common cancers, and their markedly higher mortality due to all four. This fact places a demand upon public health professionals to reach out to African American individuals and communities in novel and effective ways.

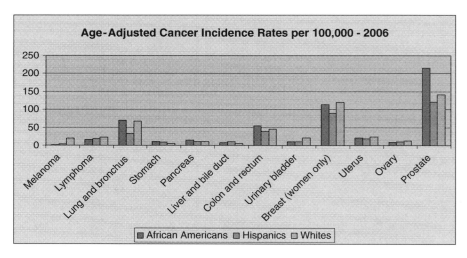

Fig. 16.1 Age-adjusted cancer incidence rates

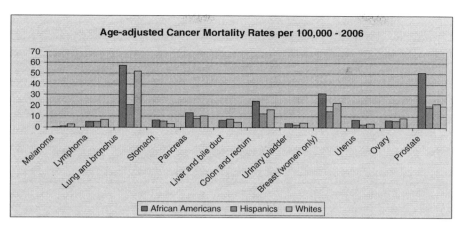

Fig. 16.2 Age-adjusted cancer mortality rates

Why Work with African American Churches to Influence Cancer Health Disparities

The church is the strongest institution in the lives of many African Americans. Weekly church attendance is higher among African Americans than for either other major racial/ethnic group, and exceeds the national average by 6% (for women, 37% vs. 31%; for men, 29% vs. 23%) (McLanahan & Garfinkel, 2000). African American churches have been central for community organization through the civil rights era, and still fulfill a vital role in the social and political, as well as spiritual, lives of their members.

African American churches frequently hold social events following services, as well as at other times, and many churches prioritize use of space and volunteer time for service programs geared toward members of different ages, including youth programs, health fairs, and assistance to elderly or disabled members. In addition, the church pastor often functions as a role model in health matters as well as spiritual ones, wielding considerable influence with his or her congregation and motivating church members to view good health behavior as a religious responsibility (Holt & McClure, 2006). These advantages make the church an excellent resource, providing space and time for effective dissemination of health information, as well as the support needed to enable church members to make recommended behavioral changes.

Cancer Prevention and Control with African American Churches

There is an expanding literature to support the use of church-based health promotion programs among African Americans for addressing cancer prevention and control behaviors (Campbell, Resnicow, Carr, Wang, & Williams, 2007). These programs have focused on breast cancer (Erwin, Spatz, Stotts, Hollenberg, & Deloney, 1996; Husaini et al., 2002; Derose, Fox, Reigades, & Hawes-Dawson, 2000; Duan, Fox, Derose, & Carson, 2000), cervical cancer screening (Davis et al., 1994), physical activity (Prochaska, Walcott-McQuigg, Peters, & Warren, 2000; Prochaska, Walcott-McQuigg, Peters, & Li, 2000); colorectal cancer screening (Frank, Swedmark, & Grubbs, 2004); prostate cancer screening (Holt et al., 2009; Husaini et al., 2002); physical activity and nutrition (Resnicow et al., 2002); physical activity, nutrition, and colorectal cancer screening

(Campbell et al., 2004); and smoking cessation (Schorling et al., 1997; Stillman, Bone, Rand, Levine, & Becker, 1993). In one example, focusing on lung cancer, Voorhees and colleagues (1996) implemented a smoking cessation program in 22 urban Baltimore churches, comparing an intensive, culturally specific intervention with a minimal self-help intervention. Those who received the intensive intervention were significantly more likely ($p=0.04$) to progress through the stages of change, including action (quitting smoking) and maintenance (Voorhees et al., 1996).

Interventions geared toward dietary change for colorectal cancer prevention include the Black Churches United for Better Health (BCUBH) study, with 2,519 participating adults in 50 rural North Carolina churches. At 2-year follow-up, fruit and vegetable (F&V) consumption, considered an important behavior for prevention of colorectal and other cancers, had increased significantly ($p<0.0001$) (Campbell, Demark-Wahnefried, et al., 1999). The Eat for Life trial also addressed fruit and vegetable consumption, recruiting 1,011 individuals in 14 primarily urban churches who were divided into three groups: no intervention, one "cue call," and three motivational interviewing calls. Those who received the motivational interviewing calls increased F&V consumption significantly ($p<0.01$) more than either comparison group (Resnicow et al., 2001). The WATCH study intervention included diet, physical activity, and colorectal cancer screening among 587 participating members of 12 rural NC churches, and compared TPV (tailored print and video) with LHA (lay health advising). TPV significantly ($p<0.05$) increased F&V consumption and physical activity and increased fecal occult blood test (FOBT) by $p=0.08$, while LHA was not found to be effective (Campbell et al., 2004).

The Body & Soul program was a collaborative outgrowth of BCUBH and Eat for Life. A randomized effectiveness study, it combined environmental, self-help, and motivational interviewing components, and recruited 1,022 members of 15 churches in six states. Significant ($p<0.05$) increases in F&V consumption were observed (Resnicow et al., 2004). This program is now being disseminated nationally by the National Cancer Institute, and process evaluation has been completed among 11 churches, eight of which initiated a peer counseling program using motivational interviewing. Participant recall of talking with a peer counselor was associated with significantly ($p=0.02$) greater F&V consumption (Allicock et al., 2009).

Finally, promotion of screening for early detection of breast cancer has been successful in both rural and urban African American churches. The Witness Project trained cancer survivors as role models to promote screening among women in four counties in rural Arkansas. The study was primarily implemented through churches, and any secular-site programs also used hymns, prayers, biblical quotations, and statements of faith by the role models. Both breast self-examination and mammography increased significantly ($p<0.0001$ and $p<0.005$, respectively) (Erwin et al., 1996). The Los Angeles Mammography Promotion in Churches Program enrolled 1,113 participants from 30 urban churches, and found significantly ($p=0.03$) better 1-year adherence to mammography guidelines among baseline-adherent participants who received the church-based telephone counseling intervention than among controls. There was no significant difference among participants nonadherent at baseline (Duan et al., 2000).

These successes illustrate the extent to which culturally appropriate interventions can promote health behaviors likely to reduce the large disparities noted above, hopefully leading to a reduction in excess cancer mortality among African Americans (Kreuter & McClure, 2004). The rest of this chapter will review factors relevant to health communication interventions for cancer prevention and control that are targeted and tailored to members of African American churches.

Perspectives on Working with Churches

Several related perspectives have been proposed as frameworks for conducting health promotion programs with faith-based organizations. One point of view considers whether programs are faith-based or faith-placed (DeHaven, Hunter, Wilder, Walton, & Berry, 2004). Distinctive features of this approach include the level of church involvement as opposed to researcher-driven programs, and the presence or absence of spiritual/religious contextualization and/or a holistic perspective on health (mind–body–spirit connection). These factors are essential for determining whether a program is faith-based or faith-placed. Programs that derive from the church congregations themselves are referred to as "emic," e.g., programs formulated by a church's own health ministry, while those that come from outside programs and organizations are called "etic." Additionally, programs can be considered "collaborative" if they are conducted in partnership between churches and outside groups. A review of health programs in faith-based organizations found that 25% were faith-based vs. 35% collaborative and 40% faith-placed (DeHaven et al., 2004). Faith-placed programs were more likely to report outcomes. All three approaches showed significant health improvements, especially faith-placed programs (developed by professionals outside of the congregation). Faith-placed programs were more likely to have used study designs able to test efficacy. The review recommended more collaborative partnerships that would be able to evaluate and disseminate findings, and called for more programs focused on effectiveness (real world) evaluations rather than efficacy evaluations.

Others have classified working with faith-based organizations by the extent to which spiritual and religious context is featured and the church participates in formulating program and messages. Lasater and colleagues (1997), in their review of cardiovascular prevention programs among church populations, classify four levels of program types. Level I programs are those that use the church as a viable access point for participant recruitment. Church members then receive the researcher-driven intervention, and the content is secular. Level II programs use the church site as a place for delivering an intervention in which the intervention content is secular, e.g., offering educational sessions after services. Level III programs include congregants in the program delivery of a secular-based intervention, e.g., training church volunteers as lay health educators to implement a particular researcher-derived protocol. Level IV programs are ones that include spiritual program elements, such as messages and scriptures that integrate religion and health. Level III and IV programs more fully utilize the strengths of religious organizations. Additionally, working with pastors and church leadership ensures that cultural and spiritual aspects of the target population are integrated into the program design and implementation.

Another consideration in determining how to work with churches stems from the view that health promotion and health care must be practiced with cultural sensitivity. Cultural sensitivity is practiced when social and cultural characteristics of the target population inform and are incorporated into the work intended for specific groups. Individuals are said to respond to health information messages based on the beliefs and values that shape their identity, as well as the rules of behavior learned in the context of their social networks. The unique cultural backgrounds and orientations of individuals can have a powerful influence on the ways they respond to communications about cancer risks, prevention, detection, and control (Chew, Bradley, & Boyko, 2004; Kreps, 2006; Kreps & Kunimoto, 1994). Thus, health information that does not correspond with an individual's beliefs or practices can be interpreted as insensitive and maladaptive (Kagawa-Singer, 1994). This perspective has implications for whether to target or tailor health promotion programs. Resnicow and colleagues (1999) suggest that cultural sensitivity functions on two levels – surface structure and deep structure. Programs that reflect surface structure in cultural sensitivity involve matching intervention materials and messages to observable social and behavioral characteristics, such as language, places, and clothing, and using delivery channels that are familiar and appropriate to the target group (Resnicow & Braithwaite, 2001). Deep-level structure, the second level of cultural sensitivity, refers to how programs and messages reflect the ways cultural, social, psychological, environmental, and historical factors influence health behaviors differently across racial and ethnic populations. This dimension requires an understanding of how members of the target group perceive cause, course, and treatment of illness, as well as perceptions regarding the determinants of specific health behaviors. Deep structure reflects how religion, family, society, economics, and government influence target behaviors, both in perception and fact. For example, the "body-temple connection," i.e., the scriptural reference 1 Corinthians 6:19 about the body as God's temple and thus worthy of honor, is often mentioned as a reason for African American church members to engage in healthy behaviors (Baskin, Resnicow, & Campbell, 2001). Understanding this value allows the creation of meaningful programs and messages. In sum, surface structure is useful for increasing receptivity, comprehension, and acceptability of health messages (Simons-Morton, Donohew, & Crump, 1997), while deep structure conveys salience and helps to determine program impact. Resnicow and Braithwaite (2001) further posit that the rationale to target or tailor using surface or deep structure depends on three areas of ethnic and racial differences. They suggest that differences in disease prevalence rates and/or differences in the prevalence of behavioral risk factors argue for targeting health promotion and disease prevention programs. This means programs are delivered to a specific population, and surface-structure cultural sensitivity factors are applied. Alternatively, when there are differences in the predictors of health behaviors, programs and messages should be tailored (i.e., adapted for subpopulations), and deep-structure factors should be utilized.

Though many successful programs aimed at cancer prevention and/or early detection have been implemented in African American churches, few such programs utilize spiritually based cancer communication interventions. A case for using spiritually based content in cancer communication interventions has been made (Holt, Kyles, Wiehagen, & Casey, 2003; Winnett et al., 1999). For example, Voorhees and colleagues (1996) used sermons, testimony in church services, and a stop-smoking booklet to provide smoking cessation messages. Others (Yanek, Becker, Moy, Gittelsohn, & Koffman, 2001) have included scriptures in health messages, group prayer, aerobics to gospel music, and a newsletter from the pastor for a diet and physical activity newsletter. Given that religion and spirituality play a major role among African Americans, spiritually- or religiously based content may be more culturally appropriate. When religious/spiritual messages, bible texts, prayer, and other spiritual aspects are used within intervention designs and implementation, the goal is not to increase the religiosity and spirituality of congregants. Rather, the focus is to guarantee that the intervention is culturally appropriate and fits with the cultural belief systems of the target population (Holt et al., 2009). To accomplish this requires a collaborative partnership with churches in the intervention design and delivery and to ensure program sustainability (Campbell et al., 2007).

In sum, the ways in which researchers have worked with churches have included some variations. These have ranged from simply using the church as a venue for participant recruitment to fully integrated partnerships where the church leadership and members are part of the design and implementation. Key elements suggested in the literature, however, highlight the need to work in partnership to assure cultural and spiritual appropriateness, to determine the level of cultural considerations to be applied, and to utilize programs that emphasize real-world evaluations.

Why Tailor and Target Health Promotion Interventions to Reduce Health Disparities

An important consideration in the fight to reduce the cancer burden is that many cancers are deemed preventable and can be cured clinically with early diagnosis and effective treatment (Stein & Colditz, 2004; Steward & Kleihues, 2003). Tobacco use, diet, physical activity levels, alcohol consumption, and adherence to cancer screening tests have been identified as modifiable risk factors that, if addressed, show strong evidence for reducing cancer mortality (Hiatt & Rimer, 1999; Stein & Colditz, 2004; Kreps, 2006). However, to successfully reduce cancer-related deaths and suffering through prevention strategies, individuals must know which healthy behaviors are recommended and how to achieve those behavior changes. Communicating knowledge and preventive actions to alleviate known risk factors has been a critical strategy in cancer control (Hiatt & Rimer, 1999; Kreps & Vishwanath, 2001; Kreuter, 1999). Careful attention should be given to communicating clearly and accurately, and to providing motivating information addressing all aspects of the cancer continuum, from prevention to diagnosis, treatment, and continued care. It is important, as well, that messages address misinformation about causes, strategies for early detection, and optimal treatment options to avoid contributing to late diagnosis and suboptimal cancer outcomes (Kreps et al., 2007; Mayer et al., 2007; O'Hair, Kreps, & Sparks, 2007). However, there is insufficient research regarding the best ways to deliver preventive health communications aimed at vulnerable populations. Traditional health communications that rely on providing generic prevention messages have generally been viewed to be insufficient for engaging individuals to change and adopt behaviors (Neuhauser & Kreps, 2003; O'Hair et al.). As such, tailored messages have been recommended to improve health communication interventions (Neuhauser & Kreps, 2003; Rimer & Krueter, 2006; Campbell & Quintiliani, 2006). Health communications for cancer prevention and control must also focus on relevant individual factors that can enhance or detract from cancer control and prevention engagement efforts on the part of the individual. The main goals of health communications aimed at African American faith-based populations include using optimal ways of communicating with and educating individuals about actions needed to reduce cancer risk and enhance well-being by means of messages that are personally relevant.

Targeting and Tailoring Messages

Interventions developed and tested for African American congregants have used generic, targeted, and tailored approaches for cancer prevention and control. Generic or "one size fits all" approaches to health communications require no audience assessment and have no customized content (Kreuter, Strecher, & Glassman, 1999). For example, a brochure or poster in a doctor's office describing breast cancer risks fits under this category. Targeted interventions, on the other hand, usually define the audience on cultural, behavioral, and psychological characteristics common at the "group" level, and all intervention participants receive similar messages and materials. The goal is to custom-fit messages and information to the group. The assumption is that the individuals, e.g., African American church audiences, have similar enough characteristics and motivations to be influenced by the same intervention messages and materials (Kreuter et al.). Such group-level targeted interventions have been found to be more effective in changing behavior than untargeted, generic health messages (Kreuter et al.; Resnicow et al., 2001, 2005). The majority of health education interventions utilizes a targeted approach quite similar to the way in which advertisers segment and target their messages to particular audiences (Grunig, 1989). A criticism of interventions using group-level targeted messages is the lack of attention paid to individual diversity within African American populations. Recently, researchers have sought to explore other characteristics, such as ethnic identity, to account for the heterogeneity within populations (Resnicow et al., 2009). Alternatively, tailored interventions aim to reach one specific person, based on individual-level psychological, social, and behavioral factors (Kreuter, Farrell, Olevitch, & Brennan, 2000; Skinner, Campbell, Rimer, Curry, & Prochaska, 1999; Kreuter et al., 1999; Strecher, 1999). Tailoring requires assessing each individual in order to create the personalized materials. Individual message-tailoring characteristics can include personalization such as a person's name and church name, demographics such as gender and race/ethnicity, psychosocial variables such as perceived benefits and barriers to initiating, changing, or maintaining behavior, and behavioral feedback and comparisons on information such as screening status vs. the recommended guidelines. Tailoring has been found in several reviews and meta-analyses (Brug, Campbell, & van Assema, 1999; Kroeze, Werkman, & Brug, 2006; Kreuter et al.; Miller et al., 2004; Noar, Benac, & Harris, 2007; Skinner et al.) to be more efficacious for behavior change compared to targeted interventions. The effectiveness of tailored communications is explained by the level of personal relevance to the receiver. Studies using tailored messages point out that participants tend to recall more, read more, and report more personal relevance compared to nontailored materials (Brug, Oenema, &Campbell, 2003; Petty & Priester, 1994). The elaboration likelihood model (Kreuter & Wray, 2003; Petty & Cacioppo, 1986) proposes that messages are more actively processed if they are considered to be more personally applicable. For example, when an individual cares about the issue of cancer and perceives the information as personally important, more central processing and cognitive elaboration of the information occurs. When there is low involvement, the use of more peripheral cures such as colors, graphics, attractiveness, or celebrity of the message source is needed.

Program Example: The Watch Project

There is a dearth of studies testing tailored communications aimed at African Americans, and fewer still have used tailored communication to African American congregants to raise awareness, recommend actions, and provide information needed for cancer-preventive actions. The Wellness for African Americans Through Churches (WATCH) project (Campbell et al., 2004) exemplifies a church-based study using both targeted and tailored communications for cancer prevention and control among African American churchgoers. The WATCH project was aimed at improving diet, physical activity, and screening for colorectal cancer (CRC) among 587 church members in 12 rural North Carolina churches. Churches were randomized to receive a TPV (tailored print and video), a lay health advisor (LHA), a combined (TPV plus LHA), or a control intervention (health education sessions and speakers on topics of their choice not directly related to study objectives).

Tailored Print and Video (TPV) intervention. The tailoring framework for WATCH included demographic, psychosocial, behavioral, and church and community-specific resource information in a newsletter format designed to address the factors that were considered most likely to predict change in the health behaviors targeted. The TPV intervention included four personalized computer-tailored newsletters and four targeted videotapes that corresponded to the same behaviors, mailed to participants' homes bi-monthly. Each magazine was tailored using the baseline survey data and addressed each health behavior in this order: (1) fruits and vegetables, (2) physical activity, (3) colorectal screening, and (4) lowering dietary fat. Pre-intervention focus groups were used in combination with pertinent literature and expertise of the project team to develop appropriate tailoring variables, message content, language, literacy level (approximately 6th grade), and graphic design for the tailored messages. The tailored feedback was presented in newsletter format, each consisting of 4 eight-page newsletters sized 8 1/2×11 in., created from two 11×17 in. sheets that were preprinted in four colors. Tailored content was subsequently laser-printed onto both sides of the paper, which was then folded in half.

An extensive message library of text, graphics, and photographs was developed to correspond with each survey question selected for tailoring and its possible response options and response combinations. The newsletters were each personalized with names of the participant, pastor, and church. They provided individually tailored elements including behavioral feedback on fat, fruit, and vegetable consumption, physical activity level, screening status, CRC risk factors, stages of change, social support, barriers to change, beliefs, and demographics (age and gender). Computer-based tailoring algorithms were written to use the individual survey data and decision rules determined by the research team to access the appropriate messages and graphics from the message library and assemble them in a predetermined format and layout. Each tailored magazine included nine message "stories" selected from the message library (which contained approximately 400 different text files) with personalized names and generic information, such as the project title and logo. The message libraries, layout, format, and number of messages and graphics per newsletter were consistent across the health behaviors. Pretesting was conducted with a convenience sample of African American church members not included in the study, and revisions were made in the content and layout based on this feedback.

Targeting. Additional message elements were targeted to cultural, spiritual, and community factors, including church-specific pastor messages, community-specific resources, testimonials written by community members, and incorporation of scriptural passages deemed relevant to the study behaviors and motivation for change. Scriptural and religious content was reviewed and approved by several pastors. The newsletters were further targeted to appeal to an African American audience through elements such as graphic design, photographs, stories, and recipes.

Four targeted videotapes were created to complement each of the four tailored newsletters. Community members and pastors who provided testimonials in the newsletters were also featured in the videotapes, which focused on reinforcing motivation and demonstrating/modeling skills to perform each behavior. For example, the fruit and vegetable videotape showed how to prepare healthy fruit and vegetable dishes, included testimonials and a pastor delivering a sermon devoted to healthy eating and CRC risk, and provided information about serving sizes and the 5-a-Day goal recommended at the time by the National Cancer Institute and numerous health organizations (Havas, Heimendinger, Reynolds, 1994). The videotapes were produced by a professional videographer and were targeted to an African American church audience.

As noted above, TPV significantly ($p<0.05$) increased F&V consumption (0.6 servings), increased physical activity (2.5 metabolic task equivalents per hour), and among those 50 and older ($n=287$), achieved a 15% increase in fecal occult blood testing screening ($p=0.08$), while LHA was not found to be effective (Campbell et al., 2004). The findings showed that the tailored intervention was effective across multiple behaviors. Few studies have studied the impact of tailoring on multiple behavior changes (Emmons, 1997). The effect on fruit and vegetable intake is comparable to outcomes of research studies that only focused on that one behavior (Buller et al., 1999; Havas et al., 1994; Marcus et al., 2001). The additional impact on recreational physical activity and CRC screening rates suggests that tailoring to multiple behaviors is feasible and effective. It was not possible to separate the relative effects of the tailored newsletters vs. the targeted videos. The purpose of adding the videos was to provide additional motivating messages and modeling/skills demonstration in order to enhance and complement the personalized information in the tailored newsletters. The resultant mailed, tailored newsletters cost approximately $20 per person (not including development costs), and therefore could be feasible for widespread dissemination. In addition, the tailoring protocol used the baseline survey to tailor all newsletters, rather than recontacting people to tailor each newsletter. This approach reduced participant burden as well as production costs.

Overview of Tailored Interventions and Cancer

A list of eight studies is included in Table 16.1. These studies may not represent an exhaustive list, but highlight experimental and quasi-experimental study designs testing targeted and tailored interventions. We identified an initial list of approximately 70 papers published in 1990 or later, and selected articles that had an appropriate comparison group and had reported outcome data and statistics. Papers that were descriptive reports of interventions, small pilot studies, and one-group pretest–posttest studies with no appropriate comparisons were excluded. Some studies were difficult to evaluate. For example, the term "culturally appropriate" was sometimes used without an adequate description of how the materials and/or intervention used were culturally or spiritually targeted. Other studies provided outcomes related to nonbehavioral measures. For example, the Praise Project, which included 60 African American churches and 1,300 participants in eight North Carolina counties in a randomized control design with 1-year follow-up, used a culturally sensitive intervention that included tailored bulletins and other targeted intervention components to improve outcomes for dietary fat, fruits and vegetables, and fiber. This study reported on the community member's trust, benefit, satisfaction, and burdens associated with participation in the intervention, but did not report impact on nutrition outcomes.

Table 16.1 Church-based tailored and targeted communication to promote cancer prevention and control among African Americans

Authors	Sample	Design	Behavior	Intervention	Outcome
Campbell, Demark-Wahnefried, et al. (1999)	2,519, African Americans, 50 rural churches in 10 eastern North Carolina counties-(Black Churches United for Better Health)	Randomized at county level, 2-year follow-up	Fruit and vegetable (F&V) consumption	Individualized tailored bulletins, lay health advisors, church-led education activities, community coalitions and events, pastor support, food events, and gardening vs. control	Intervention group consumed 0.85 servings of F&V more than control group at 2-year follow-up ($p<0.0001$)
Campbell et al. (2004)	587 African Americans, 12 rural North Carolina churches	2×2 factorial randomized, 1-year follow-up	Fruit and vegetable consumption, physical activity, colorectal cancer screening	Tailored print and targeted videos (TPV) only; lay health advisor (LHA) only; combined intervention (TPV plus LHA); or control	TPV significantly improved ($p<0.05$) F&V consumption (0.6 servings) and physical activity (2.5 METS/h) and, among those 50 and older ($n=287$), had a 15% increased in fecal occult blood testing screening ($p=0.08$)
Erwin, Spatz, Stotts, and Hollenberg, (1996)	204 African American women in Mississippi river delta region, The Witness Project	Quasi-experimental pretest and posttest design in 11 churches and 5 community groups	Breast self-exam and mammography	Intervention group received mammography education from African American breast and cervical cancer survivors, biblical quotations, prayer; hymns, and statements of faith included in the presentation. Controls were women in counties that did not receive the intervention	Intervention group participants significantly increased their practice of self breast exams ($p<0.0001$) and mammography ($p<0.005$) compared to control participants
Holt and Klem (2005)	108 African American women from six churches	Church-level random assignment to intervention or control, 1-month follow-up	Knowledge and perceived barriers to mammography	Targeted, spiritually based booklet to encourage breast cancer screening vs. demographically targeted booklet with no spiritual content	Both groups had significant increases in knowledge about treatment and lowered perceived barriers. Spiritually-based group had increased knowledge about mammograms

Holt et al. (2009)	49 African American men from 2 churches	Pre-post randomized controlled trial	Decision-making for prostate cancer screening	Trained community health advisors provided spiritually-based or non-spiritually-based education	Statistically significant increases in knowledge scores for and amount read by spiritually-based intervention group
Husaini et al. (2002)	430 African American men from 45 churches	Quasi-experimental delayed control with randomization at the church level, 3 waves	Prostate cancer knowledge, attitudes, and screening	Culturally tailored education program with video and a question and answer session with African American physician	Knowledge, perceived threat, and screening prevalence increased significantly. Knowledge at wave 2 associated with greater odds of having a digital rectal exam and only for early intervention at wave 3. Early intervention twice as likely to have talked with physician about screening at wave 3
Powell, Carter, Bonsi, Johnson, Williams, et al. (2005)	192 African American women in 13 churches in Alabama	Quasi-experimental and churches randomly divided into three groups: full program, partial program, or delayed (control), 3-month follow-up	Mammography attainment	Video and group discussion (partial); plus home visit by home health educator who reviewed video content, provided training in self breast exam, provided culturally appropriate print materials, and assisted with obtaining a mammogram (full)	Participants in full intervention had a 38% increase in mammography attainment; and reduced barriers for women who had not had mammogram at follow up
Resnicow et al. (2004)	1022 African American adults in 15 churches 6 states	Randomization at church level to intervention or control with 6-month follow up	Fruit and vegetable intake	Intervention: two motivational interviewing calls by trained lay counselor, health fairs, cookbook, printed health materials, educational sessions and cooking class	Intervention group had greater fruit and vegetable consumption than comparison group. Adjusted pos-test difference was 0.7 servings/daily for the two-item measure and 1.4 servings for the 17-item fruit and vegetable measure. Statistically significant changes in fat intake, motivation, social support, and self-efficacy were reported

The studies listed in Table 16.1 addressed breast cancer (Erwin et al., 1996; Holt & Klem, 2005; Powell et al., 2005); nutrition behaviors (Campbell, Bernhardt, et al., 1999; Campbell et al., 2004; Resnicow et al., 2004); colorectal cancer (Campbell et al.); and prostate cancer (Holt et al., 2009; Husaini et al., 2002). Only two studies used tailored interventions (Campbell, Bernhardt, et al.; Campbell et al.) all the others were targeted. Generally, the studies provided self-help print materials (Campbell, Bernhardt, et al.; Campbell et al.; Holt & Klem, 2005); videos (Campbell et al.; Husaini et al., 2002; Powell et al., 2005; Resnicow et al.); and education via community participants (Campbell, Bernhardt, et al.; Campbell et al.; Erwin et al., 1996; Holt et al., 2009; Husaini et al., 2002; Powell et al., 2005; Resnicow et al.) that were culturally targeted and/or individually tailored. These studies demonstrate that faith-based interventions have tremendous potential to be effective in achieving behavior changes relevant to cancer prevention and control. However, most studies did not specify any theoretical framework and did not assess program sustainability.

Health Communications: Issues to Consider

As highlighted in this chapter, African American churches are important partners to engage in efforts to reduce cancer health disparities. Research continues to support the use of tailored and targeted health communication interventions with church-based populations. With the substantial role that African American churches have played in the past, it is important to consider both current and emerging issues related to cancer communications and the church that may impact how ongoing health concerns among this population are addressed.

Degree of Spiritual Tailoring. The integration of spiritually based content as part of cancer communication interventions is considered culturally appropriate (Holt et al., 2003; Winnett et al., 1999). However, even working within a faith-based institution, there may exist some diversity about the need for, appropriateness of, and sophistication of religious content. It should not be assumed that all participating church members hold the same preferences for religious and spiritual content regarding cancer health information. Formative research with four focus groups from an ongoing project, ACTS, has served to highlight this fact. ACTS (Action through Churches in Time to Save Lives) of Wellness, is a current church-based research project designed to encourage colorectal cancer screening, healthy eating, and physical activity in an effort to increase colorectal cancer-preventive activities among African Americans [CDC, Special Interest Project: 3-U48-DP000059-02S1]. Participants in 19 African American churches in North Carolina and Michigan have been randomized to intervention and control conditions. Intervention churches receive four personalized, tailored newsletters and a variable number of targeted DVDs about colorectal cancer prevention and physical activity (one DVD for the church and one for each participant out of compliance with CRC screening). Control churches receive Body & Soul, an evidence-based fruit and vegetable intervention (Campbell et al., 2007; Resnicow et al., 2004). Results from the focus groups to pilot test messages and graphical content of the tailored newsletters indicated that participants had discrete preferences for whether visual images and written communications were presented in a secular or religious context. Based on this feedback, we included a question on the baseline survey to solicit participant preference for either secular or religious tailoring. Others have suggested that the diversity among African Americans may call for tailoring on other culturally relevant constructs such as religiosity, collectivism, racial pride, and time orientation (Kreuter et al., 2005), as well as ethnic identity (Resnicow et al., 2009). Positive outcomes using these variations in tailoring have been observed (Kreuter et al.; Resnicow et al.). Additionally, Holt and colleagues (2009) have suggested ways for developing spiritually based content for addressing colorectal cancer screening behaviors. Intervention development phases include soliciting advice from an advisory panel, distilling core content from focus groups, and doing additional pilot testing and cognitive testing of materials.

Message Framing. Many theories and models exist that suggest how best to communicate messages, explain the underlying processes between message exposure and behavior change prediction, and for understanding message source, recipient, and other contextually relevant variables that are beyond the scope of this chapter. We highlight two relevant factors for consideration when developing health communications to address cancer disparities. First, how race-specific mortality data is framed may have implications for subsequent screening. Nicholson and colleagues (2008), in a double-blind randomized study, compared the emotional and behavioral reactions to four versions of the same colon cancer information in mock news articles to 300 African American adults. Findings indicated that reports about African Americans improving over time regarding cancer disparities (increasing screening and decreasing mortality) produced a more positive effect on intention to be screened compared to reports emphasizing the higher risks for African Americans. The authors concluded that cancer information that emphasized racial disparities may serve to undermine prevention and control efforts among African Americans, especially those with high levels of medical mistrust.

A second consideration involves the source of the message. Campbell and colleagues (1999) tested the effect of message source on message recall and perceived credibility in the Black Churches United for Better Health Study (Campbell, Bernhardt, et al., 1999a). They compared an expert-oriented (EXP) bulletin with a spiritual and pastor-oriented (SPIR) bulletin and a control group, and found that message trust was higher in the SPIR group ($p < 0.05$). The EXP group reported higher trust of health and nutrition information coming from scientific research ($p < 0.01$), and the SPIR group reported higher trust of information coming from the pastor ($p < 0.05$). This study emphasized the need to identify credible sources that may influence recall and trust of health messages, and to use sources that church members consider trustworthy to enhance source credibility and thus positively impact health promotion efforts.

Loss of Social Cohesion. African American faith communities have a rich history of meeting the needs of their congregants within and beyond the church, including addressing the health concerns of church members. However, in the last few decades, several factors may challenge how churches operate in partnership to solve health dilemmas. First, there may be a reduction, or even a loss, of social cohesion within churches. With congregants living farther away from their churches, there may be time constraints for traveling to and from church, decreased time spent at church activities, and less use of the church as a network for extending and strengthening social ties. Process evaluation from a recently completed study (Allicock et al., 2009) indicated that attending church activities was challenging for members due to increased distances between church and home location.

The shifting structure of churches may need to be studied to examine influences on social cohesion and ways to execute health promotion programs in the current environment. Churches that now incorporate multiple services to better serve the needs of larger or multisector congregations may require more resources and increased frequency of programs presented. Congregants may also have the option of attending services via online or televised broadcasts, and thus may miss out on health-promotion activities delivered at the church. Individuals may also be turning to other social networks, such as online interactions (e.g., Facebook), for information and social connections, reducing the role of the church as a social network for providing information. Relatively little is known about the challenges to implementing research programs within the multilayered and complex organizational structures of the modern church.

Conclusion

Tailoring health promotion programs to the specific ethnic, racial, sociodemographic, and spiritual needs of African Americans is important for reducing cancer health disparities. Factors important for working in African American churches are unique to such churches, and it cannot be assumed that these qualities are transferable to other faith-based programs in other populations. Programs designed and structured for other congregations must undergo extensive formative research to ensure that they fit the needs of those congregations.

References

Allicock, M., Campbell, M. K., Valle, C. G., Barlow, J. N., Carr, C., Meier, A., et al. (2009). Evaluating the implementation of peer counseling in a church-based dietary intervention for African Americans. *Patient Education and Counseling*. doi:10.1016/j.pec.2009.11.018.

Baskin, M., Resnicow, K., & Campbell, M. K. (2001). Conducting health interventions in black churches: A model for building effective partnerships. *Ethnicity & Disease, 11*(4), 823–833.

Bowen, D. J., Beresford, S., Vu, T., Shu, J., Feng, Z., Tinker, L. F., et al. (2004). Design and baseline findings for a randomized intervention trial of dietary change in religious organizations. *Preventive Medicine, 39*(3), 602–611.

Brug, J., Campbell, M. K., & van Assema, P. (1999). The application and impact of computer-generated personalized nutrition education: A review of the literature. *Patient Education and Counseling, 36*, 145–156.

Brug, J., Oenema, A., & Campbell, M. K. (2003). Past, present, and future of computer-tailored nutrition education. *The American Journal of Clinical Nutrition, 77*(4 Suppl.), 1028S–1034S.

Buller, D. B., Morrill, C., Taren, D., Aickin, M., Sennott-Miller, L., Buller, M. K., et al. (1999). Randomized trial testing the effect of peer education at increasing fruit and vegetable intake. *Journal of the National Cancer Institute* 1, *91*(17), 1491–1500.

Campbell, M. K., James, A. S., Hudson, M. A., Carr, C., Jackson, E. J., Oates, V., et al. (2004). Improving multiple behaviors for colorectal cancer prevention among African American church members. *Health Psychology, 23*(5), 492–502.

Campbell, M. K., Resnicow, K., Carr, C., Wang, T., & Williams, A. (2007). Process evaluation of effective church-based diet intervention: Body & Soul. *Health Education & Behavior, 34*(6), 864–880.

Campbell, M. K., Hudson, M. A., Resnicow, K., Blakeney, N., Paxton, A., & Baskin, M. (2007). Church-based health promotion interventions: Evidence and lessons learned. *Annual Review of Public Health, 28*, 213–234.

Campbell, M. K., Demark-Wahnefried, W., Symons, M., Kalsbeeck, W. D., Dodds, J., Cowan, A., et al. (1999). Fruit and vegetable consumption and prevention of cancer: The Black churches united for better health project. *American Journal of Public Health, 89*(9), 1390–1396.

Campbell, M. K., Bernhardt, J. M., Waldmiller, M., Jackson, B., Potenziani, D., Weathers, B., et al. (1999). Varying the message source in computer-tailored nutrition education. *Patient Education and Counseling, 36*, 157–169.

Campbell, M. K., & Quintiliani, L. M. (2006). Tailored interventions in public health: Where does tailoring fit in interventions to reduce health disparities? *The American Behavioral Scientist, 49*(6), 1–19.

Chew, L. D., Bradley, K. A., & Boyko, E. J. (2004). Brief questions to identify patients with inadequate health literacy. *Family Medicine, 36*, 588–594.

Clegg, L. X., Li, F. P., Hankey, B. F., Chu, K., & Edwards, B. K. (2002). Cancer survival among US whites and minorities: A SEER (surveillance, epidemiology, and end results) Program population-based study. *Archives of Internal Medicine, 162*(17), 1985–1993.

Chu, K. C., Lamar, C. A., & Freeman, H. P. (2003). Racial disparities in breast carcinoma survival rates. *Cancer, 97*, 2853–2860.

Davis, D. T., Bustamante, A., Brown, C. P., Wolde-Tsadik, G., Savage, E. W., Cheng, X., et al. (1994). The urban church and cancer control: A source of social influence in minority communities. *Public Health Reports, 109*, 500–506.

DeHaven, M. J., Hunter, I. B., Wilder, L., Walton, J. W., & Berry, J. (2004). Health programs in faith-based organizations: Are they effective? *American Journal of Public Health, 94*(6), 1030–1036.

Derose, K. P., Fox, S. A., Reigades, E., & Hawes-Dawson, J. (2000). Church-based telephone mammography counseling with peer counselors. *Journal of Health Communication, 5*, 175–188.

Duan, N., Fox, S. A., Derose, K. P., & Carson, S. (2000). Maintaining mammography adherence through telephone counseling in a church-based trial. *American Journal of Public Health, 90*, 1468–1471.

Emmons, K. (1997). Maximizing cancer risk reduction efforts: Addressing multiple risk factors simultaneously. *Cancer Causes & Control, 8*(Suppl. 1), 31–34.

Eng, E., Hatch, J., & Callan, A. (1985). Institutionalizing social support through the church and community. *Health Education Quarterly, 12*, 81–92.

Erwin, D. O., Spatz, T. S., Stotts, R. C., Hollenberg, J. A., & Deloney, L. A. (1996). Increasing mammography and breast self-examination in African American women using the witness project model. *Journal of Cancer Education, 11*, 210–215.

Frank, D., Swedmark, J., & Grubbs, L. (2004). Colon can cer screening in African American women. *Association of Black Nurses Forum Journal, 15*, 67–70.

Grunig, J. (1989). Publics, audiences, and market segments: Segmentation principles for campaigns. In C. Salomon (Ed.), *Information campaigns: Balancing social values and social change* (pp. 199–228). Newbury Park, CA: Sage.

Havas, S., Heimendinger, J., Reynolds, K., Baranowski, T., Nicklas, T. A., Bishop, D., et al. (1994). 5-a-Day for better health: A new research initiative. *Journal of the American Dietetic Association, 94*, 32–36.

Hiatt, R. A., & Rimer, B. K. (1999). A new strategy for cancer control research. *Cancer Epidemiology, Biomarkers & Prevention, 8*(11), 957–964.

Holt, C. L., Roberts, C., Scarinci, I., Wiley, S. R., Eloubeidi, M., Crowther, M., et al. (2009). Development of a spiritually based educational program to increase colorectal cancer screening among African American men and women. *Health Communications, 24*, 400–412.

Holt, C. L., Kyles, A., Wiehagen, T., & Casey, C. (2003). Development of a spiritually based breast cancer educational booklet for African Americans women. *Cancer Control, 10*, 37–44.

Holt, C. L., & Klem, P. R. (2005). As you go, spread the word: Spiritually based breast cancer education for African American women. *Gynecology Oncology, 99*(3 Suppl. 1), S141–S142.

Holt, C. L., & McClure, S. M. (2006). Perceptions of the religion-health connection among African American church members. *Qualitative Health Research, 16*(2), 268–281.

Husaini, B. A., Sherkat, D. E., Levine, R., Bragg, R., Cain, V. A., Emerson, J. A., et al. (2002). The effect of a church-based breast cancer screening program on mammography rates among African American women. *Journal of the National Medical Association, 94*, 100–106.

Kagawa-Singer, M. (1994). Today's reality: Research issues in underserved populations. In *Nursing Research and Underserved Populations* (pp. 1–17). Atlanta, GA: American Cancer Society.

Kreps, G. (2006). One size does not fit all: Adapting communications to the needs and literacy levels of individuals. *Annals of Family Medicine* [online]. Retrieved from http//:www.annfammed.org/cgi/eletters/6/7/2006

Kreps, G. L., Gustafson, D., Salovey, P., Perocchia, R. S., Wilbright, W., Bright, M., et al. (2007). The NCI digital divide pilot projects: Implications for cancer education. *Journal of Cancer Education, 22*(Suppl. 1), S56–S60.

Kreps, G. L., & Kunimoto, E. (1994). *Effective communication in multicultural health care settings*. Newbury Park, CA: Sage.

Kreps, G. L., & Vishwanath, W. (2001). Foreword. Communication intervention and cancer control: A review of the National Cancer Institute's Health Communication Intervention Research Initiative. *Family & Community Health, 24*, ix–xiii.

Kreuter, M. W. (1999). Dealing with competing and conflicting risks in cancer communication. *Journal of the National Cancer Institute. Monographs, 25*, 27–35.

Kreuter, M. W., Farrell, D., Olevitch, L., & Brennan, L. (2000). *Tailoring health messages: Customizing communication with computer technology*. Mahwah, NJ: Erlbaum.

Kreuter, M. W., & McClure, S. M. (2004). The role of culture in health communication. *Annual Review of Public Health, 25*, 439–455.

Kreuter, M. W., Sugg-Skinner, C., Holt, C. L., Clark, E. M., Haire-Joshu, D., Fu, Q., et al. (2005). Cultural tailoring for mammography and fruit and vegetable intake among low-income African American women in urban public health centers. *Preventive Medicine, 41*, 53–62.

Kreuter, M. W., Strecher, V. J., & Glassman, B. (1999). One size does not fit all: The case for tailoring print materials. *Annals of Behavioral Medicine, 21*, 273–283.

Kreuter, M. W., & Wray, R. J. (2003). Tailored and targeted health communication: Strategies for enhancing information relevance. *American Journal of Health Behavior, 27*, S227–S232.

Kroeze, W., Werkman, A., & Brug, J. (2006). A systematic review of randomized trials on the effectiveness of computer-tailored education on physical activity and dietary behaviors. *Annals of Behavioral Medicine, 31*(3), 205–223.

Lasater, T. M., Becker, D. M., Hill, M. N., & Gans, K. M. (1997). Synthesis of findings and issues from religious-based cardiovascular disease prevention trials. *Annals of Epidemiology, 7*(57), s47–s53.

Mayer, D. K., Terrin, N. C., Kreps, G. L., Menon, U., McCance, K., Parsons, S. K., et al. (2007). Cancer survivors and information seeking behaviors: A comparison of survivors who do and don't seek information. *Patient Education and Counseling, 65*(3), 342–350.

Marcus, A. C., Heimendinger, J., Wolfe, P., Fairclough, D., Rimer, B. K., Morra, M., et al. (2001). A randomized trail of a brief intervention to increase fruit and vegetable intake: A replication study among callers to the CIS. *Preventive Medicine, 33*(3), 204–216.

McLanahan, S., & Garfinkel, I. (2000). The fragile families and well-being study. Retrieved March 28, 2010, from http://www.pbs.org/wnet/religionandethics/week908/Wilcox_Data.pdf

Miller, S. M., Bowen, D. J., Campbell, M. K., Diefenbach, M. A., Gritz, E. R., Jacobsen, P. B., et al. (2004). Current research promises and challenges in behavioral oncology: Report from the American Society of Preventive Oncology Annual Meeting, 2002. *Cancer Epidemiology, Biomarkers & Prevention, 13*, 171–180.

National Cancer Institute. (2006). Fast Stats: An interactive tool for access to SEER cancer statistics. Surveillance Research Program, National Cancer Institute. Retrieved April 5, 2010, from http://seer.cancer.gov/faststats

Neuhauser, L., & Kreps, G. L. (2003). Rethinking communication in the e-health era. *Journal of Health Psychology, 8*, 7–22.

Nicholson, R. A., Kreuter, M. W., Lapka, C., Wellborn, R., Clark, E. M., Sanders-Thompson, V., et al. (2008). Unintended effects of emphasizing disparities in cancer communication to African Americans. *Cancer Epidemiology, Biomarkers & Prevention, 17*(11), 2947–2952.

Noar, S., Benac, C. N., & Harris, M. S. (2007). Does tailoring matter? Meta-analytic review of tailored print health behavior change interventions. *Psychological Bulletin, 133*(4), 673–693.

O'Hair, H. D., Kreps, G. L., & Sparks, L. (Eds.). (2007). *Handbook of communication and cancer care*. Cresskill, NJ: Hampton Press.

Petty, R. E., & Cacioppo, J. T. (1986). *Communication and persuasion: Central and peripheral routes to attitude change*. New York: Springer.

Petty, R. E., & Priester, J. R. (1994). Mass media attitude change: Implication of the elaboration likelihood model of persuasion. In J. Bryant & D. Zillman (Eds.), *Media effects: Advances in theory and research* (pp. 91–122). Hillsdale, NJ: Lawrence Erlbaum.

Powell, M. E., Carter, V., Bonsi, E., Johnson, G., Williams, L., Taylor-Smith, L., et al. (2005). Increasing mammography screening among African American women in rural areas. *Journal of Health Care Poor Underserved, 16*(4 Suppl. A), 11–21.

Prochaska, T. R., Walcott-McQuigg, J., Peters, K., & Warren, J. S. (2000). Sources of attrition in a church-based exercise program for older African Americans. *American Journal of Health Promotion, 14*, 380–385.

Prochaska, T. R., Walcott-McQuigg, J., Peters, K. E., & Li, M. (2000). Recruitment of older African Americans into church-based exercise programs. *Journal of Mental Health and Aging, 6*, 53–66.

Resnicow, K., Braithwaite, R., Ahluwalia, J., & Baranowski, T. (1999). Cultural sensitivity in public health: Defined and demystified. *Ethnicity & Disease, 9*, 10–21.

Resnicow, K., Campbell, M. K., Carr, C., McCarty, F., Wang, T., Periasamy, S., et al. (2004). Body and soul. A dietary intervention conducted through African American churches. *American Journal of Preventive Medicine, 7*(2), 97–105.

Resnicow, K., Jackson, A., Braithwaite, R., DiIorio, C., Blisset, D., Rahotep, S., et al. (2002). Healthy body/healthy spirit: A church-based nutrition and physical activity intervention. *Health Education Research, 17*, 562–573.

Resnicow, K., Jackson, A., Wang, T., De, A. K., McCarty, F., Dudley, W. N., et al. (2001). A motivational interviewing intervention to increase fruit and vegetable intake through Black churches: Results of the Eat for Life trial. *American Journal of Public Health, 91*(10), 1686–1693.

Resnicow, K., & Braithwaite, R. (2001). Cultural sensitivity in public health. In R. Braithwaite & S. Taylor (Eds.), *Health issues in the Black community* (2nd ed., pp. 516–542). San Francisco: Jossey-Bass.

Resnicow, K., Davis, R., Zhang, N., Strecher, V., Tolsma, D., Calvi, J., et al. (2009). Tailoring a fruit and vegetable intervention on ethnic identity: Results of a randomized study. *Health Psychology, 28*(4), 394–403.

Resnicow, K., Jackson, A., Blissett, D., Wang, T., McCarty, F., Rahotep, S., et al. (2005). Healthy body/health spirit: Design and evaluation of a church-based nutrition and physical activity intervention using motivational interviewing. *Health Education Research, 17*, 562–573.

Rimer, B. K., & Krueter, M. W. (2006). Advancing tailored health communications: A persuasion and message effects perspective. *The Journal of Communication, 93*(4), 78–82.

Schorling, J. B., Roach, J., Siegel, M., Baturka, N., Hunt, D. E., Guterbock, T. M., et al. (1997). A trial of church-based smoking cessation interventions for rural African Americans. *Preventive Medicine, 26*, 92–101.

Simons-Morton, B. G., Donohew, L., & Crump, A. D. (1997). Health communication in the prevention of alcohol, tobacco, and drug use. *Health Education & Behavior, 24*(5), 544–554.

Skinner, C. S., Campbell, M. K., Rimer, B. K., Curry, S., & Prochaska, J. O. (1999). How effective is tailored print communication? *Annals of Behavioral Medicine, 21*, 290–298.

Stein, C. J., & Colditz, G. A. (2004). Modifiable risk factors for cancer. *British Journal of Cancer, 90*(2), 299–303.

Stillman, F. A., Bone, L. R., Rand, C., Levine, D. M., & Becker, D. M. (1993). Heart, body, and soul: A church-based smoking-cessation program for urban African Americans. *Preventive Medicine, 22*, 335–349.

Steward, B. W., & Kleihues, P. (2003). *World cancer report*. Geneva: World Health Organization, International Agency for Research on Cancer.

Strecher, V. J. (1999). Computer-tailored smoking cessation materials: A review and discussion. *Patient Education and Counseling, 36*, 107–117.

U.S. Cancer Statistics Working Group. United States Cancer Statistics: 1999–2007 *Incidence and Mortality Web-based Report*. Atlanta: U.S. Department of Health and Human Services, Centers for Disease Control and Prevention and National Cancer Institute; 2010. Retrieved from www.cdc.gov/uscs/6/8/2011

Voorhees, C. C., Stillman, F. A., Swank, R. T., Heagerty, P. J., Levine, D. M., & Becker, D. M. (1996). Heart, Body, and soul: Impact of church-based smoking cessation interventions on readiness to quit. *Preventive Medicine, 25*(3), 277–285.

Welsh, A. L., Sauaia, A., Jacobellis, J., Min, S. J., & Byers, T. (2005). The effect of two church-based interventions on breast cancer screening rates among Medicaid-insured Latinas. *Preventing Chronic Disease, 2*(4), A07.

Winett, R. A., Anderson, E. S., Wojcik, J. R., Winett, S. G., & Bowen, T. (2007). Guide to health: Outcomes of a group-randomized trial of an Internet-based, health behavior intervention in churches. *Annals of Behavioral Medicine, 33*(3), 251–261.

Winnett, R. A., Anderson, E. S., Whiteley, J. A., Wojcik, J. R., Rovniak, L. S., Graves, K. D., et al. (1999). Church-based health behavior programs: Using social cognitive theory to formulate interventions for at-risk populations. *Applied and Preventive Psychology, 8*, 129–142.

Yanek, L. R., Becker, D. M., Moy, T. F., Gittelsohn, J., & Koffman, D. M. (2001). Project Joy: Faith based cardiovascular health promotion for African American women. *Public Health Reports, 116*, 68–81.

Chapter 17
Process Evaluation of a Nursing Support Intervention with Rural African American Mothers with Preterm Infants

Margaret Shandor Miles, Suzanne Thoyre, Linda Beeber, Stephen Engelke, Mark A. Weaver, and Diane Holditch-Davis

Introduction

High-risk premature infants, those weighing less than 1,500 g or requiring mechanical ventilation, are at risk for increased neonatal morbidities and long-term neuro-developmental problems (Allen, 2008; Hack et al., 2000; Hoekstra, Ferrara, Couser, Payne, & Connett, 2004; Nosarti, Murray, & Hack, 2010). These developmental delays in cognitive, language, and motor development become evident by late preschool or early school age (Brooks-Gunn, Klebanov, Liaw, & Spiker, 1993; Engelke, Engelke, Helm, & Holbert, 1995; Hoekstra et al., 2004; Thompson et al., 1997). African Americans are not only more likely to give birth prematurely (Giscombe & Lobel, 2005; Jesse, Swanson, Newton, & Morrow, 2009), but their premature infants are also at greater risk for these developmental problems than other prematures (Brooks-Gunn, Kelbanov, & Duncan, 1996; Engelke et al., 1995; Holditch-Davis, Bartlett, & Belyea, 2000; Vohr, 2010; Zahr, 1999). Thus, prematurity and associated developmental problems are a health disparity for African American infants.

Poor developmental outcomes in prematurely born children result from multiple complex risk factors, including both biological risks (intrauterine, genetic, and postneonatal complications associated with prematurity) and environmental risks (Allen, 2008; Candelaria, O'Cnnell, & Teti, 2006; Nosarti et al., 2010; Thompson et al., 1997; Vohr, 2010). Two critical interrelated social/environmental factors associated with developmental outcomes in premature infants are poverty and the quality of parenting (Brooks-Gunn et al., 1996). Many African American mothers are single and have limited or no support from the father (Dickerson, 1995; Wilson, 1991). In the rural South, high poverty levels, low-wage jobs, low education levels, and inadequate housing are particularly difficult for African American mothers with vulnerable infants (Economic Research Service, 2003; Harris & Zimmerman, 2003; Holditch-Davis et al., 2001). Cumulative psychosocial risk associated with maternal poverty may predict parenting stress (Candelaria et al., 2006) and African American mothers are known to have high levels of and greater susceptibility to stress (Giscombe & Lobel, 2005). Despite the many cultural strengths of African American mothers (Ipsa, Thornburg, & Fine, 2006), the challenges of poverty along with maternal stress may compete with a mothers' ability to focus on infant needs (Hendrickson, Baldwin, & Allred, 2000; Singer, Daviller, Bruening, Hawkins,

M.S. Miles (✉)
School of Nursing, University of North Carolina at Chapel Hill, Chapel Hill, NC, USA
e-mail: mmiles@email.unc.edu

A.J. Lemelle et al. (eds.), *Handbook of African American Health: Social and Behavioral Interventions*, DOI 10.1007/978-1-4419-9616-9_17, © Springer Science+Business Media, LLC 2011

& Yamashita, 1996). In addition, access to adequate health care can be challenging and many African Americans distrust and are uncomfortable with the health care system as a result of experiences of discrimination or poor care (American Academy of Pediatrics Committee on Pediatric Research, 2000; Hausman, Jeong, Bost, & Ibrahim, 2008; Smedley, Stith, & Nelson, 2003). Thus, the follow-up health care of premature infants, especially in rural communities, may be inadequate (Engelke et al., 1995; Hendrickson et al., 2000; Leventhal, Brooks-Gunn, McCormick, & McCarton, 2000; Newacheck, Hughes, & Stoddard, 1996).

Parenting by African American mothers of premature infants may also be altered due to maternal trauma and distress related to the infant's birth and hospitalization. High-risk premature infants experience prolonged hospitalizations where they are treated for a multitude of complications. Mothers are stressed by seeing their tiny, frail infants surrounded by technology and undergoing invasive treatments (Miles, Burchinal, Holditch-Davis, Brunssen, & Wilson, 2002; Reichman, Miller, Gordon, & Hendricks-Munoz, 2000). Mothers are also challenged in taking on their maternal role due to the infant's fragile medical state and prolonged hospitalization that necessitates separation (Black, Holditch-Davis, & Miles, 2009). They must share parenting with nurses and experience delays in taking on basic maternal roles such as holding, feeding, and bathing (Miles & Frauman, 1993). After discharge, mothers have concerns about parenting issues such as feeding the infant, continued health problems, infections, and sleep patterns (Gennaro, Zukowsky, Brooten, Lowell, & Visco, 1990; Miles, Holditch-Davis, Thoyre, & Beeber, 2005; Thoyre, 2007).

Memories of the infants' illness and hospitalization may continue long after discharge (Affleck, Tennen, Rowe, & Higgins, 1990; Holditch-Davis & Miles, 2000; Wereszczak, Miles, & Holditch-Davis, 1997) and African American mothers' perceptions of their premature infants during hospitalization affects their views of the infants after discharge (Teti, Hess, & O'Connell, 2005). Furthermore, maternal distress, particularly anxiety and depressive symptoms, may be long lasting (Garel, Dardennes, & Blondel, 2007; Holditch-Davis, Miles, Weaver, Black, et al., 2009; Miles, Holditch-Davis, Schwartz, & Sher, 2007; Peebles-Kleiger, 2000). Some mothers may even experience post-traumatic stress symptoms long after the baby has gone home (Holditch-Davis, Bartlett, Blickman, & Miles, 2003; Shaw et al., 2009).

This maternal distress may impact on the mother–infant relationship (Garel et al., 2007; Pierrehumbert, Nicole, Muller-Nix, Forcada-Guex, & Ansermet, 2003; Zelkowitz, Bardin, & Papageorgiou, 2007). A number of researchers have identified negative effects of continued maternal distress on the maternal interactions with their infants (Feeley, Gottlieb, & Zelkowitz, 2005; Holditch-Davis et al., 2000; Pierrehumbert et al., 2003; Singer et al., 2003). Our previous research found that African American mothers parenting 3-year-old prematurely born children viewed their children as vulnerable and were protective, while at the same time, they wanted to see their infants as healthy, rather than as needing ongoing developmental and health services (Miles & Holditch-Davis, 1995). In some families, this resulted in delays in seeking needed developmental or health care for the infant (Huber, Holditch-Davis, & Brandon, 1993). In summary, rural poverty of African American mothers coupled with their distress related to the infants' hospitalization may not only interfere with use of services for premature infants but also with the mothers' abilities to parent in ways that promote child development. Yet, despite these challenges faced by low-income, rural African American mothers with preterm infants, no intervention studies have focused on this population.

Interventions with high-risk mothers that are provided in the home have been found to be effective in improving maternal psychological well-being, parenting, and developmental outcomes of the children (Astuto & Allen, 2009; Luthar & Suchman, 1999; Olds et al., 2004). In addition, early intervention programs with at-risk infants such as premature-infants became a mandated federal program, although access to these services can be limited due to state budget constraints (Herrick & Farel, 1995; Meisels, 1989). A number of studies of home interventions developed for mothers and their preterm infants have been conducted over the past two decades (Infant Health and Development Program, 1990; Kang et al., 1995; Meyer et al., 1994; Resnick, Armstrong, & Carter, 1988). A critical factor in successful intervention programs has been a strong relationship-based approach in helping mothers.

Purpose and Framework

This chapter describes a Preterm Maternal Support Intervention we designed for rural, African American mothers with preterm infants and our process evaluation of the intervention (feasibility, acceptability, and helpfulness to mothers). The aim of the nursing intervention was to improve maternal psychological well-being, enhance parenting, and improve infant developmental outcomes. The dynamic systems view of the mother–infant dyad was the theoretical framework for the intervention (Cairns, Elder, & Costello, 1996; Lewis, 2000; Miles & Holditch-Davis, 2003). Figure 17.1 displays the framework model. In this framework, infant development is a function of the infant's innate capabilities, the mother, and mother–infant interactions. The mother and infant also are imbedded in the family system, which can provide parenting support or be a source of stress. Our key assumption was that to make a significant impact on the mother–infant system, attention must be paid to maternal well being and build on her personal and cultural strengths (Barnard, Snyder, & Spietz, 1991; DeJoseph, Norbeck, Smith, & Miller, 1996; Heinicke et al., 1999 Luthar & Suchman, 1999, 2000).

Methods

African American mothers of premature infants were recruited for this clinical trial from neonatal intensive care units (NICUs) of two tertiary care university hospitals in the Southeast. Both served families from small towns and rural areas of the state. These NICUs were staffed by neonatologists, neonatal nurse practitioners, pediatric surgeons, and other subspecialists.

Mothers and Infants

African American mothers of preterm infants who weighed less than 1,500 g or required mechanical ventilation were recruited. Both singleton infants and twins were included (one infant was randomly selected from each twin set). Infants with congenital neurological problems, who were symptomatic

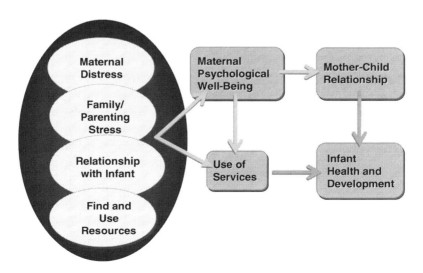

Fig. 17.1 Ecological, dynamic systems framework

Table 17.1 Demographics of the mothers

Demographic characteristics	Control mothers, $n=90$	Intervention mothers, $n=87$
Mean age (SD)*	24.9 (6.2)	26.8 (6.7)
% Married	25.8	27.5
% First time mothers	28.8	22.9
Mean years education (SD)	12.5 (1.9)	12.7 (1.8)
% C-section	52.8	55.8
% Public assistance	52.2	53.5

*$p<0.05$

from substance exposure, who were hospitalized longer than 2 months postterm, or who were part of a higher order multiple set were excluded. Mothers were randomized into either the support intervention ($n=87$) or a control group who received usual care ($n=90$). Table 17.1 describes the sample of mothers and infants.

Description of the Intervention

The aim of the intervention was to improve maternal psychological well-being by (a) processing the mothering experience with mothers to resolve distress related to preterm birth and hospitalization, (b) supporting them as they developed their relationship with their babies, (c) guiding them in reducing daily stress, and (d) strengthening their ability to identify and use family support and community and health resources. Advanced practice nurses used a Guided Discovery approach (Luthar & Suchman, 2000) to provide the intervention via hospital, home, and phone contacts until the infant was 18 months corrected age. A hospital contact was made when the infant was stable and usually in intermediate care. Home visits were made at approximately 1–2 weeks after discharge and when the infant was 5, 10, and 15 months corrected age. Telephone contacts were made in between these in-person contacts and until 18 months to maintain contact with the mothers, evaluate their situation, and problem solve issues that the mothers identified.

Guided Discovery builds on the cultural strengths of the mother and places her in control by responding to her concerns (Luthar & Suchman, 2000). Rather than teaching the mother, the nurses used insight-oriented skill facilitation to help mothers explore issues of concern, identify her strengths and resources, examine her strategies, and guide her toward developing optimal approaches to deal with the concern or find acceptable resources. Six steps were used: (a) focusing on the mother and her needs within the broader family context; (b) encouraging the mother to fully explore her concerns; (c) acknowledging her strengths and capabilities, reinforcing positive outcomes, and showing trust in her ability to manage concerns; (d) joining with the mother in examining any limitations of her strategies and guiding her in developing new approaches; (e) assisting the mother to develop her plan of action and to identify any additional skills she might need; and (f) at a later contact, helping the mother evaluate her plans and actions.

Critical to Guided Discovery was the establishment of a therapeutic relationship based on mutual trust with the mother. Studies have found that a trusting, positive relationship in which the woman feels emotionally safe is pivotal in effectively intervening with African American women (Combs & Gonzalez, 1994; Heinicke et al., 1999; Ivey & Ivey, 1999; Luthar & Suchman, 1999). Four keys to establishing this relationship were (a) maintaining professional behaviors, such as being trustworthy and nonjudgmental, maintaining confidentiality, and showing professional competence; (b) interacting with the mother in a way that she felt valued, understood, and cared about; and (c) facilitating mutuality by working collaboratively with the mother to achieve her parenting and personal goals.

Another essential approach involved understanding and respecting the mothers' rural African American culture and building on her cultural strengths (Beeber et al., 2007; Boyd-Franklin, 1989;

Cross, Bazron, Dennis, & Issacs, 1989; Ipsa et al., 2006; Yoos, Kitzman, Olds, & Overacker, 1995). Strategies included acknowledging the importance of the maternal role and respecting her parenting style. Nurses explored the role of the larger kinship network with the mother, including the mothers' relationship with the father, and were sensitive to potential maternal role stress due to their tendency to focus on the needs of others in the family. Respect was shown for the cultural strengths of the mother, such as their personal spirituality, as resources in times of stress (Polzer & Miles, 2008; Wilson & Miles, 2001). In addition, the nurses were sensitive to barriers these rural, African American mothers might face in accessing services such as pediatricians or early intervention because of past experiences with racism or poor care (American Academy of Pediatrics Committee on Pediatric Research, 2000; Newacheck et al., 1996).

Therapeutic interviewing strategies were used as part of the Guided Discovery approach. For example, active listening and directive exploration helped mothers fully identify their feelings and concerns. Reflective comments helped mothers feel understood. Summarization helped them identify common threads in feelings and concerns. Encouragement and positive responses fostered their strengths and enhanced self-esteem. Normalization helped mothers understand that other mothers of preterm infants have similar experiences or feelings. Skill development also focused on strategies such as time management, problem solving, self-affirmation strategies, and advocacy skills (Combs & Gonzalez, 1994; Heinicke et al., 1999; Ivey & Ivey, 1999; Luthar & Suchman, 1999).

Specific Intervention Goals and Strategies

Using the Guided Discovery approach, the intervention nurses' interactions with the mothers focused on four specific strategies: processing the mothering experiences, supporting the maternal relationship with the infants, reducing stress, and selecting and fitting resources.

Processing the mothering experience. One goal of the intervention was to help mothers process the mothering experience to reduce distress related to the birth and hospitalization of a premature infant. The nurse guided the mother to talk about her pregnancy, birth, and NICU experience; acknowledged and normalized her feelings; explored her family response to the infant's birth; and helped her reframe the story by recalling positive memories and her strengths in coping with the experience. Mothers were given a baby album to record information and keep mementos about the baby's birth, hospitalization, homecoming, and development. This included photos of the mother and her infant taken by the nurse at each contact. At the 10-month home visit, nurses began co-constructing with mothers a birth story that included not only stressful memories but also positive meanings and memories. The mother then chose photos to be included in a story and picture book given to her at the end of the study.

Supporting the maternal relationship with the infant. Another goal was to support the mother in developing her relationship with her infant and meeting complex infant health and developmental needs. Mothers were offered an opportunity to share their experiences and concerns in relating to and caring for their infants. The nurse listened for feelings, accomplishments, and concerns about parenting such as those related to feeding, sleeping, development, health, and behavioral management. Principles of Guided Discovery were used to explore the concerns, reinforce the mother's strengths in handling them, guide her to identify limitations of her current strategies, and assist her in exploring new approaches. The nurse also observed the mother playing with her baby, pointed out aspects of the babies' needs or behavior, and gave positive affirmation for responsive maternal behaviors. Sessions with the mother were supplemented by reinforcing the use of a manual about the care of premature infants provided in this state to all parents of preterm infants. Additional pamphlets and handouts were provided as needed.

Reducing stress. A third goal was to help the mother identify and reduce stress related to work, family life, and family relationships. Attentive listening and questioning were used to help the mother explore these stressors and share and acknowledge emotional states such as depression and worry. Using a Guided Discovery process, the nurse helped the mother process at least one area of stress by exploring the source of stress, examining strengths and limitations of strategies used, identifying new approaches and resources, and developing or strengthening skills. For example, time-management skills might help a mother set priorities and organize her day, and advocacy skills might help her seek support from others in her kin or friendship network. Strategies to minimize stressful interpersonal interactions and improve relationships might be discussed. Emphasis was placed on the importance of self-care in order to have energy to care for the baby.

Selecting and fitting resources. A final intervention goal was to empower the mother to find and use resources for her infant and herself. Mothers were guided in determining resources needed by her infant, particularly pediatric care, early intervention, and child services coordination with public health nurses; assisted in exploring where to obtain services that were acceptable to her; provided guidance in strengthening advocacy skills to access services; and encouraged to use these resources. While exploring the mothers' views of services, the nurses were sensitive about her beliefs or experiences with racism or poor care that might cause her to hesitate in using certain agencies or providers. Strategies were identified to make visits more effective such as writing down concerns and desired outcomes, communicating requests clearly, acknowledging responses, and repeating requests if not heard. Role play was used as needed to help the mother gain necessary skills. As part of the process, barriers such as distance, transportation, work, babysitting, waiting for appointments, and cost were explored, and the mother was guided toward identifying solutions. The intervention nurses did not have direct contact with the public health nurse or other providers, unless requested by the mother, as the goal of the intervention was to empower mothers to access and use resources.

Training of the Intervention Nurses

Advanced practice nurses with experience in neonatal, maternal–child, public health, pediatric or psychiatric/mental health nursing conducted the intervention. Training included didactic lectures, seminar discussion, case studies, films, readings, and role play. A major focus was on maternal response to preterm birth and parenting of premature infants. Neonatal nurse clinicians and an early intervention specialist met with the team to inform them about the infant services available such as early intervention programs and developmental evaluation centers. Training also included an in-depth discussion of cultural proficiency. The nurses read literature on African American families and parenting. An African American mother with a prematurely born child joined the team to assist with cultural competency and to consult with the nurses. The principles of Guided Discovery and therapeutic communication were emphasized. In addition, an investigator with psychiatric-mental health expertise provided training in handling intense emotional distress. This included a review of protocols for handling child neglect or abuse, mental health crises or domestic abuse, and suicide screening. Throughout the intervention supervision meetings were used to review cases, critique intervention strategies, and provide guidance for future contacts.

Intervention Procedures

The study was approved by the institutional review board of each university. Mothers were recruited by staff on the NICU units. They were told about the study by staff. If they were interested in learning more about it, their name was given to the research team. The recruitment team then gave mothers full information about the study and mothers signed a consent form for their and their infant's participation in the study. After consent procedures, mothers were randomized into the control or intervention group and enrollment data were collected. If in the intervention group, the intervention nurse contacted the mother to schedule the first hospital contact. Mothers in the control group received the usual care provided by the hospital follow-up team and any community services they were eligible to receive.

Process Evaluation

Our process evaluation examined: (a) feasibility, (b) acceptability, and (c) helpfulness to mothers. Outcome data regarding the effectiveness of the intervention, which focused on maternal psychological well-being, mother–infant interaction, and child health and developmental outcomes, are described elsewhere (Holditch-Davis et al., 2010; Holditch-Davis, Miles, Weaver, Black, et al., 2009, Holditch-Davis, Miles, Weaver, Thoyre, et al., 2009).

Feasibility

Feasibility included an evaluation of recruitment, retention, and dosage. We also critically analyze the challenges faced and share strategies used to meet these challenges. Data regarding recruitment were obtained from records kept by the recruitment team. Data regarding retention and dosage were collected from intervention nurse log sheets. On the logs, nurses recorded each visit, the time spent at each contact with the mother, including phone interventions, phone calls from the mother, and hospital and home visits. Missed appointments or difficulty making appointments were recorded in the field notes.

Recruitment, retention, and dosage. One hundred and seventy-seven rural African American mothers were recruited in the study with 90 randomized to the control group and 87 to the intervention group. The mothers were on the average about 27 years of age and had at least a high school education (87%). A majority of mothers were unmarried (73%), were first time mothers (74%), and about half were on public assistance (49%). Table 17.1 shows the maternal demographics and Table 17.2 the infant characteristics by control and intervention group.

Most of the intervention mothers ($n=66$; 76%) completed the study, while three were never located after enrollment. The causes of intervention dropouts with the remaining 18 mothers were death of the infant ($n=1$), relocation out of state ($n=2$), request of the mother ($n=1$), and difficulty maintaining contact ($n=14$).

The dosage of the intervention, measured by the number of in-person contacts, was affected by attrition as well as delays in making contacts or missed appointments. In addition, some mothers with special needs had more visits or phone calls. Twenty-one mothers had a limited dose (1.33 in-person

Table 17.2 Infant characteristics

	Control infants	Intervention infants
% Male	44.4	41.3
Mean gestational age (SD)	28.2 (3.0)	28.5 (2.8)
Mean birth weight (SD)	1,105 (409)	1,100 (376)
Mean neurological insults (SD)	3.0 (2.9)	2.5 (2.4)
Mean days on mechanical ventilation (SD)	17.4 (28.6)	11.7 (17.2)
% Intraventricular brain hemorrhage	28.2	15.0
% Patent ductus arteriosis*	46.1	31.0

*$p<0.05$

contacts, 2.05 phone contacts), 27 had a moderate dose (2.72 in-person contacts, 3.38 phone contacts), and 36 completed all or most of the 18-month long intervention (3.77 in-person contacts, 6.67 phone contacts). Mothers were clustered into distress groups based on their levels of NICU stress, depressive symptoms, anxiety, and daily hassles (see Holditch-Davis, Miles, Weaver, Black, et al., 2009). There was no difference in dosage of the intervention by level of distress.

Challenges faced. A number of challenges affected maintaining contact with the intervention mothers. One was the technological advances leading to increased mobile phone use in rural areas. Over time, the number of mothers who had landline phones decreased and cell phones created numerous challenges. Since cell phone calls are charged for both incoming and outgoing calls, even brief calls to make or verify appointments for home visits cost the mothers money. In addition, cell phones were often cut off during the month when the paid cell phone time was used up, and mothers then could not be reached until the beginning of the next month. Cell phones were sometimes shared among family members or with the baby's father or friends who could serve as gatekeepers for calls. This also limited privacy. One solution we tried was prepaid phone cards, but these were only rarely used probably because of limitations in access to landlines and difficulty finding pay phones in a confidential, quiet area.

Another issue for maintaining contact was that a number of mothers moved during the study and were difficult to reach in their new residences. A few mothers moved out of state or to a distant city beyond the study range. These numbers were higher than past studies of mothers that we had conducted in these rural areas (Holditch-Davis et al., 2000; Miles et al., 2007). We hypothesized that the economic downturn in the rural South over the past 5–10 years with loss of industry and jobs and the scarce and inadequate housing in the rural South influenced these moves (Harris & Zimmerman, 2003).

Distance from the university research site to the women's rural homes was another challenge. This problem was inevitable in a study of rural mothers since only a small number of premature infants were located in any one town. Nurses often had to travel very long distances (up to 4 h one way) to meet with many of the mothers. When a mother did not show for an appointment, making a return trip was difficult. Too, making extra visits for mothers with special needs was sometimes difficult to carry out due to time and budget constraints.

Design challenges. The longitudinal nature of the intervention which spanned over 18 months coupled with the infrequency of home visits and the long intervals between visits (four home visits at intervals between 4 and 6 months) presented a number of challenges affecting dosage. For one thing, it may have affected the mothers' investment in and interest in the intervention over time. As noted earlier, phone contacts in between home visits, intended to maintain contact, were effective for some mothers but were not always feasible.

The length of the intervention also may have intersected with changing maternal needs and focus. As the preterm infants stabilized and mothers returned to work or school, the focus of the mothers was more on their daily hassles and economic survival than on issues related to their infants and their own mental health. This was particularly true for single mothers who were extremely busy.

Given the length of the intervention, we also experienced nurse turnover as nurses (two full-time and two part-time nurses moved or found other positions). Nurse turnover clearly was a factor in subject loss. For each case that was incomplete when the nurse left the study, steps were taken for transitioning to the new nurse. This included informing the mother before the final visit by the first nurse and double visits in some cases by both nurses. Nevertheless, the newly assigned nurses often had difficulty reaching the mother to continue the intervention or mothers' discontinued the study shortly after the new nurse began. In addition, we found that full time nurses were more committed to the project.

The skills and sensitivity of the nurses also varied and probably affected retention as well as other aspects of implementing the intervention. Personality, experience, neonatal background, and expertise in counseling were interrelated factors. Cultural match may have been another factor.

This included matching based on sensitivity to the rural Southern culture and to the African American culture of the mothers. Finding advanced practice nurses who were minorities was difficult. We had one African American nurse and, because of difficulty in finding others, we hired an African American mother who had a prematurely born child to consult with the nurses and contact select mothers with special needs. We found that the most salient characteristic of effective intervention nurses was their skill in listening, caring, and showing sensitivity to the culture of the women.

Strategies used. Approaches used to strengthen retention included phone calls and notes. Phone calls were used to maintain a relationship with the mother between in-person contacts. As noted earlier, due to challenges with phones and the mothers' busy schedules, these were not always as frequent as desired. On the other hand, some mothers liked phone contacts more than home visits since they were less disruptive of routines, and they readily used the phone contacts to share ongoing concerns. After each home visit, the nurse wrote a personal note to the mother to thank her for the visit, summarize key issues that were discussed, provide brief information about anticipated developmental changes in the infant over the next few months, and note the timing of the next contact. Photos were often put into the notes.

For mothers whom the nurses could not reach for appointments or who did not show for an appointment, carefully and sensitively worded "concern" letters were mailed. The nurse mentioned the difficulty reaching the mother, reminded her of the study and its goals, and included the 1–800 number for them to call should they wish to resume the intervention. The notes also indicated that they were free to withdraw if they wished. These letters were effective in helping many mothers return to the intervention. If mothers did not respond to the "concern" letter, another similarly sensitive letter was sent to the mother indicating that because of our difficulty reaching her, she would no longer be in the intervention program. Several mothers responded to this final letter and re-engaged.

Acceptability

Acceptability focused on the salience of the four intervention goals and the strategies used to achieve these goals. Content analysis and team discussion of field notes were used in analysis. These notes were written immediately after each contact using a macro on the computer. Field notes included a description of the setting, the presence and level of involvement of family members in the intervention, and observations of the mother, infant, and mother–infant interactions. An in-depth description was written about how each aspect of the intervention was conducted (relationship building, processing mothering, stress reduction, maternal relationship with the infant, resource identification, and closure). Verbal and nonverbal responses of the mother and any concerns were recorded, along with plans for the next visit. Brief case reports of several cases are presented as examples at the end of the chapter. Note that these case reports focus on only one aspect of the mothers' intervention.

Process the mothering experience. One goal of the intervention was to help the mother process the mothering experiences and distress related to the infant's birth and hospitalization. The chief strategy for achieving this goal was helping the mother share her experiences and explore her feelings, as well as helping her focus on her strengths in coping with this difficult period. Sharing of the story was most salient at the first contact in the hospital and, to some extent, the first home visit. At the 10-month visit, mothers were offered opportunities to retrospectively recall their experiences. While this was salient for some mothers, many had moved on to other aspects of their lives and did not respond. A few mothers said that they did not want to think about the stress surrounding their child's birth and hospitalization. Most mothers, however, did take up the opportunity to co-create with the nurse a story and photo book that focused on positive memories and on her strength as a mother. See Box 17.1.

Box 17.1 Natasha

Natasha shared with the nurse her long-term denial of the unplanned pregnancy and her avoidance of prenatal care because she was fearful of another preterm birth from preeclampsia. Indeed, when she finally had a prenatal visit, she was immediately admitted to the hospital. Faced with a decision to have a caesarian section, she argued with the doctor because she was scared due to frightening stories her sister told her. Finally, she agreed only after she was told there was a 50% chance she or the baby could die. Her son subsequently had many complications and a long hospitalization which delayed opportunities to take on mothering roles. With three other children at home, she was unable to visit often and the staff began nagging her about her infrequent visiting patterns. The nurse helped Natasha identify staff she could trust to talk about her challenges in visiting. Throughout the course of the intervention, the mother increasingly shared with the nurse her experiences in the NICU, including her intense reaction to being told that she might die, leaving her children without a mother, or that her baby might die. Sharing with the nurse and writing her experiences in the baby book helped her process the hard times and recall some good memories. At the end of the study, Natasha was preparing to take the baby back to the NICU to see the nurses and donate clothing for other babies.

Box 17.2 Joana

Joana was a single mom who had been abandoned by her mother in infancy. She was living with her aunt and uncle when her preterm infant was born. Her aunt was supportive but her uncle was verbally abusive and sexually threatening. The father of the baby was not involved. The pregnancy was not planned and she felt guilty because she tried several times to cause a miscarriage. However, once her daughter was born she quickly became very attached as she wanted to give her the mothering she had never received. The baby had many complications and a long hospitalization and discharge was delayed because of poor weight gain and reflux. Since the baby had previously had feeding problems and reflux, the nurse guided the mother in successfully breast feeding the baby. Joana also had questions about other aspects of infant nutrition and childcare throughout the intervention. At the time of discharge, the nurse guided the mother as she needed to secure many needed services such as the Women, Infants, and Children nutrition program, aid to dependent children, early intervention, and pediatric follow-up. An important intervention was helping the mother see that although she articulated what she needed and who she was going to contact for services, she frequently did not follow through with her plans. Two of Joana personal goals were to attend cosmetology school and find housing apart from her aunt and uncle. By the end of study, she had achieved these goals and was feeling successful in mothering her daughter.

Mother–infant relationship and parenting. An ongoing goal of the intervention was to help mothers as they developed their relationship with their infant and their parenting skills. Mothers particularly responded to positive feedback from the nurse about their relationship with the baby and their parenting. They also used the nurses to identify strategies for parenting issues such as feeding the baby, sleeping behaviors, and concerns about infections (Miles et al., 2005). Another major issue was finding appropriate childcare when the mother returned to work. While some mothers wanted guidance in developmental stimulation or shared concerns about development, many were unaware of or not concerned about developmental delays that are not yet obvious in the first year of life. See Box 17.2.

Box 17.3 Kalia

Kalia was an 18-year-old mother whose preterm infant was born via caesarian section after Kalia started bleeding at school during her 27th week of pregnancy. When she first saw her baby, she was shocked and cried for several days. Her baby had a difficult course in the NICU and Kalia first held her just before she went to the operating room for heart surgery. The baby came home with a heart monitor and a gastrostomy tube due to a paralyzed vocal cord. The nurse helped Kalia share her concerns during this time and supported her in learning new skills in caring for a baby as well as mothering a sick infant. Kalia's major source of distress during the intervention revolved around her relationship with the baby's father who left her soon after birth for another woman. Kalia became particularly distraught when the father told her that he wished God would take the baby away. He and his girlfriend accused Kalia of causing the early labor and threatened her with hateful comments. At one point, Kalia and the other woman had a fist fight that involved authorities. This was extremely stressful to Kalia. The nurse, along with the African American mother on our team, provided intensive support to the mother and helped her seek counseling for her ensuing depression from an acceptable professional (a previous mental health professional had severely upset her). With the help of her supportive parents and the research team, Kalia eventually learned to cope with her status as a single mother and with managing mothering and school work. By the end of the study, she had finished high school and was accepted in the nursing program at the local university.

Maternal stress. Another goal of the intervention was to reduce maternal stress. Most of the mothers brought up stressors related to poverty, housing, and jobs. Keeping food on the table with minimal income and finding jobs that paid an adequate wage were constant struggles. Many mothers had issues related to housing. Some lived in very crowded conditions with various relatives or friends and often moved seeking more privacy and space. Others lived in very poor rental housing and had dreams of living in their own home. The nurses helped the mothers problem-solve and strategize regarding how to overcome these issues and find resources in their communities. However, jobs, housing, and other resources were often hard to find in these rural communities.

A considerable number of mothers shared distress associated with interpersonal relationships with grandparents, other family members, and friends. Of particular note was conflicts in their relationship with the baby's father (Miles et al., 2008). Conflicts with the father were more common in unmarried couples who were not living together. These conflicts revolved around (a) relationship issues including domestic violence, desire for a romantic or more supportive relationship, and anger regarding other women in his life; (b) his relationship with the baby and assistance with childcare including child support; and (c) social issues such as drug use or imprisonment. Interventions with the mothers included strategies such as helping her to explore the sources of the conflict, to develop skills in asking for what they wanted, and to be assertive about breaking off an undesired relationship. See Box 17.3.

Find and use resources. Throughout the intervention, a goal was helping the mothers to find and use needed resources for themselves and for their infant. One common issue was finding acceptable primary care for the baby in the local community. Some mothers felt providers were not familiar with the special needs of preterm infants. When mothers were not satisfied with care, the nurse helped the mother advocate for her child or change providers. For example, a nurse helped one mother who distrusted her pediatrician to assess her concerns, identify her goal, and help her find a more satisfactory primary care physician in a nearby community. See Box 17.4.

Box 17.4 Lakea

Lakea was a mother with a history of drug abuse. Two of her previous children were in the custody of her mother due to drug use. During the first home visit, the mother shared her intense fear of losing custody of her prematurely born-son and her determination to be a good mother to him. The nurse also noted that Lakea was severely depressed and was concerned about the possible return to drug abuse to cope with the sadness. Hence a major goal for this mother was to listen to her concerns, help her identify support systems, and to get her into mental health therapy. This mother lived with the father of her baby and the nurse helped the mother see that, although he was not a romantic partner or good communicator, he was an important part of her support system because he was a wonderful father to the baby. Since no agency would see her without funding and the mother was unable to contact Medicaid herself, the nurse directly helped her follow-through with the application process and identified an appropriate agency for therapy. The nurse also helped her to find a community program to obtain her GED and assisted her in identifying child care services when she was ready to work. At the end of the study, the mother was proud of her son, now a thriving toddler. She even took him back to the NICU to show all the nurses. However, she still talked about her fear of losing custody of her son.

A major goal of the intervention was to support mothers in obtaining and keeping their infant in early intervention services. However, the availability of these services was greatly reduced due to state budget cuts, shifts in policies, and reorganization of state and county services. Thus, helping mothers learn to advocate agencies for needed services was critical.

Mothers who had issues with the father were helped to find resources such as legal action to obtain child support and shelters and agencies to help with domestic violence. Mothers in need of mental health services were helped in finding acceptable health and mental health resources for themselves.

Maternal Perceptions of the Helpfulness of the Intervention

At the end of the study mothers in both the control and intervention group completed a helpfulness survey. Because both control and intervention mothers completed this survey, the instrument referred to the "study" rather than the "intervention." Mothers were asked to use a 4-point rating scale to rate the helpfulness of 14 strategies that were integral to the intervention. This included learning about the baby, sharing feelings, thinking about caring for myself, and talking about the pregnancy and birth of the infants. In presenting these data, we compare the control and intervention group outcomes.

Mothers in the intervention group had significantly higher helpfulness scores than control mothers ($p \leq 0.01$). The mean total helpfulness scores for intervention mothers was 33.41 (SD = 11.44) and for the control mothers was 26.64 (SD = 13.02). Table 17.3 shows the items rated as most helpful for mothers in each group. Sharing feelings, learning about the baby, learning how to play with the baby, and assistance in how to talk with doctors and nurses were the areas of the intervention rated as most helpful by intervention mothers. Interestingly, control mothers rated feeling good as a mother slightly higher than intervention mothers, suggesting that the experience of data collection and contact with the data collection team was, in and of itself, helpful. The items with lowest endorsement were learning how to reduce stress and finding ways to ask family and friends for support.

Table 17.3 Perception of the study: helpfulness

Survey item	Intervention mothers (%)	Control mothers (%)
The study was helpful to me in:		
Learning about baby's needs	84	75
How to play with/teach baby	82	63
How to talk with doctors/nurses	82	62
Sharing feelings	80	66
Feeling good as a mother	78	80
Remember positive things about birth/hospitalization	78	70
Know my coping strengths	78	63
Answer to questions about parenting	76	58
Think about caring for myself	76	53
Talk about pregnancy/birth	76	64

Mothers also rated how much they changed as a person and as a mother as a result of being in the study on 3-point scale ranging from "I did not change" to "I changed a lot." Most intervention mothers indicated that they had changed as a person "some" (49%) or "a lot" (34%). Scores for the control mothers were significantly lower but still a majority had indicated that they changed. Both mothers in the intervention and control group indicated that they had changed as a mother but at slightly lower levels ("some" = 49% and "a lot" = 22%).

Comments from the mothers as recorded by the nurses in field notes are also revealing. One intervention mother noted: "I've grown physically and mentally. I didn't let this early birth stop my dreams. I've finished college and now I'm a certified teacher." Another mother focused proudly on her increased sense of responsibility in caring for her infant: "As a mother I realized the great responsibility that I had to take on. I had to become aware of her medical problems, keep all appointments, make sure I was on time, [and] make sure everything was accurate."

Control mothers also revealed change. One mother indicated that she had "changed as a person by being able to deal with my inner feelings and put them in perspective." Another learned better ways to cope with different issues associated with the baby. One clue about why control mothers reported change is found in a comment made my one control mother: "[The] questions let me know what I needed to work on."

Discussion and Implications for Practice

Our process evaluation of the Preterm Maternal Support intervention provides insight into successes and challenges in providing an in-home intervention with rural low-income mothers. The intervention strategies were helpful to mothers in sharing the distress associated with their premature delivery and hospitalization of their small preterm infant, in developing their relationship with and parenting their prematurely born-child, in managing related to work, family life, and family relationships, and in identifying and using resources to support them and their child. Mothers' needs for support related to each goal changed over time and it differed among mothers. Early contacts with mothers tended to focus more on the mother's experiences during hospitalization and early maternal caregiving. As mothers adjusted to their maternal caregiving role, they began to focus more on other stressors in their lives such as managing school and work, financial concerns, and, for some mothers, interpersonal conflicts with the father and the extended family. Helping mothers identify their need for support and resources, find such resources, and advocate to obtain them was a consistent theme throughout, although the resources needed changed over time. This holistic approach, coupled with our individualized strategies, allowed the mother to focus on her concerns and needs rather than having a scripted intervention guide.

The Guided Discovery approach along with development of a therapeutic relationship of mutual trust with the mothers was critical. As noted by Beeber et al. (2007), a therapeutic relationship is especially important for mothers who are depressed. Furthermore, it was important to respect the mothers' cultural and personal strengths (Ipsa et al., 2006). This approach has been found helpful in other similar studies (Barnard et al., 1991; Beeber et al., 2007; Heinicke et al., 1999; Luthar & Suchman, 1999, 2000). To accomplish this, intervention staff must be chosen based on their cultural sensitivity; their ability to be accepting, caring, and patient; and their experience in counseling and/ or working with the population of interest. While cultural matching is important, these characteristics of staff are the most important attributes of a successful intervener. Too, intensive training before and during such interventions is critical.

One approach to enhance cultural sensitivity, while also providing access to professional evaluation, advice, and therapeutic counseling, might be joint intervention by a professional such as a nurse and a local mother who has successfully reared a preterm infant. This would also address the distance barrier allowing the nurse to intervene less frequently or through guiding the lay mother. Indeed, our African American mother who had a prematurely born-son was effective, in collaboration with the nurse in helping some of our most complicated mothers. They often shared things with her that they did not share with the nurse.

The challenges that we encountered in retention of mothers in our longitudinal intervention have been reported by other parenting interventions with low-income mothers who have busy lives (Barnard et al., 1991; Beeber et al., 2007; Garvey, Julion, Fogg, Kratovil, & Gross, 2006). Low-income mothers have many pressures including maintaining a household with minimal finances, caring for other children or family members, and keeping up with work or school. Additionally, life events and crises add to the struggle to manage many competing demands. Our mothers also had the demand of caring for a prematurely born-infant some of whom had special health and developmental needs. As noted by Garvey et al. (2006), low-income mothers who are struggling with immediate problems use their energies to focus on current crises rather than future worries, such as future developmental outcomes of their preterm infant.

Too, many mothers lived with other family members, the baby's father, or others under crowded conditions. This challenged their privacy during home calls and visits. While phone calls are a cost-effective approach to reaching rural mothers (Muender, Moore, Chen, & Sevick, 2000), many mothers did not have reliable phone access. Cell phones were both helpful and a deterrent to connecting with mothers, as they were often disconnected when they ran out of minutes. Nevertheless, phone interventions were very helpful for certain mothers in the study who found home visits less desirable. Learning more about effective ways to reach rural mothers using telephones and other upcoming technology is needed.

Triangulation of the maternal rating of the intervention with the field notes provides insight into how the intervention worked for mothers. It is interesting that the opportunity to share, learn about her infant's needs, and how to talk with doctors and other health professionals were rated the highest. This supports the data from field notes that three of the goals of the intervention – processing feelings about the birth and hospitalization of the infant, helping mothers establish their relationship with and care of their infant, and accessing resources were helpful to the mothers. It is interesting that fewer mothers found the goal of maternal stress reduction as helpful. This suggests that future interventions should encompass a stronger stress reduction component that might include more structured strategies such as use of music, meditation, bible reading, and prayer to reduce feelings of stress.

It is interesting that a high percentage of control group mothers also rated aspects of the study as helpful. This suggests that more attention must be paid in design and analysis to what the control groups get from being in a study. In our longitudinal descriptive study of parenting by HIV positive African Americans, we asked at the end of study what they thought about their participation and whether they had changed as a result of being in the study. Many mothers indicated that they had become a better parent. They learned about parenting from answering the questionnaires which made them think about parenting, from watching the staff conducting developmental assessments of their children, and from sharing their stories with the interviewers (Mallory, Miles, & Holditch-Davis, 2002). We also learned from these mothers that they stayed in the study because they were gaining something from the study and also because they felt they were helping the researchers by contributing to understanding the needs of mothers like them. This concept of reciprocity in research needs further exploration. We strongly recommend that participants at the end of a longitudinal study be asked what they thought about the study and how they changed as a result of participating. In addition, a brief survey assessing the helpfulness of aspects of the intervention is a useful way of evaluating the impact of an intervention study on control and intervention participants.

Our study reinforces current knowledge about prematurity as a health disparity. African American mothers are at risk of having a premature birth. Health problems such as hypertension and social issues such as stress and racism may contribute to this health disparity. In addition, rural mothers may have inadequate access to or may not take advantage of prenatal care. This health disparity continues for their prematurely born-children who are at risk of health and developmental problems. Poverty, maternal stress, and inadequate infant day care for these high risk infants also impact on the health and development of these vulnerable infants. The overall goal of our intervention was to prevent or reduce developmental and health problems by supporting and improving the parenting of the children and by helping the mothers find and use resources such as pediatric care and early intervention. Unfortunately, federal and state funds for early intervention have been drastically reduced and fewer infants are accessing these important services. Health policies and resources need to be made available to rural mothers with preterm children during the critical preschool years of development. This includes developmental surveillance and stimulation, special nutritional needs, high quality child care, parenting information, and support to mothers such as job training to achieve satisfactory income, and housing. Rural health care and early intervention professionals working with these preterm infants and their mothers also need improved training into the special issues and needs of prematurely born-infants.

Acknowledgments The authors acknowledge members of the research team – Beth Black, Brigit Carter, Virginia Gamble, Edna Merrill, Jackie Pilgrim, Christine Raines, Shannon Wong, Diane Yorke, Janice Werezczak, Carol Hubbard, Paula Anderson, Lindsay Baird, Martha Ferebee, Donna Harris, Zhaowei Hua, James Gregory Lewis, HyeKyun Rhee, Donna Smart, William Wooten, and Tara Wright – and mothers who participated in our study. This study was supported by Grant R01 NR035962 from the National Institute for Nursing Research, NIH, to the last author.

References

Affleck, G., Tennen, H., Rowe, J., & Higgins, P. (1990). Mothers' remembrances of newborn intensive care: A predictive study. *Journal of Pediatric Psychology, 15*, 67–80.

Allen, M. C. (2008). Neurodevelopmental outcomes of preterm infants. *Current Opinion in Neurology, 21*, 123–128.

American Academy of Pediatrics Committee on Pediatric Research. (2000). Race/ethnicity, gender, socioeconomic status-research exploring their effects on child health: A subject review. *Pediatrics, 105*, 1449–1351.

Astuto, J., & Allen, L. (2009). Home visitation and young children: An approach worth investing in? *Social Policy Report, 23*(4), 3–18.

Barnard, K. E., Snyder, C., & Spietz, A. (1991). Supportive measures for high-risk infants and families. In K. Barnard, P. Brandt, B. Raff, & P. Carroll (Eds.), *Social support and families of vulnerable infants* (pp. 291–329). White Plains, NY: March of Dimes Birth Defects Foundation.

Beeber, L. S., Cooper, C., Van Noy, B. E., Schwartz, T. A., Blanchard, H. C., Canuso, R., et al. (2007). Flying under the radar: Engagement and retention of depressed low-income mothers in a mental health intervention. *Advances in Nursing Science, 30*, 221–234.

Black, B. P., Holditch-Davis, D., & Miles, M. (2009). Life Course Theory as a framework to examine becoming a mother of a medically fragile preterm infants. *Research in Nursing and Health, 32*, 38–49.

Boyd-Franklin, N. (1989). *Black families in therapy: A multisystem approach*. New York: Guilford.

Brooks-Gunn, J., Kelbanov, P. K., & Duncan, G. J. (1996). Ethnic differences in children's intelligence test scores: Role of economic deprivation, home environment, and maternal characteristics. *Child Development, 67,* 396–408.

Brooks-Gunn, J., Klebanov, P. K., Liaw, F., & Spiker, D. (1993). Enhancing the development of low-birthweight, premature infants: Changes in cognition and behavior over the first three years. *Child Development, 64,* 736–753.

Cairns, R. B., Elder, G. H., & Costello, E. J. (1996). *Developmental science.* Cambridge, UK: Cambridge University.

Candelaria, M. A., O'Connell, M. A., & Teti, D. M. (2006). Cumulative psychosocial and medical risk as predictors of early infant development and parenting stress in an African American preterm sample. *Journal of Applied Developmental Psychology, 27,* 588–597.

Combs, A. W., & Gonzalez, D. M. (1994). *Helping relationships: Basic concepts for the helping professions.* Boston: Allyn and Bacon.

Cross, T., Bazron, B., Dennis, K., & Issacs, M. (1989). *Towards a culturally competent system of care* (Vol. 1). Washington, DC: National Technical Assistance Center for Children's Mental Health.

DeJoseph, J. F., Norbeck, J. S., Smith, R. T., & Miller, S. (1996). The development of a social support intervention among African American women. *Qualitative Health Research, 6,* 283–297.

Dickerson, B. J. (1995). *Black single mothers: Understanding their lives and families.* Thousand Oaks, CA: Sage.

Economic Research Service. (2003). *Rural income, poverty, and welfare: Rural child poverty.* United States Department of Agriculture. Retrieved January 2010, from http://www.ers.usda.gov/Briefing/incomepovertywelfare/ChildPoverty/

Engelke, S. C., Engelke, M. K., Helm, J. M., & Holbert, D. (1995). Cognitive failure to thrive in high-risk infants: The importance of the psychosocial environment. *Journal of Perinatology, 15,* 325–329.

Feeley, N., Gottlieb, L., & Zelkowitz, P. (2005). Infant, mother, and contextual predictors of mother-very low birth weight infant interaction at 9 months of age. *Journal of Developmental and Behavioral Pediatrics, 26,* 24–33.

Garel, M., Dardennes, M., & Blondel, B. (2007). Mothers' psychological distress 1 year after every preterm childbirth. Results of the EPIPAGE qualitative study. *Child Care, Health, and Development, 33,* 137–143.

Garvey, C., Julion, W., Fogg, L., Kratovil, A., & Gross, D. (2006). Measuring participation in a prevention trial with parents of young children. *Research in Nursing and Health, 29,* 212–222.

Gennaro, S., Zukowsky, K., Brooten, D., Lowell, L., & Visco, A. (1990). Concerns of mothers of low birthweight infants. *Pediatric Nursing, 16,* 459–462.

Giscombe, C. L., & Lobel, M. (2005). Explaining disproportionately high rates of adverse birth outcomes among African Americans: The impact of stress, racism, and related factors in pregnancy. *Psychological Bulletin, 131,* 662–683.

Hack, M. M., Wilson-Costello, D., Friedman, H., Taylor, G. H., Schluchter, M., & Fanaroff, A. A. (2000). Neurodevelopment and predictors of outcomes of children with birthweights of less than 1000g: 1992–1995. *Archives of Pediatric and Adolescent Medicine, 134,* 725–731.

Harris, R. P., & Zimmerman, J. N. (2003). *Children and poverty in the rural South.* Southern Rural Development Center. http://srdc.msstate.edu/publications/srdcpolicy/harris_zimmerman.pdf. Accessed Jan 2010.

Hausmann, L. R., Jeong, K., Bost, J. E., & Ibrahim, S. A. (2008). Perceived discrimination in health care and health status in a racially diverse sample. *Medical Care, 46,* 905–914.

Heinicke, C. M., Fineman, N., Rodning, C., Ruth, G., Recchia, S., & Guthrie, D. (1999). Relationship based intervention with at-risk mothers: Outcome in first year of life. *Infant Mental Health Journal, 20,* 349–374.

Hendrickson, S., Baldwin, J. H., & Allred, K. W. (2000). Factors perceived by mothers as preventing families from obtaining early intervention services for their children with special needs. *Children's Health Care, 29,* 1–17.

Herrick, H., & Farel, A. (1995). Statewide coverage of very low birthweight infants and teenage mothers (less than 15 years of age) in North Carolina's child services coordination program: 1991 and 1993. *State Center for Health and Environmental Statistics, 94,* 1–9.

Hoekstra, R., Ferrara, T. B., Couser, R. J., Payne, N. R., & Connett, J. E. (2004). Survival and long-term neurodevelopmental outcome of extremely premature infants born at 23–26 weeks gestational age at a tertiary center. *Pediatrics, 113,* e1–e6.

Holditch-Davis, D., & Miles, M. S. (2000). Mothers' stories about their experiences in the neonatal intensive unit. *Neonatal Network, 19*(3), 13–21.

Holditch-Davis, D., Bartlett, T. R., & Belyea, M. (2000). Developmental problems and the interactions between mothers and their three-year-old prematurely born children. *Journal of Pediatric Nursing, 15,* 157–167.

Holditch-Davis, D., Bartlett, T. R., Blickman, A. L., & Miles, M. S. (2003). Post-traumatic stress symptoms in mothers of premature infants. *Journal of Obstetric, Gynecologic, and Neonatal Nursing, 32,* 161–171.

Holditch-Davis, D., Miles, M. S., Burchinal, M., O'Donnell, K., McKinney, R., & Lim, W. (2001). Parental caregiving and developmental outcomes in infants of mothers with HIV. *Nursing Research, 50,* 5–14.

Holditch-Davis, D., Miles, M. S., Weaver, M. A., Black, B. P., Beeber, L. S., & Engelke, S. (2009). Patterns of distress in African American mothers of preterm infants. *Journal of Behavioral and Developmental Pediatrics, 30,* 193–205.

Holditch-Davis, D., Miles, M. S., Weaver, M., Thoyre, S., Beeber, L., Black, B. P., & Engelke, S. (2009, February). *Maternal psychological well-being and the mother-child relationship effects of the nursing support intervention for African American mothers*. Presented at the 23rd annual meeting of the Southern Nursing Research Society, Baltimore.

Holditch-Davis, D., Miles, M. S., Weaver, M., Thoyre, S., Beeber, L., Black, B. P., & Engelke, S. (2010, February). *The Nursing Support Intervention for African American mothers of prematures: Infant health and development effects*. Presented at the 24th annual meeting of the Southern Nursing Research Society, Austin, TX.

Huber, C., Holditch-Davis, D., & Brandon, D. (1993). High-risk preterms at three years of age: Parental response to the presence of developmental problems. *Children's Health Care, 22*, 107–122.

Infant Health and Development Program. (1990). Enhancing the outcomes of low-birth-weight premature infants: A multisite, randomized trial. *Journal of the American Medical Association, 263*, 3035–3042.

Ipsa, J. M., Thornburg, K. R., & Fine, M. A. (2006). *Keepin' on: The everyday struggles of young families in poverty*. Baltimore, MD: Brookes.

Ivey, A. E., & Ivey, M. B. (1999). *Intentional interviewing and counseling: Facilitating client development in a multicultural society*. New York: Brooks/Cole.

Jesse, D. E., Swanson, M. S., Newton, E. R., & Morrow, J. (2009). Racial disparities in biopsychosocial factors and spontaneous preterm birth among rural low-income women. *Journal of Midwifery & Women's Health, 54*, 35–42.

Kang, R., Barnard, K., Hammond, M., Oshio, S., Spencer, C., Thibodeaux, B., et al. (1995). Preterm infant follow-up project: A multi-site field experiment of hospital and home intervention programs for mothers and preterm infants. *Public Health Nursing, 12*, 171–180.

Leventhal, T., Brooks-Gunn, J., McCormick, M. C., & McCarton, C. (2000). Patterns of service use in preschool children: Correlates, consequences, and the role of early intervention. *Child Development, 71*, 802–819.

Lewis, M. D. (2000). The promise of dynamic systems approaches for an integrated account of human development. *Child Development, 71*, 36–43.

Luthar, S. S., & Suchman, N. E. (2000). Relational psychotherapy mothers' group: A developmentally informed intervention for at-risk mothers. *Development and Psychopathology, 12*, 235–253.

Luthar, S., & Suchman, N. (1999). Developmentally informed parenting interventions: The Relational Psychotherapy Mothers' Group. In D. Cicchetti & S. Toth (Eds.), *Rochester Symposium on Developmental Psychopathology* (Developmental approaches to prevention and intervention, Vol. 9, pp. 271–309). Rochester, NY: University of Rochester.

Mallory, C. M., Miles, M. S., & Holditch-Davis, D. (2002). Reciprocity and retention with African American women. *Applied Nursing Research, 15*, 35–41.

Meisels, S. J. (1989). Meeting the mandate of Public Law 99–457: Early childhood intervention in the nineties. *American Journal of Orthopsychiatry, 59*, 451–459.

Meyer, E. C., Garcia Coll, C. T., Lester, B. M., Boukydis, C. F. Z., McDonough, S. M., & Oh, W. (1994). Family-based intervention improves maternal psychological well-being and feeding interaction of preterm infants. *Pediatrics, 93*, 241–246.

Miles, M. S., & Holditch-Davis, D. (1995). Compensatory parenting: How mothers describe parenting their 3-year-old prematurely born children. *Journal of Pediatric Nursing, 10*, 243–253.

Miles, M. S., & Holditch-Davis, D. (2003). Enhancing nursing research with children and families using a developmental science perspective. *Annual Review of Nursing Research, 21*, 1–20.

Miles, M. S., Burchinal, P., Holditch-Davis, D., Brunssen, S., & Wilson, S. (2002). Perceptions of stress, worry, and support of black and white mothers of hospitalized medically fragile infants. *Journal of Pediatric Nursing, 17*, 82–88.

Miles, M. S., & Frauman, A. (1993). Barriers and bridges: Nurses' and parents' negotiation of caregiving roles with medically fragile infants. In S. Funk, E. M. Tornquist, M. T. Champagne, & R. A. Wiese (Eds.), *Key aspects of chronic illness care: Home and hospital* (pp. 239–250). New York: Springer.

Miles, M. S., Holditch-Davis, D., Schwartz, T. A., & Sher, S. (2007). Depressive symptoms in mothers of prematurely-born-children. *Journal of Developmental and Behavioral Pediatrics, 28*, 36–44.

Miles, M. S., Holditch-Davis, D., Thoyre, S., & Beeber, L. (2005). Rural African American Mothers parenting prematurely-born infants: An ecological systems perspective. *Newborn and Infant Nursing Reviews, 5*, 142–148.

Miles, M. S., Thoyre, S., Beeber, L., Holditch-Davis, D., Song, H., & Engelke, S. C. (2008, April). *Patterns of relationships between low-income, rural African American mothers and the fathers of their preterm infants*. Poster presented at the International Conference on Infant Studies, Vancouver, Canada.

Muender, M. M., Moore, M. L., Chen, G. J., & Sevick, M. A. (2000). Cost-benefit of a nursing telephone intervention to reduce preterm and low-birthweight births in an African American clinic population. *Preventive Medicine, 30*, 271–276.

Newacheck, P. W., Hughes, D. C., & Stoddard, J. J. (1996). Children's access to primary care: Differences by race, income, and insurance status. *Pediatrics, 97*, 26–32.

Nosarti, C., Murray, R., & Hack, M. I. (2010). *Neurodevelopmental outcomes of preterm birth: From childhood to adult life*. Cambridge, UK: Cambridge University Press.

Olds, D. L., Robinson, J., Pettitt, L., Luckey, D. W., Holmberg, J., Ng, R. K., et al. (2004). Effects of home visits by paraprofessionals and by nurses: Age 4 follow-up results of a randomized trial. *Pediatrics, 114*, 1560–1568.

Peebles-Kleiger, M. J. (2000). Pediatric and neonatal intensive care hospitalization as a traumatic stressor: Implications for intervention. *Bulletin of the Menninger Clinics, 64*, 257–280.

Pierrehumbert, B., Nicole, A., Muller-Nix, C., Forcada-Guex, M., & Ansermet, F. (2003). Parental post-traumatic reactions after premature birth: Implications for sleeping and eating problems in the infant. *Archives of Disease in Childhood: Fetal and Neonatal Edition, 88*, F400–F404.

Polzer, R., & Miles, M. S. (2008). Spirituality: A cultural strength for African American mothers with HIV. *Clinical Nursing Research, 17*, 118–132.

Reichman, S. R. F., Miller, A. C., Gordon, R. M., & Hendricks-Munoz, K. D. (2000). Stress appraisal and coping in mothers of NICU infants. *Children's Health Care, 29*, 279–293.

Resnick, M. B., Armstrong, S., & Carter, R. L. (1988). Developmental intervention program for high-risk premature infants: Effects on development and parent-infants interactions. *Journal of Developmental and Behavioral Pediatrics, 9*, 73–78.

Shaw, R. J., Bernard, R. S., DeBlois, T., Ikuta, L. M., Ginzburg, K., & Koopman, C. (2009). The relationship between acute stress disorder and posttraumatic stress disorder in the neonatal intensive care unit. *Psychosomatics, 50*, 131–137.

Singer, L. T., Daviller, M., Bruening, P., Hawkins, S., & Yamashita, T. S. (1996). Social support, psychological distress, and parenting of very low birthweight infants. *Family Relations, 45*, 343–350.

Singer, L. T., Fulton, S., Davillier, M., Koshy, D., Salvator, A., & Baley, J. E. (2003). Effects of infant risk status and maternal psychological distress on maternal-infant interactions during the first year of life. *Journal of Developmental and Behavioral Pediatrics, 24*, 233–241.

Smedley, B. D., Stith, A. Y., & Nelson, A. R. (Eds.). (2003). *Unequal treatment: Confronting racial and ethnic disparities in health care.* Washington, DC: The National Academies.

Teti, D. M., Hess, C. R., & O'Connell, M. (2005). Parental perceptions of infant vulnerability in a preterm sample: Prediction from maternal adaptation to parenthood during the neonatal period. *Journal of Developmental and Behavioral Pediatric, 26*(4), 283–292.

Thompson, R. J., Gustafson, K. E., Oehler, J. M., Catlett, A. T., Brazy, J., & Goldstein, R. F. (1997). Developmental outcome of very low birth weight infants at four years of age as a function of biological risk and psychosocial risk. *Journal of Developmental and Behavioral Pediatrics, 18*, 91–96.

Thoyre, S. (2007). Feeding outcomes of extremely preterm infants after neonatal care. *Journal of Obstetric, Gynecologic, and Neonatal Nursing, 36*, 366–376.

Vohr, B. R. (2010). Cognitive and functional outcomes of children born preterm. In C. Nosarti, R. Murray, & M. I. Hack (Eds.), *Neurodevelopmental outcomes of preterm birth: From childhood to adult life* (pp. 141–163). Cambridge, UK: Cambridge University Press.

Wereszczak, J., Miles, M. S., & Holditch-Davis, D. (1997). Maternal recall of the neonatal intensive care hospitalization of a preterm infant. *Neonatal Network, 16*, 33–40.

Wilson, M. N. (1991). The context of the African American family. In J. E. Everett, S. S. Chipungu, & B. R. Leashore (Eds.), *Child welfare: An Afrocentric perspective* (pp. 85–118). New Brunswick, NJ: Rutgers University.

Wilson, S., & Miles, M. S. (2001). Expressions of spirituality by African American mothers with seriously ill infants. *Journal of the Society of Pediatric Nurses, 6*, 116–122.

Yoos, H. L., Kitzman, H., Olds, D. L., & Overacker, I. (1995). Child rearing beliefs in the African American community: Implications for culturally competent pediatric care. *Journal of Pediatric Nursing, 10*, 343–353.

Zahr, L. K. (1999). Predictors of development in premature infants from low-income families: African Americans and Hispanics. *Journal of Perinatology, 19*, 284–289.

Zelkowitz, P., Bardin, C., & Papageorgiou, A. (2007). Anxiety affects the relationship between parents and their very low birth weight infants. *Infant Mental Health Journal, 28*, 296–313.

Chapter 18
Interventions to Provide More Equitable Health Care: Emerging Evidence and Next Steps

Marcia J. Wilson, Bruce Siegel, Vickie Sears, Jennifer Bretsch, and Holly Mead

Introduction

Multiple studies have shown that racial and ethnic minorities often experience lower quality of health care when compared with white patients (Institute of Medicine [IOM], 2002). Even after taking into account various factors like differences in access to care and disease severity, racial and ethnic disparities in care remain, and are often associated with worse health outcomes (IOM; Mead et al., 2008). Disparities are particularly pervasive in cardiac care (Kaiser Family Foundation [KFF], 2002). While the overall performance of certain national cardiac quality measures has improved recently (Bradley et al., 2006; Jencks, Huff, & Cuerdon, 2003; Williams, Schmaltz, Morton, Koss, & Loeb, 2005), disparities in health care persist (IOM, 2009).

Disparities among African Americans as compared to other groups are well documented particularly in the Institute of Medicine (IOM) landmark report *Unequal Treatment: Confronting Racial and Ethnic Disparities in Health Care* (2002). Even a more recent report, the *National Healthcare Disparities Report*,[1] shows that 50% of the time African Americans receive poorer quality of care than do Whites for measures of quality in multiple conditions (e.g., cancer, diabetes, end stage renal disease) (AHRQ, 2008). Evidence also exists documenting disparities for African Americans in cardiac care. For example, African American patients suffering a heart attack experience longer door-to-balloon times relative to other groups, which includes Whites, Hispanics, American Indians, and Asians (Bradley et al., 2004). African Americans are also at risk of not receiving therapies such as revascularization and implementation of cardioverter-defibrillators (Jha, Fisher, Zhonghe, Orav, & Epstein, 2005; Thomas et al., 2007).

Given the substantial body of evidence documenting disparities in health care for African Americans, what do we know about the strategies or interventions that can help reduce these disparities? *Unequal Treatment* (2002) recommends that health systems consider equity as an essential element of quality and reduce health disparities through consistency in care. These recommendations include the regular use of evidence-based guidelines (e.g., those guidelines for care that have shown to be effective) and the accurate collection of patients' race, ethnicity, and language to monitor the quality of care that is provided to all patients (IOM, 2002). Research in recent years has

---

[1] The National Healthcare Disparities Report is an annual report by the Agency for Healthcare Quality and Research that provides a national overview of disparities data in both quality of care and access (AHRQ, 2008).

M.J. Wilson (✉)
Center for Health Care Quality, The George Washington University, Washington, DC, USA
e-mail: marcia.wilson@gwumc.edu

A.J. Lemelle et al. (eds.), *Handbook of African American Health: Social and Behavioral Interventions*,
DOI 10.1007/978-1-4419-9616-9_18, © Springer Science+Business Media, LLC 2011

shown the ability of guidelines and related quality improvement tools (e.g., standard orders) to improve overall care for patients (Eagle et al., 2002; LaBresh, Ellrodt, Gliklich, Liljestrand, & Peto, 2004; Mehta et al., 2002; Schwamm et al., 2008). Other work has shown that the use of these approaches may also eliminate racial or ethnic disparities (Sehgal, 2003).

What we know about the specific interventions that have been shown to reduce disparities in the health care setting, however, is limited. A recent review of the literature from 1995 to 2006 revealed only 62 cardiovascular interventions that had been rigorously evaluated (Davis, Vinci, Oksuosa, Chase, & Huang, 2007). Less than half of the interventions were applicable to the health care setting, while the remainder focused on the management of risk factors, e.g., controlling hypertension through diet and exercise. All the interventions were evaluated within an individual minority population and few formally assessed changes in disparities as a primary outcome. While much is known about disparities in health care for African Americans, much less is known about specific interventions that might narrow these gaps and lead to more equitable care.

The purpose of this chapter is threefold. First, we seek to understand the steps or activities necessary to develop additional interventions that will address disparities in health care, specifically those interventions most germane to health care organizations such as hospitals. Next we will share the experiences from a recent hospital collaborative designed to improve the quality of cardiac care for minority Americans. Funded by the Robert Wood Johnson Foundation and led by the authors of this chapter, *Expecting Success: Excellence in Cardiac Care* (Expecting Success) charged ten hospitals serving high numbers of African American and/or Latino patients with reducing any identified disparities in cardiac care through the implementation of quality improvement strategies. Finally, we will discuss the implications for policy based on the current evidence and the lessons learned from Expecting Success. While disparities for African Americans exist in many areas, we explore this issue primarily within the context of disparities in cardiac care in the hospital setting.

Background

In August 2009, the IOM released *Race, Ethnicity and Language Data: Standardization for Health Care Improvement* that examines the issue of how data on patient race, ethnicity, and language are collected in various contexts and makes recommendations on standardizing categories for these variables. Within the report, the IOM describes a framework found in successful initiatives (like Expecting Success) addressing disparities. This framework outlines four fundamental steps including (1) the collection of standardized patient race, ethnicity, and language data; (2) the stratification of performance measures by race, ethnicity, and language to determine if disparities exist; (3) the design and implementation of interventions to target specific populations or to raise overall quality; and (4) reanalysis of stratified data to evaluate the impact of the interventions (IOM, 2009). While the collection of R/E/L data is an important first step, using the data to look for potential disparities and to develop interventions to address any disparities are equally important. The collection and use of data are both essential components in moving toward more equitable care.

Provider Perceptions About Disparities in Care

Prior surveys of US acute care hospitals regarding the current practices in the collection of patient R/E/L data reveal that not all hospitals believe that data collection is necessary (Hasnain-Wynia, Pierce, & Pittman, 2004; Regenstein & Sickler, 2006). In a 2006 survey, one in five hospitals reported that they saw no need to collect patients' data regarding R/E/L (Regenstein & Sickler, 2006). Perhaps these hospitals believed that the limited diversity within their patient population precluded any need for data collection, i.e., few of their patients are members of different racial and ethnic groups so there is no need to look for disparities among their patients.

Other research suggests two alternative reasons as to why hospital leaders see no reason to collect patient R/E/L data – hospital leaders believe that disparities are a result of factors outside the hospital walls or they believe that all their patients are receiving the same quality of care, even in the absence of data. While designing the Expecting Success collaborative, interviews with 38 hospital and health systems leaders revealed that disparities in health care were not an organizational priority for US hospitals (Siegel, Bretsch, Sears, Regenstein, & Wilson, 2007). The interviews revealed that hospital leaders perceive disparities as a function of social and economic conditions beyond their control, e.g., lack of insurance.

Additionally, hospital leaders reported that they did not believe that there were disparities in the quality of care they provided among the different populations that they served even though the hospital had never looked at any data to verify this statement. Similar perceptions were found in interviews with senior leaders in public hospitals (Siegel, Regenstein, & Jones, 2007). Senior leaders perceived that disparities are driven by factors outside the hospital walls (e.g., socioeconomic status) while believing that all the hospitals' patients are receiving the same level of care.

Hospital and health system leaders are not the only ones that think disparities exist but not within their own organizations. A survey of more than 300 cardiologists revealed that, while almost two-thirds of the cardiologists rated the evidence about disparities as "strong" or "very strong," few thought disparities existed in the care of their own patients (Lurie et al., 2005). Only one-third of the cardiologists surveyed agreed that disparities existed in care overall in the US health care system; a similar percentage believed that disparities existed in cardiac care. When asked whether they believed that disparities existed within their own hospital setting or in their own practices, the percentage of cardiologists agreeing dropped to 12 and 5%, respectively (Lurie et al., 2005). While a relatively low percentage of cardiologists accept that disparities in health care exist, an even smaller percentage of cardiologists believe that disparities could be an issue within their own practice. Similar to hospital and health system leaders, cardiologists believe that disparities are something that happens "out there," beyond the walls of their organization or practice.

Most Hospitals Collect Patient Race, Ethnicity, and Language Data but Few Use the Data

While hospital and health system leaders may not believe that disparities exist within their organizations, research has shown that most US hospitals collect patient race, ethnicity, and/or language data to varying degrees and that the percentage of hospitals collecting the data is increasing. A 2006 survey (Regenstein & Sickler, 2006) showed that just over three-quarters of hospitals collected race data while 2008 hospital data show that almost 90% of hospitals collect race and ethnicity data (IOM, 2009). Similarly, the percentage of hospitals reporting the collection of language has increased from 50% in 2006 (Regenstein & Sickler, 2006) to almost 80% in 2008 (IOM).

Even though a high percentage of hospitals collect patient R/E/L data, few use the data for quality improvement purposes. A 2006 survey shows that fewer than one in five hospitals used the patient R/E/L data to compare quality of care, health outcomes, or patient satisfaction (Regenstein & Sickler, 2006). A similar finding occurred among the 122 hospitals that applied to Expecting Success. Data from the hospitals' applications revealed that most (96.7%) of the hospitals reported collecting data on patients' race and ethnicity and more than two-thirds of the hospitals reported being able to stratify their performance measures using these variables. Less than 5% of all applicant hospitals, however, indicated that they had planned or implemented formal quality improvement initiatives specifically designed to address racial or ethnic disparities (Siegel, Regenstein, & Jones, 2007).

Historically, hospitals have collected race data to ensure compliance with civil rights provisions (IOM, 2009) so initially a culture of using patients' data to drive quality improvement interventions did not exist. As previously discussed, hospitals may not have made stratifying performance measures a priority because they assume that they provide the same equitable care to all their patients. This "assumed equity" may be one reason that available data are not used for stratifying performance measures. In effect, hospitals may be sitting on a treasure trove of data that are not used, i.e., data are never transformed into actionable information.

Another explanation for why hospitals fail to use the R/E/L data they collect may be a lack of trust in the quality of the data. Hospital practices for data collection vary widely as do the racial and ethnic classifications used (Hasnain-Wynia & Baker, 2006). Hospital staff often determines race and ethnicity by observing (e.g., "eyeballing") the patient rather than asking the patient directly (Hasnain-Wynia et al., 2004; Regenstein & Sickler, 2006). If clinicians and hospital staff do not believe that the R/E/L data collected accurately represents the patients that the hospital serves, then any analysis using that data will be subject to criticism and ultimately dismissed as not useful.

In the next section of the chapter, we introduce Expecting Success, a collaborative intended to identify and address disparities in cardiac care. We describe the collaborative's design and explain how the structure of Expecting Success allowed participating hospitals to identify and address disparities in care.

Expecting Success

In 2005, the Robert Wood Johnson Foundation (RWJF) built upon the existing body of evidence in disparities and quality improvement and launched *Expecting Success: Excellence in Cardiac Care*, a hospital collaborative aimed at improving cardiac care for racial and ethnic minority populations in the USA. The Expecting Success project had four goals: to improve cardiovascular care for African Americans and Latinos; to develop effective, replicable quality improvement strategies, models, and resources; to encourage the spread of those strategies and models to clinical areas outside of cardiac care; and to share relevant lessons with health care providers and policy makers. RWJF chose the George Washington University School of Public Health and Health Services (GW) to manage the Expecting Success project.

The 32-month hospital collaborative included five phases designed to move the hospitals from initial orientation and planning to sustaining equitable high-quality care with hard-wired data collection systems. Expecting Success represented a modified "breakthrough series" collaborative model structure developed by the Institute for Healthcare Improvement (IHI), which focuses on engaging teams from health care organizations in a short-term learning experience that includes training opportunities, face-to-face meetings, and shared resources (Asch et al., 2005; IHI, 2003).

A Structure for Addressing Disparities

The Expecting Success activities focused on three essential components that foreshadowed the IOM framework presented in 2009. First, participating hospitals implemented the standardized collection of patient R/E/L data throughout the organization. Second, hospitals reported select cardiac performance measures monthly stratified by R/E/L. Finally, hospitals developed and tested quality improvement interventions that would improve the quality of care to their patients with specific emphasis on the reduction of any identified disparities.

Standardized R/E/L data collection. A core component of the Expecting Success project was the standardization of patient R/E/L data collection as prior work had demonstrated the frequent unreliability of this data (Hasnain-Wynia et al., 2004; Hasnain-Wynia & Baker, 2006; Regenstein & Sickler, 2006). Early in the planning process, the project designers, RWJF and GW, elected to use the expertise of the Health Research & Educational Trust (HRET) of the American Hospital Association to train all project hospitals on state-of-the-art techniques to ensure that the hospitals collected high-quality R/E/L data for all patients at registration (Hasnain-Wynia et al., 2007).

Standardizing data collection requires that (1) patients are asked their race, ethnicity, and language and (2) hospitals use standard categories for race and ethnicity adopted by the U.S. Office of Management and Budget (OMB) (Office of Management & Budget, 1997). Project designers added categories for patients that declared more than one race (multiracial) or that were unable to provide R/E/L data or that declined to answer. The project designers also added to the OMB categories by defining the minimum language categories to be collected (English, Spanish, and other). These categories allowed the stratification of all quality measures by patient R/E/L characteristics.

Collection of performance measures stratified by R/E/L. Twenty-one quality measures were selected for use in the project. Most are used by the Centers for Medicare & Medicaid Services (CMS) for public reporting nationally including four heart failure (HF) measures and eight acute myocardial infarction (AMI) measures. These measures were selected to simplify reporting for hospitals while making the project relevant to their current environment. In addition, the project designers also included two bundled measures that showed whether patients with HF or AMI had received all of the core components of care that they were eligible to receive. These composite measures reflect the national move toward bundling individual measures in order to capture multiple aspects of treatment for a specific condition (IOM, 2006). Hospitals submitted aggregate de-identified data to GW for all patients eligible for public reporting under national requirements.

Developing quality improvement interventions. Expecting Success hospitals could access a limited number of tools and resources that would be useful in their improvement work from the beginning of the collaborative. The initial resources provided to all participants included tools such as standard forms used when patients are admitted to the hospital, evidence-based clinical practice guidelines and diet and medication guidelines developed by the American College of Cardiology and the American Heart Association for use with patients with AMI or HF. Each hospital was expected to develop and contribute additional materials to these initial resources over the course of the project.

Selected Hospitals

All US general acute care hospitals were eligible to apply for inclusion in the collaborative. Over 120 hospitals applied to Expecting Success and 10 hospitals were eventually selected to join the project. As project designers sought to have any lessons gleaned by participating institutions be replicable by the broadest possible array of hospitals, the selection process yielded a diverse set of hospitals (see Table 18.1). The final ten hospitals varied in their ownership (e.g., public hospitals, not-for-profits, and one for-profit) as well as teaching status (e.g., academic medical centers, teaching hospitals, and community hospitals). Hospitals ranged in size from just over 300 beds to more than 1,000 beds. While representing a diverse group of organizations, the hospitals selected shared several common traits: each had a large cardiovascular service line, high numbers of African Americans and/or Latino patients, and a strong record in quality improvement efforts. For participating in the collaborative, each hospital received a modest grant to help defray project-related costs.

Table 18.1 Characteristics of *Expecting Success* collaborative hospitals

Institution	Location	Hospital ownership	Discharges[a] 2005	Percent of AMI/HF patients race=black 2006[b]	Percent of AMI/HF patients ethnicity=hispanic 2006[b]
Del Sol Medical Center	El Paso, TX	Investor-owned	14,493	1	85
Delta Regional Medical Center	Greenville, MS	Public	8,729	68	<1
Duke University Hospital	Durham, NC	Not-for-profit	37,738	35	<1
Memorial Regional Hospital	Hollywood, FL	Public	32,180	24	16
Montefiore Medical Center	Bronx, NY	Not-for-profit	57,587	24	34
Mount Sinai Hospital Medical Center	Chicago, IL	Not-for-profit	19,877	83	11
Sinai-Grace Hospital	Detroit, MI	Not-for-profit	21,151	87	<1
University Health System	San Antonio, TX	Public	21,869	9	65
University of Mississippi Health Care	Jackson, MS	Public	27,332	71	1
Washington Hospital Center	Washington, DC	Not-for-profit	44,841	62	1

[a]Source: CMS HCRIS file, FY2005 Medicare cost report data, from first quarter 2009 release
[b]Source: Data reported by the *Expecting Success* hospitals to the GW project office based on those patients eligible for AMI and HF project measures in 2006

The Collaborative Structure

During the first 6 months of the collaborative, hospitals received training on rapid-cycle improvement techniques, which allowed hospitals to quickly identify areas where the quality of care needs to be improved, to test different strategies or interventions, and to determine if measures of care have improved. HRET also trained hospital registration staff and other key personnel in the standardized collection of patient R/E/L data, which included a day-long site visit. Early in the collaborative, each hospital formed a multidisciplinary team to oversee all Expecting Success activities. While team membership varied among the hospitals, most teams had a similar composition that included a senior administrative leader (e.g., chief operating and/or nursing officer), senior clinical leadership (e.g., chief of cardiology), director of quality improvement, information technology staff, managers responsible for patient registration, nurse managers overseeing cardiac units, and emergency department staff. Including representatives from the clinical, registration, and administrative staff ensured that the hospital could address clinical improvement goals as well as the necessary changes to the patient registration and information systems to accommodate the accurate collection of patient R/E/L data.

Six months after the start of the collaborative, most project hospitals had begun collecting standardized R/E/L data at the time of patient registration while some of the larger hospitals took slightly longer to implement standardized data collection. Hospitals reported aggregate data on select cardiac measures by patient R/E/L via a password protected Web site in the first quarter 2006. Analysis of the performance measure data by GW gave the Expecting Success hospitals information they could then use to identify patients that were receiving suboptimal care and, after developing interventions targeting areas for improvement, monitor progress once interventions had been implemented.

Lessons Learned

During the course of the collaborative, the ten Expecting Success hospitals were able to improve care for patients with AMI and HF significantly. From the first quarter to the last quarter of the collaborative, the median percentage of patients with heart failure receiving all recommended therapies increased from 41 to 78% (The Robert Wood Johnson Foundation, 2008a). The improvement in the percentage of patients with AMI that received all the recommended therapies was less dramatic but still significant with the change from the first to the last quarter improving from 74 to 86% (Expecting Success Final Report). This improvement is reflected in composite measures that capture whether patients with HF or AMI received all recommended therapies, a more comprehensive standard of care than any single measure. These hospitals that were treating large numbers of minority patients were able to make dramatic improvements in the overall quality of care that thousands of patients were receiving.

The following highlights important lessons learned by Expecting Success hospitals that can provide guidance for other organizations that want to engage in addressing disparities. Further, Expecting Success demonstrates that the framework described in the 2009 IOM report offers a clear set of steps for addressing disparities within any health care organization, which can be translated into "on the ground" action by hospitals regardless of their size, location, or teaching status.

Gaining Buy-In from Senior Leadership Is Key

Getting buy-in from senior leadership is an essential first step if equitable care is going to become a priority for the hospital (The Robert Wood Johnson Foundation, 2008a; Mehta et al., 2002). Engaging senior leadership is critical for multiple reasons. Support from senior leadership is a signal that providing equitable care is an important if not fundamental value for the hospital. Senior leadership can help overcome institutional barriers (e.g., making necessary information system changes a priority) and allocate needed resources (e.g., dedicating employee time for working on the change process).

The Expecting Success CEOs offer several key points for engaging senior leadership (The Robert Wood Johnson Foundation, 2008b). Data can be a powerful motivator. If the data show that the hospital is not consistently providing high quality care, for example, as measured by the publicly reported cardiac care measures, senior leadership can use the data as a call to action for the organization. Serving large numbers of minority patients may mean that providing equitable care is a stated value embedded in the hospital's mission statement. A program to improve care and reduce disparities helps the hospital meet that mission. Committing to such a program is also a way to engage not only senior leadership but board members as well. Improving overall care for the hospital's patients and ensuring the same quality of care for all patients are a success that can be celebrated at all levels of the organization. Finally, the ten Expecting Success hospitals have now proven that a diverse group of institutions could improve the quality of cardiac care they were providing to their patients; positive change is possible.

Based on the experience of the Expecting Success hospitals, we suggest one modification to the IOM framework (IOM, 2009). The IOM framework as presented assumes that the hospital has already made a commitment to addressing disparities, i.e., the organization is ready to collect patient race, ethnicity, and language (R/E/L) data and use that data to identify and address any possible disparities. We assert that the initial steps in the framework should include building awareness of the possibility of disparities within the hospital and gaining buy-in from senior leadership. While other staff (e.g., clinicians, registration staff, information systems staff) will ultimately need to accept addressing as an important undertaking, the commitment of senior leadership (e.g., the CEO) to making equitable care on organizational priority is critical. The lack of senior leadership involvement in organization-wide efforts to address disparities decreases the likelihood that those efforts will be successful.

Standardized Collection of R/E/L Data Is Feasible

All ten project hospitals were able to standardize the collection of patient R/E/L data. At the beginning of the collaborative, all participating hospitals anticipated resistance to collecting these data from both staff and patients and noted this resistance as a potential barrier to moving forward. Staff was concerned about having to ask patients about their R/E/L and assumed that patients would not want to answer the questions, i.e., patients would be uncomfortable answering these questions and wonder why the questions were being asked. This perceived anxiety was addressed through a combination of training and tools designed to educate and inform both staff and patients. For example, staff received training in how to ask patients about R/E/L data in a uniform manner and also how to respond to patient questions or concerns. The Expecting Success hospitals developed materials (e.g., posters and patient handouts) that explained to patients why the hospital was collecting R/E/L data and hospitals shared these materials with patients before and during the registration process. Recognizing and addressing the potential anxiety of staff and patients allowed the implementation of standardized R/E/L data collection to move forward with few problems; Expecting Success hospitals reported that pushback from the patients did not materialize as expected. All ten hospitals were able to collect R/E/L data in the same manner, thus providing each of them with accurate, reliable data.

Following Standards of Care Improved Care for All Patients

In achieving their results, the Expecting Success hospitals designed and implemented a variety of interventions (The Robert Wood Johnson Foundation, 2008b). While the project required the collection and reporting of specific performance measures, the hospitals had considerable latitude in designing interventions that would best fit their organization's culture and available resources. Interventions ranged from the fairly simple (e.g., designing a checklist or reminder as training tools for staff) to the more complex (e.g., redesigning organizational-wide processes of care). For example, one hospital looked at reducing the time it took for patients coming to the hospital with a heart attack to receive a needed procedure. The hospital broke down the process into each of the different steps and then used data to determine how to improve the individual steps.

Many of the hospitals focused on developing standard forms, such as order sets (for when the patient is admitted to the hospital) and discharge instructions (for when the patient is sent home) as prior evidence has shown that the use of such standard forms improves adherence to quality measures (Mehta et al., 2002). The Expecting Success hospitals considered the implementation of standardized forms to be "high-leverage" interventions, i.e., those interventions that the hospitals considered having a high degree of effectiveness toward achieving the hospitals' goals.

Having Data Broadens the Disparities Discussion

It is important to note that the Expecting Success collaborative focused on reducing disparities in cardiac care; however, hospitals collected R/E/L data on all their patients making R/E/L data available for all patients regardless of diagnosis or condition. Consequently, the hospitals had access to data that created a powerful analytic advantage with which they could examine any clinical condition for variations in quality by R/E/L. Discussing disparities and inequities in care can be difficult given the many reasons why disparities occur. The experience of the Expecting Success hospitals was no exception. However, having relevant data on the hospital's performance measures allowed senior leadership to have forthright and meaningful conversations about disparities with clinicians and staff in terms of providing the same quality of care to all patients.

For example, during the collaborative, one of the hospitals looked at readmission rates by R/E/L for multiple conditions. While the hospital had not found any disparities in its cardiac care measures, the hospital did identify disparities in readmission rates for different conditions. The data provided the hospital with a new set of questions to explore in order to understand more clearly what disparities exist in readmission rates and how the hospital might address those disparities through specific interventions. The important lesson to draw from this experience is that even with the lack of disparities in one condition, senior leadership continued to explore other areas of care and broadened its search for disparities.

As it has been noted, standardized data collection allowed the Expecting Success hospitals to look for disparities beyond the cardiac care performance measures and collaborative hospitals continue to use their R/E/L data even after the end of the project. One of the Expecting Success hospitals recently explored the role of race and ethnicity in self-reported pain by patients in the emergency department with suspected long-bone fracture (Bernstein, Gallagher, Cabral, & Bijur, 2009). The authors found that race and ethnicity did not affect baseline self-report of pain, thus contributing to the body of evidence examining the multifaceted reasons for disparities in the use of analgesics for pain management. This new knowledge also provides the hospital with more questions to explore to understand more clearly the variables that can affect disparities in pain management.

Discussion

While there have been many hospital collaboratives focusing on a variety of issues, Expecting Success may well be the first collaborative to focus on equity, one of the Institute of Medicine's domains of quality (IOM, 2001). All ten Expecting Success hospitals implemented the standardized collection of patient R/E/L data. This process went more smoothly than expected despite staff anxiety and anticipated pushback from the patients, which did not materialize. Asking patients about their race, ethnicity, and language in the health care setting is certainly feasible and the ability of ten hospitals to make this change in a relatively short period of time is encouraging. Using standardized patient R/E/L data, the Expecting Success hospitals moved to data-driven decision making to design and implement quality improvement interventions that resulted in improved care for their patients.

Expecting Success hospitals serve large numbers of minority patients, particularly African Americans and Latinos. By improving overall HF and AMI measures, the hospitals were able to improve care for thousands of minority patients. These results were primarily accomplished through the regular use of standard order sets and discharge instructions and redesigned processes of care. For hospitals that are underperforming in cardiac measures, quality improvement interventions involving adherence to evidence-based guidelines can result in a significant improvement in select performance measures overall. In those hospitals treating minority patients, these improvements translate into gains that result in improved care for minority patients. Quality improvement efforts such as those implemented by the Expecting Success hospitals can make a substantial difference, but are not the complete answer for reducing disparities. For example, addressing disparities in cardiac procedures (Jha et al., 2005) may require a better understanding of the variables driving the disparities that leads to targeted interventions designed for specific patient populations. It is reasonable to expect that addressing disparities in all aspects of health care will require disease-specific solutions tailored to all segments of minority patients.

During the collaborative, the Expecting Success hospitals implemented a variety of quality improvement interventions in their efforts to improve performance in the cardiac care measures. The hospitals could trend changes in each of the collaborative performance measures by the broad OMB categories, allowing them to track their progress and to look for differences in their various patient populations. Using the data to monitor the hospitals' performance before and after making any changes to patient care processes was an essential part of improving performance. However, the hospitals were unable to measure specifically how much of a difference each individual intervention made. The nature of hospital collaboratives is that multiple interventions are implemented at any given point in time, which makes it difficult to attribute results to a specific intervention. The findings from the collaboratives suggested which interventions had been most effective, but results could not be linked back to a single intervention. As hospitals continue to explore their performance by comparing various segments of their patient population and to identify possible disparities in care, hospitals will need to know about interventions that have proven effective for specific patient populations and that mitigate the factors contributing to any identified disparity.

The paucity of literature identifying which specific interventions will reduce disparities for which minority populations points to a strong need for additional research. One such endeavor is *Finding Answers: Disparities Research for Change* (2007), an RWJF-funded program designed to encourage, evaluate, and disseminate new interventions to reduce disparities (Chin, Walters, Cook, & Huang, 2007). More specifically, Finding Answers focuses on interventions to address disparities within cardiovascular disease, depression, and diabetes. Currently, Finding Answers is funding the evaluation of 28 interventions around the USA and will be disseminating the results of those evaluations broadly (RWJF). This initiative is filling an important gap in the body of evidence that demonstrates how we can move toward more equitable health care.

Building upon the lessons learned of Expecting Success will be critically important given the direction of current and future legislation in this area at both the federal and state levels. Lawmakers have begun to recognize the importance of addressing equity and are laying the critical foundational steps in terms of additional future data collection requirements. The Medicare Improvements for Patients and Providers Act of 2008 (MIPPA) requires the evaluation of methods for ongoing data collection and the measurement and evaluation of disparities as well as the assessment of performance according to patients' race, ethnic background, and sex (MIPPA, 2008).

The American Recovery and Reinvestment Act of 2009 (ARRA) creates the Health Information Technology for Economic and Clinical Health Act, which will make recommendations on the development of electronic data-collection methods that provide for the collection of data on patients' race, ethnic background, primary language, and sex (ARRA, 2009). ARRA also establishes Medicare and Medicaid reimbursement incentives for physician and hospital providers for the meaningful use of electronic health records (EHR). The final rule defining meaningful use, targeted for publication in mid-2010, is expected to include a requirement that providers collect R/E/L data consistent with OMB race and ethnicity categories to be eligible for incentive payments (ARRA). The expanded adoption of EHR throughout the provider community will facilitate and support further collection of standardized R/E/L data collection.

Activity involving R/E/L data collection and use at the state and local level is growing and Massachusetts, for example, has been a leader in this area. Recent regulations mandate that hospitals in both Boston and throughout the state collect and report patient race and ethnicity data beginning in January 2007 (Weinick, Caglia, Friedman, & Flaherty, 2007). Hospitals report standardized race and ethnicity categories that are granular enough to capture the diversity of the state's population (IOM, 2009). These regulations grew out of a task force in Boston and a state-wide commission that recognized the need to make addressing disparities in health care a priority.

In addition to federal and state legislation, outside regulatory bodies are also moving forward in efforts to advance R/E/L data collection and use. The Joint Commission, an independent, not-for-profit organization that accredits and certifies more than 17,000 health care organizations and programs in the USA including hospitals, recently revised its requirements regarding R/E/L data collection (Joint Commissions Perspectives, 2010). Effective no sooner than January 1, 2011, hospitals will be required to document the patient's race and ethnicity (a new requirement) as well as the patient's preferred language for discussing health care (a modified requirement) in the patient's medical record. These requirements are designed to improve patient-provider communication and lay the foundation for additional future requirements regarding the use of R/E/L data.

The evidence documenting disparities in health care is compelling and pervasive and now the IOM (2009) has provided a framework that health care organizations can use in identifying and addressing disparities in care. Evidence from the Expecting Success collaborative demonstrates that the IOM framework serves as a strong foundation upon which health care organizations can build in order to provide more equitable care for their patients. With further research to determine which interventions will be most effective for specific minority populations, the body of evidence will shift from documenting the existence of disparities to documenting interventions that will reduce disparities and improve care for all.

References

American Recovery and Reinvestment Act of 2009, Pub. L. 111–5, 123 Stat. 467 (2009, Feb. 17).

Asch, S. M., Baker, D. W., Keesey, J. W., Broder, M., Schonlau, M., Rosen, M., et al. (2005). Does the collaborative model improve care for chronic heart failure? *Medical Care, 43*(7), 667–675.

Bernstein, S. L., Gallagher, J., Cabral, L., & Bijur, P. (2009). Race and ethnicity do not affect baseline self-report of pain severity in patients with suspected long-bone fracture. *Pain Medicine, 10*(1), 106–110.

Bradley, E. H., Curry, L. A., Webster, T. R., Mattera, J. A., Roumanis, S. R., Radford, M. J., et al. (2006). Achieving rapid door-to-balloon times: How top hospitals improve complex clinical systems. *Circulation, 113,* 1079–1085.

Bradley, E. H., Herrin, J., Wang, Y., McNamara, R. L., Webster, T. R., Magid, D. J., et al. (2004). Racial and ethnic differences in time to acute reperfusion therapy for patients hospitalized with myocardial infarction. *JAMA, 292,* 1563–1572.

Chin, M. H., Walters, A. E., Cook, S. C., & Huang, E. S. (2007). Interventions to reduce racial and ethnic disparities in health care. *Medical Care Research and Review, 64,* 7S–28S.

Davis, A. M., Vinci, L. M., Okwuosa, T. M., Chase, A. R., & Huang, E. S. (2007). Cardiovascular health disparities: A systematic review of health care interventions. *Medical Care and Review, 64*(5), 29S–100S.

Eagle, K. A., Gallogly, M., Mehta, R. H., Baker, P. L., Blount, A., Freundl, M., et al. (2002). Taking the national guideline for care of acute myocardial infarction to the bedside: developing the Guideline Applied in Practice (GAP) initiative in southeast Michigan. *Joint Commission Journal on Quality Improvement, 28*(28), 5–19.

Hasnain-Wynia, R., & Baker, D. (2006). Obtaining data on patient race, ethnicity, and primary language in health care organizations: Current challenges and proposed solutions. *Health Services Research, 41,* 1501–1518.

Hasnain-Wynia, R., Pierce, D., Haque, A., Hedges Greising, C., Prince, V., & Reiter, J. (2007). Health Research and Educational Trust Disparities Toolkit. http://www.hretdisparities.org. Accessed 22 Jan 2009.

Hasnain-Wynia, R., Pierce, D., & Pittman, M. A. (2004). Who, when and how: The current state of race, ethnicity, and primary language data collection in hospitals. The Commonwealth Fund, May, 2004.

Institute for Healthcare Improvement. (2003). *The Breakthrough Series: IHI's collaborative model for achieving breakthrough improvement, IHI Innovation Series white paper.* Boston: Institute for Healthcare Improvement.

Institute of Medicine. (2009). *Race, ethnicity, and language data: standardization for health care quality improvement.* Washington, DC: National Academies.

Institute of Medicine. (2006). *Performance measurement: Accelerating Improvement.* Washington, DC: The National Academies Press.

Institute of Medicine. (2002). *Unequal treatment: Confronting racial and ethnic disparities in healthcare.* Washington, DC: National Academies.

Institute of Medicine. (2001). *Crossing the quality chasm.* Washington, DC: National Academies.

Jencks, S. F., Huff, E. D., & Cuerdon, T. (2003). Change in the quality of care delivered to Medicare beneficiaries, 1998–1999 to 2000–2001. *JAMA, 289*(3), 305–312.

Jha, A. K., Fisher, E. S., Zhonghe, L., Orav, E. J., & Epstein, A. M. (2005). Racial trends in the use of major procedures among the elderly. *New England Journal of Medicine, 353,* 683–691.

Joint Commission Perspectives (2010). New and revised hospital requirements [Internet]. http://www.Jcinc.com/common/PDFs/fpdfs/pubs/pdfs/JCReqs/JCP-01.S8.pdf. Accessed 31 Jan 2010.

Kaiser Family Foundation. (2002). *Racial/ethnic differences in cardiac care: The weight of the evidence.* Menlo Park, CA: The Henry J. Kaiser Family Foundation.

LaBresh, K. A., Ellrodt, A. G., Gliklich, R., Liljestrand, J., & Peto, R. (2004). Get with the Guidelines for cardiovascular secondary prevention: Pilot results. *Archives of Internal Medicine, 164*, 203–209.

Lurie, N., Fremont, A., Jain, A. K., Taylor, S. L., McLaughlin, R., Peterson, E., et al. (2005). Racial and ethnic disparities in care: The perspectives of cardiologists. *Circulation, 111*, 1264–1269.

Medicare Improvements for Patients and Providers Act of 2008, Pub. L. 110–275, 122 Stat. 2494 (2008, Jul. 15).

Mehta, R. H., Montoye, C. K., Gallogy, M., Baker, P., Blount, A., Faul, J., et al. (2002). Improving quality of care for acute myocardial infarction: The Guidelines Applied in Practice (GAP) initiative. *JAMA, 287*, 1269–1276.

Mead, H., Cartwright-Smith, L., Jones, K., Ramos, C., Woods, K., & Siegel, B. (2008). Racial and ethnic disparities in U.S. Health Care: A chartbook. The Commonwealth Fund, March 2008.

Office of Management and Budget (1997). Revisions to the Standards for the Classification of Federal Data on Race and Ethnicity. Federal Register Notice (1997, October).

Regenstein, M., & Sickler, D. (2006). *Race, ethnicity and language of patients: Hospital practices regarding collection of information to address disparities in health care.* Oakland, CA: National Public Health and Hospital Institute.

Schwamm, L. H., Fonarow, G. C., Reeves, M. J., Pan, W., Frankel, M. R., Smith, E. E., et al. (2008). Get with the Guidelines – Stroke is associated with sustained improvement in care for patients hospitalized with acute stroke or transient ischemic attack. *Circulation, 107*, 107–115.

Sehgal, A. R. (2003). Impact of quality improvement efforts on race and sex disparities in hemodialysis. *JAMA, 289*, 996–1000.

Siegel, B., Bretsch, J., Sears, V., Regenstein, M., & Wilson, J. (2007). Assumed equity: Early observations from the first hospital disparities collaborative. *Journal of Healthcare Quality, 29*(5), 11–15.

Siegel, B., Regenstein, M., & Jones, K. (2007). Enhancing public hospitals' reporting of data on racial and ethnic disparities in care. The Commonwealth Fund, May, January 2007.

The Robert Wood Johnson Foundation. (2008a). Expecting Success Final Report. http://www.rwjf.org/pr/product. jsp?id=36189.

The Robert Wood Johnson Foundation. (2008b). Expecting Success Toolkit. http://www.rwjf.org/pr/product. jsp?id=28433.

The Robert Wood Johnson Foundation. (2007). Finding Answers – Disparities research for change. http://www. solvingdisparities.org/home.

Thomas, K. L., Al-Khatib, S. M., Kelsey, R. C., Bush, H., Brosius, L., Velazquez, E. J., et al. (2007). Racial disparity in the utilization of implantable-cardioverter defibrillators among patients with prior myocardial infarction and an ejection fraction of ≤35%. *American Journal of Cardiology, 100*, 924–929.

U.S. Department of Health and Human Services, Agency for Healthcare Research and Quality [AHRQ] (2008). 2007 National healthcare disparities report [Internet]. http://www.ahrq.gov/qual/Nhdr05/nhdr05.pdf. Accessed 27 Dec 2008.

Weinick, R. M., Caglia, J. M., Friedman, E., & Flaherty, K. (2007). Measuring racial and ethnic health care disparities in Massachusetts. *Health Affairs, 26*(5), 1293–1302.

Williams, S. C., Schmaltz, S. P., Morton, D. J., Koss, R. G., & Loeb, J. M. (2005). Quality of care in U.S. hospitals as reflected by standardized measures, 2002–2004. *New England Journal of Medicine, 353*(3), 255–264.

Index

A.J. Lemelle et al. (eds.), *Handbook of African American Health: Social and Behavioral Interventions*,
DOI 10.1007/978-1-4419-9616-9, © Springer Science+Business Media, LLC 2011

Made in the USA
Middletown, DE
17 January 2017